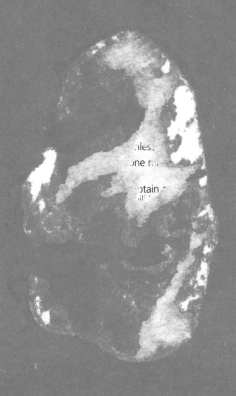

Aesthetics and Cosmetic Surgery for Darker Skin Types

Pearl E. Grimes, MD

Clinical Professor
Division of Dermatology
David Geffen School of Medicine
University of California, Los Angeles
Los Angeles, California
and
Director,
Vitiligo and Pigmentation Institute of Southern California

with 27 contributing authors

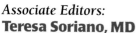

Associate Editors:

Teresa Soriano, MD
Assistant Clinical Professor
Division of Dermatology
David Geffen School of Medicine
University of California, Los Angeles;
Co-director UCLA Dermatologic
* Surgery and Laser Center*
Los Angeles, California

Doris M. Hexsel, MD
Former Professor of Dermatology
Department of Internal Medicine
School of Medicine of the
* University of Passo Fundo;*
Member of Clinical Body
Hospital Moinhos de Vento
Porto Alegre, Brazil

Jenny Kim, MD, PhD
Assistant Professor
Division of Dermatology
David Geffen School of Medicine
University of California, Los Angeles;
Chief, Department of Dermatology
Greater Los Angeles Healthcare
* Services Veterans Affairs*
Los Angeles, California

Wolters Kluwer | Lippincott Williams & Wilkins
Health

Philadelphia • Baltimore • New York • London
Buenos Aires • Hong Kong • Sydney • Tokyo

Acquisitions Editor: Susan Rhyner
Managing Editor: Nancy Winter
Developmental Editor: Franny Murphy
Project Manager: Alicia Jackson
Senior Manufacturing Manager: Benjamin Rivera
Associate Director of Marketing: Adam Glazer
Design Coordinator: Stephen Druding
Cover Designer: Stephen Druding
Production Service: Aptara, Inc.
Printer: Gopsons Paper Ltd.

Printed in India

Library of Congress Cataloging-in-Publication Data

Aesthetics and cosmetic surgery for darker skin types / [edited by] Pearl E. Grimes.
       p. ; cm.
   Includes bibliographical references and index.
   ISBN-13: 978-0-7817-8403-0
   ISBN-10: 0-7817-8403-4
  1. Surgery, Plastic. 2. Human skin color.   I. Grimes, Pearl E.
   [DNLM: 1. Cosmetic Techniques. 2. Reconstructive Surgical Procedures—methods.
   3. Continental Population Groups. 4. Skin Pigmentation. WO 600 A2545 2008]
   RD119.A396 2008
   617.9'5—dc22

                                                    2007010769

Care has been taken to confirm the accuracy of the information presented and to describe generally accepted practices. However, the authors, editors, and publisher are not responsible for errors or omissions or for any consequences from application of the information in this book and make no warranty, expressed or implied, with respect to the currency, completeness, or accuracy of the contents of the publication. Application of the information in a particular situation remains the professional responsibility of the practitioner.

The authors, editors, and publisher have exerted every effort to ensure that drug selection and dosage set forth in this text are in accordance with current recommendations and practice at the time of publication. However, in view of ongoing research, changes in government regulations, and the constant flow of information relating to drug therapy and drug reactions, the reader is urged to check the package insert for each drug for any change in indications and dosage and for added warnings and precautions. This is particularly important when the recommended agent is a new or infrequently employed drug.

Some drugs and medical devices presented in the publication have Food and Drug Administration (FDA) clearance for limited use in restricted research settings. It is the responsibility of the health care provider to ascertain the FDA status of each drug or device planned for use in their clinical practice.

To purchase additional copies of this book, call our customer service department at (800) 638-3030 or fax orders to (301) 223-2320. International customers should call (301) 223-2300.

Visit Lippincott Williams & Wilkins on the Internet: at LWW.com. Lippincott Williams & Wilkins customer service representatives are available from 8:30 am to 6 pm, EST.

10 9 8 7 6 5 4 3 2 1

Dedication

To Ephriam and Ruby Grimes, my parents, educators, and visionaries. Through them I have learned focus, dedication, resilience, and tenacity. To my loving daughter, Ashley, who is always there with endless love, support, and encouragement. To the late John A. Kenney Jr., MD, my mentor, eminent dermatologist extraordinaire, and "godfather" of ethnic dermatology. To the late Harold Pierce, MD, my mentor and trailblazer in ethnic cosmetic surgery. And lastly, to all the unsung heroes and pioneers of aesthetics and cosmetic surgery in darker racial ethnic groups.

Contributors

Marc R. Avram MD
Clinical Associate Professor of Dermatology
Department of Dermatology
Weill-Cornell Medical Center/New York
    Presbyterian Hospital
New York, New York

Mathew M. Avram, MD, JD
Department of Dermatology
Harvard Medical School
Director, MGH Dermatology Laser &
    Cosmetic Center
Department of Dermatology
Harvard Medical School
Boston, Massachusetts

Frederick Beddingfield III, MD, PhD
Assistant Clinical Professor,
Division of Dermatology
David Geffen School of Medicine
University of California, Los Angeles
Los Angeles, California
Vice President and Therapeutic Area Head,
Allergan, Inc.
Irvine, California

David Beynet, MD
Resident
Divison of Dermatology
David Geffen School of Medicine
University of California, Los Angeles
Los Angeles, California

Leticia T. Brunetto, MD
Medical Resident
Department of Dermatology
Hospital de Clinicas de Porto Alegre
Porto Alegre, RS, Brazil

Valerie D. Callender, MD
Assistant Clinical Professor
Department of Dermatology
Howard University, College of Medicine
Washington, DC
Director
Callender Skin and Laser Center
Mitchellville, Maryland

Dafnis C. Carranza, MD
Chief Resident
Division of Dermatology
David Geffen School of Medicine
University of California, Los Angeles
Los Angeles, California

Henry H.L. Chan, MD, FRCP
Honorary Clinical Associate Professor
Division of Dermatology
Department of Medicine
The University of Hong Kong
Honorary Consultant
Division of Dermatology
Department of Medicine
Hong Kong West Cluster, Queen Mary Hospital
Hong Kong, SAR

Fran E. Cook-Bolden, MD
Clinical Assistant Professor
Department of Dermatology
College of Physicians and Surgeons
    at Columbia University
Director
Ethnic Skin Specialty Group
New York, New York

Steven C. Dresner, MD
Associate Clinical Professor
University of Southern California
Keck School of Medicine
Los Angeles, California
Director, Fellowship in Ophthalmic
    Plastic Surgery
Eyesthetica
Santa Monica, California

Melanie Ho Erb, MD
Clinical Instructor
Department of Ophthalmology
University of California-Irvine
Irvine, California
Clinical Instructor
Department of Ophthalmology
USC, Keck School of Medicine
Los Angeles, California
Eyesthetica
Santa Monica, California

Sorin Eremia, MD
Associate Clinical Professor
Director, Cosmetic Surgery Unit
Division of Dermatology
David Geffen School of Medicine
University of California, Los Angeles
Los Angeles, California
Director
Department of Plastic, Cosmetic,
    and Skin Cancer Surgery
Riverside, California

Rafael Falabella, MD
Professor
Department of Dermatology
Universidad del Valle
Chief
Department of Dermatology
Hospital Universitario del Valle
Cali, Colombia, S.A.

Pearl E. Grimes, MD
Clinical Professor
Division of Dermatology
David Geffen School of Medicine
University of California, Los Angeles
Los Angeles, California
Director
Vitiligo and Pigmentation Institute of
    Southern California

Camile L. Hexsel, MD
Clinical Research Fellow
Department of Dermatology
Henry Ford Hospital
Detroit, Michigan

Doris M. Hexsel, MD
Former Professor of Dermatology
Department of Internal Medicine
School of Medicine of University of Passo Fundo, Brazil
Passo Fundo, RS-Brazil
Member of Clinical Body
Hospital Moinhos de Vento
Porto Alegre, RS-Brazil

Julie Iwasaki, BS
Division of Dermatology
David Geffen School of Medicine
University of California, Los Angeles
Los Angeles, California

H. Ray Jalian, MD
Department of Medicine
Division of Dermatology
David Geffen School of Medicine
University of California, Los Angeles
Los Angeles, California

Reza Jarrahy, MD
Assistant Professor
Division of Plastic and Reconstructive Surgery
University of California, Los Angeles
Los Angeles, California

Michael Jones, MD
Assistant Clinical Professor
Department of Head and Neck Surgery
Columbia University
Chief, Facial Plastic Surgery
Department of Surgery
Metropolitan Hospital
New York, New York

Matthew R. Kaufman, MD
Clinical Instructor
Department of Surgery
Division of Plastic Surgery
Drexel University College of Medicine
Saint Peters University Hospital
New Brunswick, New Jersey
Plastic and Reconstructive Surgeon
The Plastic Surgery Center
Shrewsbury, New Jersey

Malcolm S. Ke, MD
Assistant Professor
Department of Dermatology
Case Western Reserve University
Cleveland, Ohio
Director, Skin Surgery, Aesthetic and Laser Center
Department of Dermatology
University Hospitals of Cleveland
Orange Village, Ohio

A. Paul Kelly, MD
Professor and Chief
Division of Dermatology
Department of Internal Medicine
Charles R. Drew University of Medicine & Science
Staff Physician
Department of Internal Medicine
Martin Luther King, Jr./Harbor Hospital
Los Angeles, California

Jenny Kim, MD, PhD
Assistant Professor
Division of Dermatology
David Geffen School of Medicine
University of California, Los Angeles
Chief
Department of Dermatology
Greater Los Angeles Healthcare Services Veterans Affairs
Los Angeles, California

Seong-Jin Kim, MD, PhD
Associate Professor
Department of Dermatology
Chonnam National University Medical School
Chonnam National Hospital
Kwangiu, South Korea

Yoon-Duck Kim, MD, PhD
Professor
Department of Ophthalmology
Sungkyunkwan University School of Medicine
Chairman
Department of Ophthalmology
Samsung Medical Center
Seoul, Korea

Daniel E. Kremens, MD, JD
Jefferson Medical College
Philadelphia, Pennsylvania

Chang-Keun Oh, MD, PhD
Chair and Associate Professor
Department of Dermatology
Pusan National University
Chief
Department of Dermatology
Pusan National University Hospital
Busan, Korea

Joyce Teng Ee Lim, MD
Consultant Dermatologist
National Skin Centre
Paragon Medical Centre
Singapore

Heather Woolery-Lloyd, MD
Assistant Professor
Department of Dermatology and
    Cutaneous Surgery
University of Miami Miller School of Medicine
Miami, Florida

Amit G. Pandya, MD
Professor
Department of Dermatology
University of Texas Southwestern
    Medical Center
Staff Dermatologist
Department of Dermatology
Parkland Memorial Hospital
Dallas, Texas

Jocelyne Papacharalambous, MD, MPH
Research Coordinator
Department of Dermatology
Ethnic Skin Specialty Group
New York, New York

Juan Pellerano, MD
Dermatology & Aesthetic Center
Boca Raton, Florida

P. Kim Phillips, MD
Assistant Professor
Department of Dermatology
Mayo Clinic College of Medicine
Consultant
Department of Dermatology
Mayo Clinic
Rochester, Minnesota

Marta I. Rendon, MD
Associate Clinical Professor
Department of Dermatology
University of Miami
Miami, Florida
Medical Director
The Dermatology and Aesthetic Center
Boca Raton, Florida

Vermén M. Verallo-Rowell, MD
Clinical Professor
Department of Dermatology
Skin and Cancer Foundation at VMV Skin Research
    Centre and Clinics
Head Dermatopathology Section
Chair, Dermatology
Departments of Dermatology / Pathology
Makati Medical Center
Makati City, Philippines

Marcio Rutowitsch, MD
Chief
Department of Dermatology
Federal University, RJ
State Civil Hospital
Rio de Janeiro–RJ, Brazil

Parrish Sadeghi, MD
Denver Dermatology Consultants
Denver, Colorado
Consultant
Department of Internal Medicine
Lutheran Medical Center Hospitals
Wheat Ridge, Colorado

Rashmi Sarkar, MD, NAMS
Assistant Professor
Department of Dermatology and Venereology
Maulana Azad Medical College
    and Lok Nayak Hospital
New Delhi, India

Quyn Sherrod, MD
Resident
Division of Dermatology
David Geffen School of Medicine
University of California, Los Angeles
Los Angeles, California

Mariana Soirefmann, MD
Fellow in Training
Federal University of Rio Grande do Sul
Porto Alegre, RS, Brazil

Teresa Soriano, MD
Assistant Professor
Division of Dermatology
University of California Los Angeles
Co-director UCLA Dermatologic Surgery
    and Laser Center
UCLA Medical Center
Los Angeles, California

Stefani Takahashi, MD
Assistant Clinical Professor
Division of Dermatology
David Geffen School of Medicine
University of California, Los Angeles
Los Angeles, California

Luiz S. Toledo, MD, FICS, TCBC, SBCP
Staff Member
Department of Plastic Surgery
Hospital Sirio-Libanes
Sao Paulo, Brazil

Cherie M. Young, MD
Director of Research
Callender Skin and Laser Center
Mitchellville, Maryland

Stephanie R. Young, BS
Division of Dermatology
David Geffen School of Medicine
University of California, Los Angeles
Los Angeles, California

"We are of course a nation of differences. Those differences don't make us weak. They're the source of our strength."

When presidential candidate Jimmy Carter said those words in 1976, he was thinking of many kinds of differences, but those differences, which are most immediately obvious, are those related to facial appearance. This wonderful book, produced by our friend Dr. Pearl Grimes and her associate editors and authors, addresses, highlights, and analyzes those similarities and differences using the concepts of balance and harmony. While there is a focus on color as in "darker skin types," in this book and in its title, the book contains valuable information which is independent of skin color or ethnicity. There are other highly relevant physical distinctions in the structure and function of eyelids with the chapter on "Blepharoplasty in Asian Eyes" as a wonderful example. The chapters on the surgical approaches best suited to management of the nasal area, face tightening, body contouring, hair restoration and removal are some of the practical backbone of this new text.

Having emphasized the broad perspectives of this book, we must commend Dr. Grimes on the wonderful wealth of material and information included that is specific to darker skin types, especially of African origin. This type of skin presents very specific problems from disorders of pigmentation, the problems associated with resurfacing, and the aging processes which are quite different from those seen in paler skin. Of course tumors, such as keloids, are a more severe problem in types V and VI skin.

Interestingly, despite the well-described differences in facial appearance between ethnic groups, anthropological and social analysis of the canons of facial beauty shows similarities throughout cultures—even in groups not even remotely communicating with other broader cultures. Dr. Grimes points out also that many African Americans are triracial descendants of African, Native American, and Northern Europeans, and many Hispanics are racial mixtures of Northern Europeans, Spaniards, and Native Americans. Their individual facial features are a blend of their particular heredities. We must be aware that despite an individual's perceived racial background (individual skin color may vary from pale to dark) there may be potential difficulties if the resurfacing physician does not recognize an individual's underlying skin type and look for this information prior to treatment. With the increasing integration of our culture, greater understanding of skin types and their variations and nuances are essential to the physician attempting to do the very best for all patients.

There is a narrow line between problems that are considered medical and those that are considered cosmetic. This book treats both with equal seriousness that we think is appropriate. There are chapters that are clearly cosmetic in focus and others that have no cosmetic material as well as some that straddle the boundary comfortably. All are absolutely relevant to the scope of this text. As in other areas, it is the very obvious comfort level which Dr. Grimes and her co-authors have achieved in addressing this large and important area of knowledge which is so impressive.

We are all indebted to Dr. Grimes for her research on topical treatments to restore normal tone and texture to darker skin types. She has worked hard for many years to help us understand the challenges inherent in darker skin types and the differences from paler skin. This new book is an expansion of her initial focus as well as a broadening, which helps us to expand our view of skin. Rather than regarding paler skin as "normal," we should now be regarding all skin as individual and managing it as such. The many factors involved in the assessment of the skin, including but not limited to pigmentation, should all be considered equally. This is the triumph of this book. Dr. Grimes and her co-authors are to be congratulated.

Wherever and whatever your practice in medicine, this book has lessons for all physicians to the benefit of all our patients and students.

ALASTAIR AND JEAN CARRUTHERS

Preface

Aesthetics and Cosmetic Surgery for Darker Skin Types has been a labor of love, passion, history, and expanding scientific knowledge. As a teacher, researcher, clinician, and mentor in dermatology and dermatologic surgery for more than 25 years, I have observed, participated, and contributed to the evolving field of cosmetic surgery in darker-racial ethnic groups.

Such individuals constitute the majority of the global population. They include Hispanics, Latinos, Africans, African Americans, Caribbeans, Native Americans, Pacific Islanders, East Indians, Pakistanis, Eskimos, Koreans, Chinese, Vietnamese, Filipinos, Japanese, Thai, Cambodians, Malaysians, Indonesians, and Aleuts. Darker racial ethnic groups are often classified as Fitzpatrick's Skin Types IV through VI and constitute a third of the United States population. Twenty percent of cosmetic procedures in the United States are performed in darker races. Current data suggest that the popularity and interest in cosmetic surgery in this group is expanding at a rapid pace.

Multiple studies have documented the unique structural and functional differences in the skin of darker skin types as compared to Caucasians. These differences can impact the choice of topical pharmacologic agents and cosmetic surgical procedures used in pigmented skin. The efficacy and outcomes of procedures vary in different racial groups. Some procedures may be extremely well tolerated in Caucasians or fair-skinned individuals but may cause myriad complications including scarring in dark skin.

There has been an explosion in new surgical techniques and technologies since the late 1990s. Despite this rapid growth, there is a dearth of published knowledge regarding cosmetic surgery in darker skin types. In addition, few textbooks have exclusively addressed this subject. To our knowledge, none have been published since W. Earle Matory Jr's "Ethnic Considerations in Facial Aesthetic Surgery" published by Lippincott in 1998.

John F. Kennedy stated: "The greater our knowledge increases the more our ignorance unfolds."

As we expand our knouledge of cosmetic surgery, it is clear that we must learn substantially more regarding techniques, outcomes, and complications of cosmetic surgery in darker racial ethnic groups.

Aesthetics and Cosmetic Surgery for Darker Skin Types was written to fill a tremendous scientific void. The intent was to provide cutting edge data, procedures, protocols, outcomes, and complications of cosmetic surgery in darker-racial ethnic groups. It was written for dermatologists, dermasurgeons, plastic surgeons, primary care physicians, medical students, interns, residents, and fellows.

This textbook is a compendium of the latest information addressing many aspects of aesthetics and cosmetic surgery, encompassing nine sections and 36 chapters by esteemed authors from around the globe. Hence, it represents and reflects a global treatise of current scientific knowledge.

Many topics of interest are addressed for the student and teacher of cosmetic surgery. The introductory chapter on beauty provides the reader with historical and societal constructs of beauty for darker skin types as compared to Caucasians. The following chapter reviews structural and physiologic differences in the skin of darker racial ethnic groups. The authors establish a paradigm for therapeutic options presented in subsequent chapters. The general textbook sections include: General considerations for cosmetic surgery; cosmeceutical and pharmaceutical agents; therapies for dyschromias; resurfacing procedures; facial tightening procedures; noninvasive wrinkle correction; correction of specific anatomic imperfections; surgical approaches for hair disorders; and benign and malignant skin tumors.

I hope that this textbook will serve as a foundation, bridge, and ladder of knowledge for any student, clinician, or scientist interested in aesthetics and cosmetic surgery in darker skin types.

Acknowledgments

I would like to thank my associate editors, Teresa Soriano, MD, Doris Hexsel, MD, and Jenny Kim, MD, for their dedication and hard work. In addition, I am indebted to all of my distinguished authors who worked tirelessly, contributing extraordinary and unique chapters to bring this scientific venture to fruition. I sincerely thank all of you. I would also like to give a very special acknowledgment of gratitude to George Rudkin, MD, Matthew Kaufman, MD, and William Rassman, MD.

This textbook would not have been possible without the relentless efforts and work of my staff, Kali Ghazali and Michael Gonzalez, and the support of my family and dearest friends. Finally, I am deeply indebted to the vision and profound commitment of the Lippincott editorial staff. Many thanks to Nancy Winter, Managing Editor; Susan Rhyner, Editor, Division of Dermatology; Franny Murphy, Development Editor; Alicia Jackson, Project Manager; and Wendy Druck, Project Manager for Aptara, Inc.

Contents

Dedication   iii
Contributors   v
Foreword   ix
Preface   xi
Acknowledgments   xiii

PART 1

General Considerations for Cosmetic Surgery 1

1 Beauty: An Historical and Societal Perspective . . . 3
PEARL E. GRIMES

2 Structural and Physiologic Differences in the Skin of Darker Racial Ethnic Groups 15
PEARL E. GRIMES, QUYN SHERROD

3 The Aging Face in Darker Racial Ethnic Groups 27
PEARL E. GRIMES, DORIS M. HEXSEL, MARCIO RUTOWITSCH

4 Outcomes in Aesthetic Surgery: Patient Satisfaction 37
PEARL E. GRIMES

5 Evaluation and Design of Cosmetic Research Studies 42
AMIT G. PANDYA

6 Cosmetic Issues of Concern for Potential Surgical Patients 49
CHANG-KEUN OH, H. RAY JALIAN, STEPHANIE R. YOUNG, SEONG-JIN KIM

7 Informed Consent and Treating the Cosmetic Patient 59
MATHEW M. AVRAM, DANIEL E. KREMENS

8 Photography in Cosmetic Surgery 62
PEARL E. GRIMES

PART 2

Use of Cosmeceuticals and Pharmacologic Agents 71

9 Skin-Lightening Agents 73
MARTA I. RENDON

10 Topical Retinoids in Ethnic Skin 82
STEFANI TAKAHASHI, JULIE IWASAKI

11 Antioxidants 92
FRAN E. COOK-BOLDEN, JOCELYNE PAPACHARALAMBOUS

12 Photoprotection 103
VERMÉN M. VERALLO-ROWELL

PART 3

Therapies for Dyschromias 115

13 Laser Therapies for Disorders of Hyperpigmentation 117
MALCOLM S. KE, TERESA SORIANO

14 Cosmetic Leukodermas: Therapeutic Approaches 125
PEARL E. GRIMES

15 Surgical Approaches for Vitiligo 133
RAFAEL FALABELLA

PART 4

Resurfacing Procedures 145

16 Microdermabrasion 147
JOYCE TENG EE LIM

17 Superficial Chemical Peels 154
PEARL E. GRIMES, MARTA I. RENDON, JUAN PELLERANO

18 Medium-Depth Chemical Peels and Deep Chemical Peels 170
RASHMI SARKAR

19 Ablative and Nonablative Resurfacing in Darker Skin 179
HENRY H. L. CHAN

PART 5

Facial Tightening Procedures 187

20 Surgical Tightening Procedures 189
MATTHEW R. KAUFMAN, REZA JARRAHY, MICHAEL JONES

21 Nonsurgical Tightening Procedures 197
SORIN EREMIA

PART 6

Noninvasive Wrinkle Correction ... 209

22 Botulinum Toxin 211
DORIS M. HEXSEL, CAMILE L. HEXSEL, LETICIA T. BRUNETTO

xv

23 Fillers in Ethnic Skin 225
FREDERICK BEDDINGFIELD III, JENNY KIM

PART 7

Correction of Specific Anatomic Imperfections 241

24 Blepharoplasty for Asian Eyes 243
YOON-DUCK KIM

25 Blepharoplasty in Blacks and Latinos 250
STEVEN C. DRESNER, MELANIE HO ERB

26 Ethnic Rhinoplasty 257
MATTHEW R. KAUFMAN, REZA JARRAHY, MICHAEL JONES

27 Reduction and Augmentation of the Breasts . . 262
MATTHEW R. KAUFMAN, REZA JARRAHY, MICHAEL JONES

28 Body-Contouring Procedures 268
LUIZ S. TOLEDO

29 Vascular Surgery in Darker Racial Ethnic Groups 276
PARRISH SADEGHI

PART 8

Surgical Approaches for Hair Disorders 285

30 Alopecias and Hair Restoration in Women . . . 287
VALERIE D. CALLENDER, CHERIE M. YOUNG

31 Hair Transplantation for Men 296
MARC R. AVRAM

32 Laser Hair Removal in Darker Racial Ethnic Groups 303
TERESA SORIANO, DAVID BEYNET, DAFNIS C. CARRANZA

PART 9

Tumors 311

33 The Pathogenesis of Keloids 313
HEATHER WOOLERY–LLOYD

34 Medical and Surgical Therapies for Keloids . . . 320
A. PAUL KELLY

35 Cosmetic Aspects of Common Benign Tumors 327
DORIS M. HEXSEL, MARIANA SOIREFMANN

36 Surgical Treatment of Skin Cancers in Darker Racial Ethnic Groups 335
P. KIM PHILLIPS

Index   347

General Considerations for Cosmetic Surgery

Beauty: An Historical and Societal Perspective

Pearl E. Grimes

HISTORICAL PERSPECTIVE

Beautiful faces are those that wear
It matters little if dark or fair
Whole-souled honesty printed there.

—"Beautiful Things" ELLEN ATHERTON

Historical definitions of beauty

If you ask patients to define "beautiful people," they will probably cite modern-day icons or historical legends renowned for their beauty. Such examples include Cleopatra, Angelina Jolie, or Halle Berry. But what do their answers tell us? White or black, Asian or Hispanic, beautiful people brought to mind probably share key attributes. For instance, virtually every culture has celebrated smooth skin, albeit a surface that is sometimes painted, tattooed, or pierced for extra appeal. Symmetry of features has long been a lure, if only subconsciously. Proportion, which represents the ratio of facial features relative to attraction, has held surprisingly steady over the centuries. Is there a recognized definition of beauty and, if so, where does it originate?

The accepted definition of beauty is based on ancient methods of quantifying beauty and applying those principles to all forms of nature. The ancient Egyptians may have been among the first to describe facial characteristics relative to beauty during the fourth and fifth centuries, but the ancient Greeks were the ones who appear to have quantified it. The artist Polykleitos, in the fifth century B.C., laid down recommended ratios for the ideal proportions in figures.[1] Those recommendations were later modified and refined. The Romans adapted the Greek canon, which developed and became known as the Golden Proportion. This ideal highlighted the connection between harmony, order, and proportion. This theme of defining beauty continued through the Middle Ages and was adapted during the Renaissance. In 1741, Père André described beauty as the balance of "Unity, order, proportion and symmetry."[2] No doubt many people would say

the same today, even if they can't articulate their attraction to certain objects.

Studies have shown that few people fit the historical canons of beauty.[3] In the 19th century, a group of anthropologists in Frankfort agreed on standard cranial measurements that have since been used to measure attractiveness in addition to the earlier canons. History has shown that certain ideals are found attractive in most societies. Certain characteristics and proportions can be seen as universal. However, different methodologies, genetic algorithms, and modern digital facial manipulations that identify and define beauty have shown that there is no clear answer to the question "What is beauty?"[4,5]

Beautiful women in society: historical icons

Beautiful women have been etched onto cave walls, carved in stone, painted on canvas, and paid homage to in song, poetry, and prose. They have been with us since the beginning of time. The Greeks had the mythology of Aphrodite; the Norse had Freya. Hindu mythology reveres Lakshmi as the goddess of beauty. The Romans called their mythological goddess Venus.

The Venus of Willendorf is one of the oldest depictions of a human woman, an icon of prehistoric art, created nearly 30,000 years ago (Fig. 1-1). She was almost certainly a celebration of procreation and nurturing. By today's Western standards, however, she would be unlikely to find herself on the cover of *Vogue, Elle,* or *Essence* magazines.

Throughout history, there are examples of mutual appreciation of beauty across ethnic divides. Nefertiti and the Queen of Sheba are renowned beauties believed to have been black Africans (Fig. 1-2). The Queen of Sheba was from present-day Ethiopia or Yemen and is well known in Jewish, Christian, and Islamic texts. In Greek mythology, there were the celebrated black figures Isis from the Nile Valley and Diana of Attica from Ethiopia.

Pocahontas, the daughter of Chief Powhatan, was reportedly a beautiful and intelligent woman who was treated as royalty. The most well-known, idealized painting of her, *The Baptism of Pocahontas,*[5] depicts her as a lighter-skinned, virginal beauty compared with the other Indians in the picture.

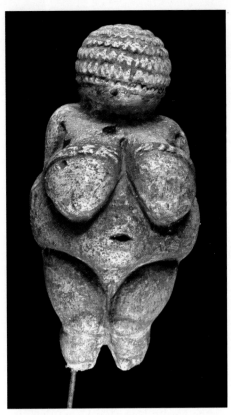

Figure 1-1 The Venus of Willendorf. (The Natural History Museum, Vienna.)

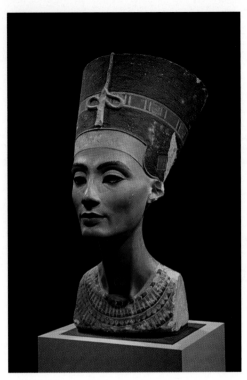

Figure 1-2 Bust of Queen Nefertiti. (Altes Museum, Berlin.)

As stated by Margaret Hungerford in 1878, "Beauty is in the eye of the beholder and David Hume in 1757, "Beauty is no quality in things themselves: It exists merely in the mind which contemplates them; and each mind perceives a different beauty." But is this true? Is everyone's idea of beauty distinctly individual, or is there a template laid down in our genes against which we measure it? How much does the ideal vary from race to race or from culture to culture? Can exposure to new ideals influence our perception of beauty?

In our multiracial, multicultural, and multimedia society, it is difficult to tease out the factors that define beauty. Instead, observation of historical or isolated populations provides clues about the perception of beauty and the way it changes over time.

GENETIC AND EVOLUTIONARY ASPECTS OF BEAUTY

From an evolutionary perspective, beauty is a gauge to measure fitness and suitability of a mate. Attractive facial features may signal sexual maturity and fertility, emotional expressiveness, or confer a cuteness that evokes a protective instinct.[6] As a "survival-of-the-fittest" instinct, avoidance of deformity and disease directs us toward mates who exude health and vitality. Symmetrical features, healthy bodies, and flawless skin are idealized. These parameters are commonly used to define physical beauty—but they also leave room for variability and interpretation.

There is clear agreement that attractiveness ratings are similar in a number of cross-cultural studies.[7,8] When considering the genetic angle of defined beauty, men are attracted to delicate jaws, large eyes, narrow waists, and full hips and lips, probably because these features signal youth and a high estrogen level, which in turn means fertility and fecundity. Women, on the other hand, are attracted to strong chins, height, broad shoulders and wide jaws, probably because they signal a high testosterone level and imply an ability to protect and feed a family.[9,10]

The pursuit of beauty is a basic instinct and a biological adaptation to help ensure the survival of our genes and, in a sense, ourselves. Research suggests that sensitivity to beauty is due to an instinct that has been shaped by natural selection.[11] For example, certain studies show that infants will stare significantly longer at faces deemed by adults to be attractive.[12] In addition, mothers of attractive newborns spend more time interacting with their babies. Studies have also shown a disproportionate number of abused children may not fit the standard canons for beauty.[12]

In other words, beautiful people are excused for everything from stupidity to serious crimes. People are more likely to help the good-looking (even if they dislike them) and are less likely to ask them for help.[13–15] A common theory even has it that beauty is the appearance of things and people that are good, meaning attractive people are judged more worthy simply because of their looks.

Beauty clearly brings ease. It is, as they say, its own reward.[14]

MEASUREMENTS FOR FACIAL AESTHETICS

Anatomical beauty is relatively easy to define and measure. Population surveys have identified the facial features that contribute to a generalized ideal. These include a full head of hair, smooth complexion, large eyes, small nose, full lips, slightly protrusive lower face, and high cheekbones. On the other hand, facial features that detract from beauty are disproportion, asymmetry, excessive size, convexity of profile, retrusion of the chin, skin laxity, thin lips, large nose, and irregular or discolored teeth.[16]

Historical tools or parameters used to measure facial aesthetics include the golden aesthetic proportions, neoclassical canons of facial proportion, the Frankfort horizontal plane, and facial shapes (Table 1-1).

The Greeks were fascinated by beauty as conveyed by the pursuit of godlike perfection in their statues. They also considered mathematics to be the unifying basis of life, art, the gods, and the universe. It is therefore no surprise that they tried to define beauty with mathematics. The divine proportion, or "golden section," was taken up by Plato as a mathematical relationship expressing universal harmony. Considered an ideal measure to govern the relationship of elements of the human body, it is expressed as 1:1.618, a ratio that occurs in many natural forms such as plants, shells, and snowflakes. Leonardo da Vinci later used the "golden section" in his portraits. The apparent importance of the ratio led Ricketts, an orthodontist, in 1982 to postulate a divine proportion for facial analysis.[17] This concept is believed to have originated with the sculptor Phidias, hence the expression *phi* in relation to the golden proportion, which has been used as an aesthetically pleasing relationship of vertical and/or horizontal structures. Ricketts indicated that this relationship seems to occur naturally in a variety of guises in the human face and body. However, in 1992, Davis and Jahnke disputed the relevance of the "golden section." They demonstrated a preference for internal facial divisions with a unitary value with bilateral symmetry.[18]

The neoclassical canons of facial proportions, described by scholars and artists of the Renaissance based on classical Greek canons, are still used for evaluation of facial features today (Table 1-1). Standard canons include the division of the face profile into thirds, with the height from the hairline to the eyebrow, from the brow to the lower edge of the nostril, and from the nostril to the chin being equal (Fig. 1-3). Other guidelines state that the height of the nose and the ear be the same, the width of the mouth be one and a half times the width of the nose, and the inclination of the nose bridge be parallel to the axis of the ear.

In 1985, Farkas et al. suggested that the facial canons did not work well when used to measure beauty in contemporary white subjects.[19] How would the canons perform

Table 1-1	
Aesthetic parameters of the face	
Aesthetic parameter	Measurements
Golden aesthetic proportions	The nasal height (A) is related to the maxillary height (B) as 1.000:0.618. The sum of nasal height and maxillary height (A + B) are related to the mandibular height (C) as 1.618:1.000
	The mandibular height (C) is related to the maxillary height (B) as 1.000:0.618
	The orofacial height (B + C) is related to the nasal height (A) as 1.618:1.000
	Note that each ratio is 1.618
Neoclassical canons of facial proportion	Nine in total: three vertical profile, four horizontal facial, and two nasoaural canons
Frankfort horizontal	Glabellar, columellar, and incisal angles
Facial shapes	Oval, heart, rectangular, other

Data from Tweed CH. The Frankfort-mandibular plane angle in orthodontic diagnosis, classification, treatment planning and prognosis. *American Journal of Orthodontics and Oral Surgery* 1946;32:175; Farkas LG, Hreczko TA, Kolar JC, et al. Vertical and horizontal proportions of the face in young adult North American Caucasians: revision of neoclassical canons. *Plast Reconstr Surg* 1985;7(3):328–338.

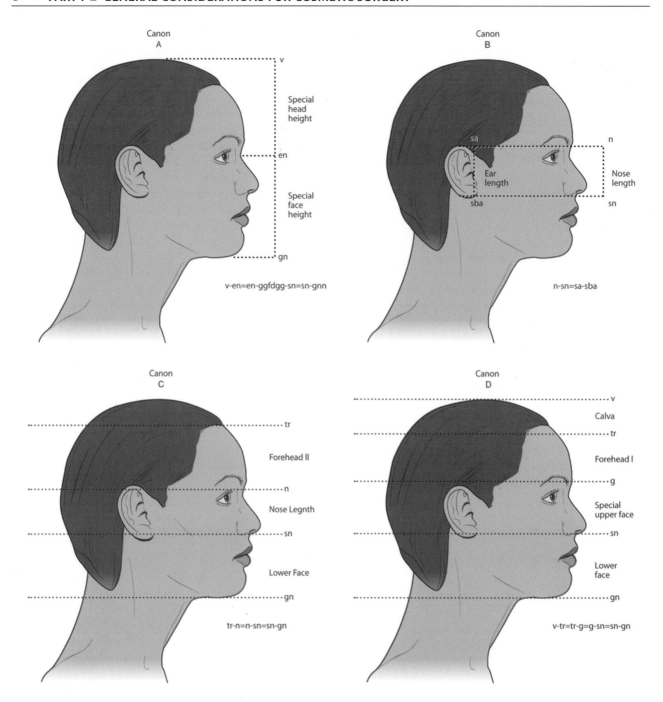

Figure 1-3 Golden Proportion and Neoclassical Canons. **A:** Two-section facial profile canon. The combined head-face height is divided into two equal parts: the special head height (vertex-endocanthion, v-en) and the special face height (endocanthion-menton, en-gn). **B:** Nasoaural proportion canon. The length of the nose (nasion-subnasale, n-sn) equals the length of the ear (supraaurale-subaurale, sa-sba). **C:** Three-section facial profile canon. The combined forehead-face height is divided into three equal parts: the forehead (trichion-nasion, tr-n), the nose (nasion-subnasale, n-sn), and the lower half of the face (subnasle-gnathion, sn-gn). **D:** Four-section facial profile canon. The combined head-face height is divided into four equal parts: the height of the calva (vertex-trichion, v-tr), the height of the forehead (trichion-glabella, tr-g), the special upper face height (glabella-subnasale, g-sn), and the height of the lower face (subnasale-gnathion, sn-gn). (Modified from Farkas LG, Hrecko TA, Kolar JC, et al. Vertical and horizontal proportions of the face in young adult North American Caucasians: revision of neoclassical canons. *Plast Reconstr Surg* 1985;75(3):328–337. Farkas LG, Forrest CR, Litsas L. Revision of neoclassical facial canons in young adult Afro-Americans. *Aest Plast Surg.* 2000;24:179–184.)

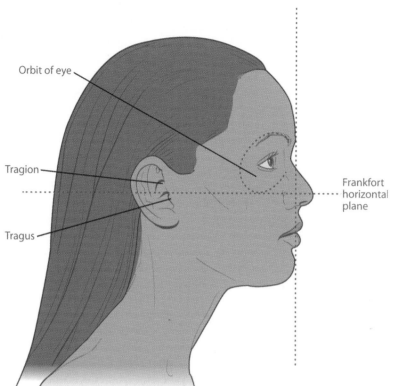

Orbit of eye

Tragion

Tragus

Frankfort horizontal plane

Figure 1-4 Frankfort horizontal scale. Standard craniometric reference used for facial surgery evaluation and photography. The position of the Frankfort horizontal line is determined by taking a lateral photograph and drawing a vertical line from just in front of the glabella to the front of the chin. A line is then drawn horizontally from right at the supratip to above the auricular canal, right above the tragus.

across ethnic boundaries? Matory assessed the applicability of various parameters of attractiveness in 400 "attractive" subjects representing different ethnic and racial groups: black Americans, Hispanic, Asian, Middle Eastern, and Caucasian.[20] The neoclassical canons were inconsistent in each of the ethnic categories. The face could be divided into three equal parts, and the face and cranium into four equal parts, in fewer than 9% and 4% of individuals, respectively.

In later work, Farkas et al. compared the validity of seven neoclassical canons in African Americans and Caucasian Americans.[3] They found that the three sections of the facial profile were not equal in either population. In the African American population, there was commonly a longer lower face height in relation to the height of the forehead and greater nose width. Farkas et al. concluded that the frequency of valid canons was greatly surpassed by their variations. In a similar study, Wang et al. compared horizontal neoclassical facial canons in Chinese and North American Caucasian populations.[21] They found that the nose corresponded to one quarter of the face in about half of Chinese subjects and approximately one third of Caucasian subjects. The Chinese mouth was significantly more often narrower than 1.5 times the nose width (71.8% of subjects), whereas the Caucasian mouth was significantly more frequently wider (60.2% of subjects).

The Frankfort horizontal plane, named in 1884, is the standard craniometric reference used for facial surgery evaluation and photography. The position of the Frankfort horizontal line is determined by taking a lateral photograph and drawing a vertical line from just in front of the glabella to the front of the chin (Fig. 1-4). Ideally, this line would be perfectly vertical, although some facial cosmetic surgeons believe the chin can be slightly behind this line in women and still look feminine and proportionate. A line is then drawn horizontally from right at the supratip to above the auricular canal, right above the tragus. Matory reported that the Frankfort horizontal was a common characteristic in African Americans with narrow and moderate features (98% and 65% of female subjects, respectively) but was less common in individuals with wide facial features (33.2% of female subjects).[20] He obtained similar results in male subjects.

In contrast to his results with neoclassical canons and the Frankfort horizontal plane, Matory found a dramatic consistency in the applicability of "golden aesthetic" proportions to the ethnic face (Table 1-1). The phi ratio of 1:1.618, as measured by the Ricketts caliper, correlated well with a number of facial relationships, including nose/eye/lip and nose/lip/chin relationships. In addition, he reported that among African Americans, the most attractive female faces are oval, diamond, or square shaped. In men, heart-shaped faces were more common. Oval faces when noted in men were considered feminizing.

Today, facial cosmetic surgeons rely on universally accepted guidelines and measurements of facial proportions to aid them in modifying facial structures and relationships.

A basic knowledge of standard reference points and their normative values is essential for computer imaging, record keeping, photography, and communication with patients and colleagues. However, these represent only basic standards for facial evaluation and analysis; there must also be an acceptance of their limitations in the clinical setting, because rigid adherence to calculated proportions may limit success in achieving a "natural" appearance.

DEFINING ETHNIC BEAUTY

The definition of a beautiful face will differ by ethnic group. Characteristic global defining features of people include skin color, hair texture, and morphologic differences in eyes, nose, and lips. Albeit there are diverse differences in the facial appearance of darker racial ethnic groups, several studies have indeed elucidated some defining features in facial structure of African Americans, Asians, and Hispanics.[3,22-25]

Most African Americans are triracial descendants of African, Native American, and Northern Europeans. Their facial features often reflect a multiracial heritage. African American skin tone can range in color from olive to light brown to brown to black. African American faces are characterized by a decreased nasal projection, broader nasal base, bimaxillary protrusion, and increased soft tissue thickness of the midface, lips, chin, orbital proptosis, and increased facial convexity (Table 1-2, Fig. 1-5).[23,26-28]

Asian populations include East Indians, Chinese, Japanese, Koreans, Vietnamese, Cambodians, Thai, Malay, Indonesians, Polynesians, and Filipinos. Some characteristic features of Asians include a wider intercanthal distance in relation to a shorter palpable fissure and a broad prominent forehead with nonptotic brows, lack of upper eyelid crease, broader nasal base, and a small mouth. Asians typically have a wider lower face with a recessed chin. In addition, wide mandibular angles and square-shaped faces are common (Table 1-3, Fig. 1-6).[23]

Many Hispanics living in North, Central, and South America are racial mixtures of Europeans, Spaniards, and Native Americans. African migration to the Americas—as well as migration of Asians and Central and Northern Europeans—has resulted in further miscegenation and given rise to the current-day Hispanic or Latino population. Variation depends on racial makeup.[29] Skin color may be white, olive, or brown. Many South American Latinos of Spanish and European ancestry have typical Caucasian facial features, whereas many Latinos in the Caribbean are of African ancestry. Common features of the Hispanic face include an increased bizygomatic distance,

Table 1-2
Features of the African American face

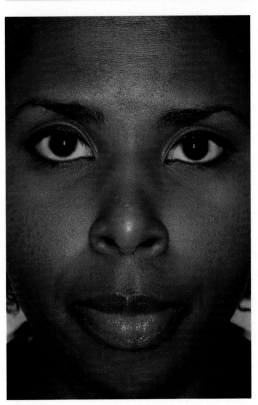

Bimaxillary protrusion

Broad nasal base

Decreased nasal projection

Orbital proptosis

Increased soft tissue of the midface

Prominent lips

Increased facial convexity

fication has come under increasing scrutiny in its lack of ability to predict minimal erythema dosing (MED), minimum melanogenic dosing (MMD) to tanning, or even constitutive skin color. Multiple investigators are examining new scales to assess ultraviolet responses as well as scales that more accurately predict cosmetic surgery outcomes.[10]

New objective technologies have evolved that facilitate objective and reproducible quantitative measures of skin color and erythema. A variety of color-measuring instruments have evolved based on two different principles of color physics. These include reflectance spectrophotometry and tristimulus colorimetry.[11] Spectrophotometer instruments use broad bands or selected wavelengths of light in the visible range and measure absorbance and reflectance. Tristimulus analysis of blue, red, and green light measures light reflection from skin structures. Convenient instruments using these principles include the Minolta Chromameter, the DermaSpectrometer, the Photovolt ColorWalk Colorimeter, the Mexameter, the DermaSpectrophotometer, and the Erythema Meter.

Grimes et al.[12] measured the ranges of skin color and erythema by reflectance spectrophotometry in a multiracial population of 160 subjects including African Americans, Caucasians, Hispanics, Asians, and East Indians. Measurements were taken during the months of November through January, when summer tans had likely faded. There was a statistically significant correlation between reflectance spectrophotometry measurements using the Meximeter MX 16 (Courage Khazaka, Electronics, GMbH) and race and Fitzpatrick's skin types (Fig. 2-2A,B). As the intensity of cutaneous pigmentation increased, measurements for melanin and erythema increased. There was no statistically significant correlation with age or sex. Additional studies

are indeed warranted to further validate the reliability of bioinstrumentation as a tool for skin typing.

MELANOCYTES, MELANIN, AND PIGMENTATION

The key feature defining races is the color of an individual's skin. Although skin color is influenced by melanin, hemoglobin in blood vessels, and dietary carotenoids, the predominant chromophore is melanin produced by melanocytes. The biologic differences observed in melanocytes and epidermal melanin have been well defined in black skin and white skin. Melanocytes are dendritic cells located in the basal layer of the epidermis (Fig. 2-3A,B). There are approximately 36 keratinocytes interfacing with 1 melanocyte, forming what is called an epidermal-melanin unit.[13] The distribution of these cells varies in different regions of the body (Fig. 2-4). Melanocytes are more numerous on the head and neck, scrotum, foreskin, and dorsal feet.

The content of melanin within keratinocytes determines skin color, with deeply pigmented skin having the highest content of epidermal melanin (Fig. 2-5). Melanin is a dense, relatively insoluble polymer of high molecular weight. It exists in two forms: eumelanin and pheomelanin. Eumelanin is a highly cross-linked dark brown to black pigment predominantly responsible for skin pigmentation. Pheomelanin is a yellow-red alkali soluble pigment derived from tyrosine, in which dopaquinone combines with glutathione or cysteine to form cysteinyl-dopa. Pheomelanin is predominantly found in auburn or red-haired fair skinned individuals.

Melanin is synthesized on melanosomes via the Raper-Mason pathway (Fig. 2-6).[14] The rate-limiting

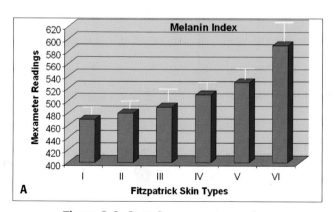

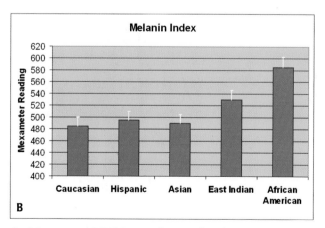

Figure 2-2 A: Reflectance spectrophotometry using the Mexameter MX16: correlation of melanin index with Fitzpatrick's skin types. There was a statistically significant correlation ($p = 0.01$) between intensity of pigmentation (melanin index readings) and Fitzpatrick's skin types.
B: Reflectance spectrophotometery utilizing the Mexameter MX16: correlation of melanin index with race/ethnicity. There was a statistically significant correlation ($p < 0.05$) between intensity of pigmentation (melanin index readings) and race.

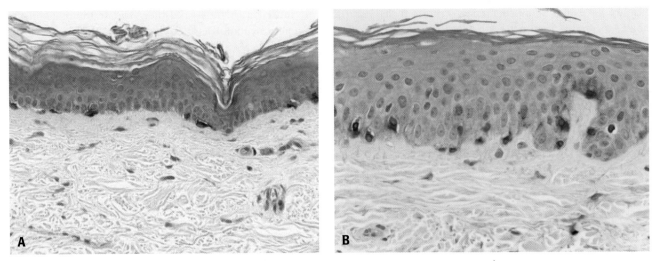

Figure 2-3 Immunohistochemical staining for melanocytes using an alkaline phosphatase detection kit and a 1:5 dilution of MEL-5 antibody after predigestion for 4 minutes with protease in **(A)** white skin and **(B)** black skin.

enzyme for this process is tyrosine. Although the precise mechanism of transfer of melanosomes to keratinocytes is unknown, suggested mechanisms include (a) fusion of melanocyte and keratinocyte plasma membranes, (b) melanosome secretion into the intercellular space followed by keratinocyte endocytosis, and (c) phagocytosis of melanocyte dendritic tips by keratinocytes.[15,16]

Melanosomes can occur as large, single membrane–bound mature melanosomes or as aggregates of smaller melanosomes. Although there are no quantitative differences

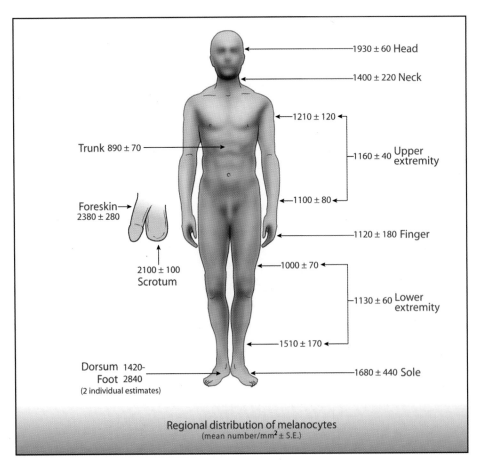

Figure 2-4 Anatomic distribution of melanocytes. (Modified from Fitzpatrick TB, Szabo G, Wick MM. Biochemistry and physiology of melanin pigment. In: Goldsmith LA, ed. *Biochemistry and Physiology of the Skin.* New York: Oxford Univ Press; 1983:112.

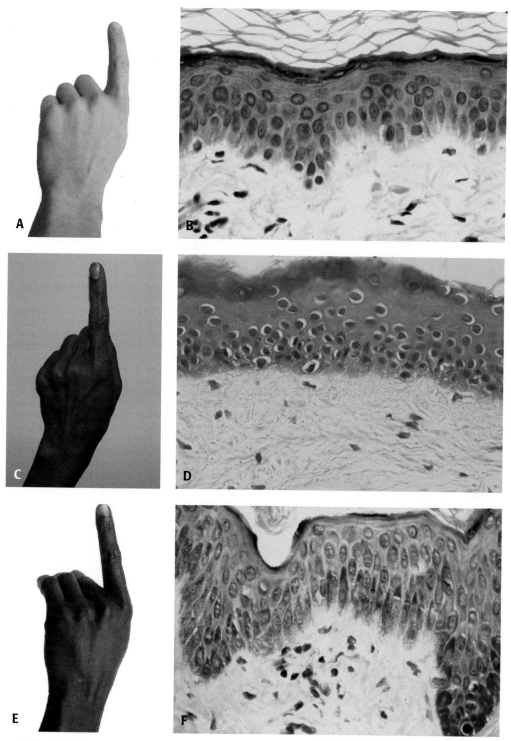

Figure 2-5 Photos and biopsies (40X magnification) taken from the hand of **(A)** and **(B)** Caucasians, **(C)** and **(D)** East Indians, and **(E)** and **(F)** African Americans. Note the progressive increase in melanin as skin pigmentation darkens. Courtesy of Jag Bhawan, MD.

in melanocytes amongst various racial/ethnic groups, the skin of blacks has an increased content of epidermal melanin and large singly dispersed melanosomes within melanocytes and keratinocytes.[17,18] Melanosomes have been identified in the entire epidermis, including the stratum granulosum,

stratum lucidum, and stratum corneum. Pigmented skin in particular black skin has more stage IV melanosomes. In contrast, in very pale white skin, few melanosomes are seen in the basal keratinocytes and malpighian layer.[19] However, darker-skinned Caucasians, upon skin exposure to sun, have

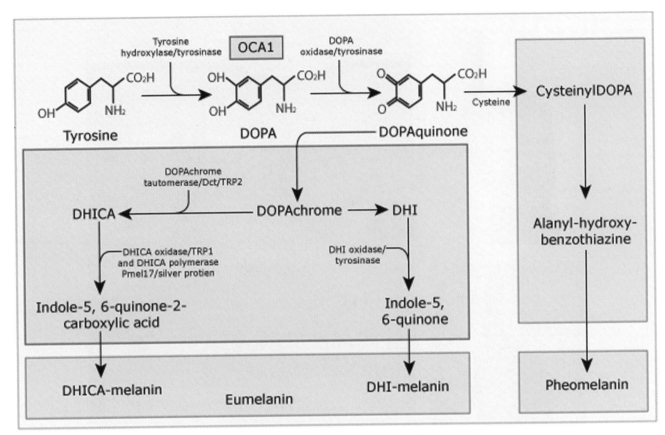

Figure 2-6 Melanin Biosynthetic Pathway.

larger nonaggregated melanosomes. Lighter-complexioned blacks have a combination of large nonaggregated and smaller aggregated melanosome.[19] In Asians, non–sun-exposed areas of skin have aggregated melanosomes, whereas sun-exposed areas have predominantly nonaggregated melanosomes.[20] Such observations support the concept of significant intraracial and interracial variations in pigmentation.

Recent work suggests that the expression and activation of protease-activated receptor-2 (PAR-2) correlates with skin color and may influence ethnic skin color phenotypes. PAR-2 receptors are expressed on keratinocytes. They have been shown to play a role in controlling melanosome ingestion and phagocytosis by keratinocytes.[21,22] In addition, PAR-2 may play a regulatory role in skin pigmentation.[23,24] Babiarz-Magee et al.[21] examined the expression of PAR-2 and its activator trypsin in human skin from individuals with different shades of pigmentation. These findings suggest PAR-2 and trypsin were expressed in higher levels in darker compared with lighter skin. In addition, darker skin showed an increase in PAR-2 specific protease cleavage ability. These findings suggested that PAR-2 expression and activity may play an important role in ethnic skin color phenotypes.

A study comparing the transmission of ultraviolet radiation (UVA and UVB) through skin samples of blacks and whites using both biologic and spectroscopic techniques found that, on average, five times as much ultraviolet light reached the upper dermis of white skin as compared with black skin.[25] Differences in transmission between the stratum corneum of blacks and of whites were far less striking. The main site of UV filtration in whites was the stratum corneum, whereas in blacks, it was the malpighian layers of the epidermis. The main UV protective factor for black epidermis was 13.14 compared with 3.4 for white skin.[25]

Rijken et al.[26] investigated the responses of black and white skin to solar-simulating radiation. In subjects with skin types I to III, 12,000 to 18,000 mJ per cm^2 of solar-simulating radiation (SSR) induced DNA damage in epidermal and dermal cells, an influx of neutrophils, active proteolytic enzymes, and diffuse keratinocyte activation. In addition, IL-10 positive neutrophils were found to infiltrate the epidermis. Except for DNA damage in the suprabasal epidermis, none of these changes was found in subjects with skin types IV to VI exposed to comparable doses of SSR. Increased skin pigmentation appeared to be the primary source of these observed differences. Hence, the increased epidermal melanin content of black skin serves as a major filter for blocking ultraviolet light transmission, further substantiating melanin's role in lowering the susceptibility to sunburn, photoaging, and skin cancer.[27,28]

In a study assessing the relationship between constitutive skin color and UV light sensitivity in Koreans, darker skin color conferred photoprotection in younger patients.[29] Similarly, an assessment of physiologic factors affecting skin susceptibility to ultraviolet radiation in Japanese women showed that darker-skinned Japanese women had less severe reactions to sun exposure.[30]

The melanocytes of darker-skinned individuals show labile, exaggerated responses to cutaneous injury.[31] A major consequence of this phenomenon is the high frequency of dyschromias, in particular melasma and postinflammatory hyperpigmentation.

EPIDERMAL STRUCTURE AND FUNCTION

Stratum corneum

There are some differences described in the epidermis in lighter compared with darker racial ethnic groups.

Differences include variations in stratum corneum thickness, water content, lipid production, and melanin (Table 2-1).

Corneocytes are key in determining cutaneous water loss and percutaneous absorption of topically applied products. Some differences have been reported in the stratum corneum of darker racial ethnic groups. Despite a scarcity of data, some of these differences are generally accepted. Weigand et al.[32] assessed cell layers and density of the stratum corneum in 25 white and 21 black subjects. The authors reported that the stratum corneum of black and white skin was of equal thickness. However, in blacks, it contains more cell layers and requires more cellophane tape strippings to remove the stratum corneum.

Corcuff et al.[33] assessed corneocyte surface area and spontaneous desquamation in blacks, whites, and Asians

Table 2-1

Comparison of epidermis of different racial groups

	White	Black	Asians*
Stratum corneum thickness	7.2 μm	6.5 μm	
Stratum corneum layers	17 layers	22 layers	
Stratum lucidum	1–2 layers; on exposure to sun becomes swollen and distinctly cellular	Remains compact and unaltered with sun exposure	
Water barrier	High	Low	
Melanosomes	Small. Grouped melanosomes in keratinocytes less dense, more numerous in stratum corneum than basal layer	Larger. Individually dispersed melanosomes in keratinocytes more numerous in basal layer	Mainly aggregated melanosomes; nonaggregated in sunlight-exposed areas
Stratum corneum lipids	Low	High	
Vitamin D production	High	Low	
Minimal Erythema Dosing	Low	High	
Photodamage	Significant changes in the epidermis	Marginal changes in the epidermis	Significant changes in the epidermis
Melanin	Has greater protective capability in the stratum corneum	Has less protective capability in the stratum corneum	
Mast cell morphology	Smaller granules. Less cathepsin G	Larger granules. More cathepsin G	

From Halder RM. *Dermatology and Dermatological Therapy of Pigmented Skins.* Boca Raton, FL: Publisher; 2006:5. With permission from CRC Press, Taylor & Francis Group.
*There is minimal published data on Asians.

of Chinese ancestry with 18 to 25 subjects in each group. They found no evidence of differences in corneocyte surface area among black, white, and Asian skin. However, black subjects were noted to have increased spontaneous desquamation compared with whites and Asians. They suggested this difference might be due to differences in the lipid composition of the intercellular cement. Other studies have also failed to show differences in stratum corneum thickness among darker skin types compared with Caucasians.[34]

Barrier function

The epidermal barrier provides an effective covering that prevents loss of body fluids while controlling absorption of infectious, toxic, or other externally applied substances. The results of studies assessing barrier function including transepidermal water loss (TEWL), conductance, sodium lauryl sulfate irritation, and pericutaneous absorption of chemicals have shown variable results among different racial-ethnic groups. Multiple investigations, including Berardesca and Maibach,[35] Wilson et al.,[36] Reed et al.,[37] Kompaore et al.,[38] Grimes et al.,[39] and others have assessed TEWL in darker-racial ethnic groups. Sample size, methodologies, and testing sites have varied.

An initial study by Berardesca and Maibach showed greater TEWL in blacks compared with whites after sodium lauryl sulfate (SLS) challenge to preoccluded, predelipidized skin of the back.[35] Subsequent studies by these investigators showed varying results.[40,41] When testing the upper back after SLS stress in seven Hispanic men and nine white men, TEWL was greater in Hispanic men but not statistically significant. A volar and dorsal forearm study in 15 blacks, 12 whites, and 12 Hispanics showed no difference between site or race at baseline. Grimes et al.[39] recently assessed TEWL from the inner forearm in 18 African American and 19 Caucasian women. No differences in TEWL were observed in baseline assessments. A subset of three African Americans and five Caucasians underwent testing after SLS challenge. No statistically significant differences were observed at 30 minutes, 24 hours, or 48 hours. In addition, Goh and Chia[42] reported no differences in TEWL at baseline and after irritation with SLS in Chinese, Malays, and Indians.

In contrast, other studies have shown increased TEWL at baseline and/or after irritation. Kampaore et al.[38] assessed TEWL after application of a vasodilator, methyl nicotinate, and after tape stripping. The study population included seven blacks, eight Caucasians, and six Asians. TEWL was greater in blacks and Asians compared with Caucasians. After tape stripping, Asians showed the most significant TEWL, followed by blacks.

Additional studies have reported a more resistant barrier in deeply pigmented skin with enhanced TEWL after tape stripping compared with lighter skin types.[43]

The differences in skin irritation were assessed in 22 Japanese and 22 German women.[44] Tests performed included forearm patch testing with SLS, measurement of TEWL, stratum corneum hydration, sebum secretion, laser Doppler flowmetry, melanin content, and erythema. No significant differences in barrier function of the stratum corneum were found between these two groups. However, stronger clinical sensory differences were evident among Japanese women.

In general, investigations assessing hydration and skin biomechanics showed variable results. Water content measured by capacitance after topical administration of the irritant sodium lauryl sulfate was compared in blacks and whites, and in Hispanics and whites.[34] There were no significant differences. Concrete variations were not observed using other methods, such as resistance, conductance, and impedance to quantify variations in hydration. However, after topical application of the vasodilator methyl nicotinate, black and Asian skin was reported to be more permeable to water than white skin measured using laser Doppler velocimetry (LDV). Studies assessing blood vessel reactivity in darker racial ethnic groups have been difficult to interpret given that different vasoactive substances were used. However, some differences in blood vessel reactivity have been noted.[45–47] Studies following well-defined protocols carried out on larger experimental and control groups are direly needed to further assess the definitive differences in water content, blood reactivity, and elastic recovery between racial groups.

Irritation

Marshall et al.[48] reported an increased frequency of irritation as assessed by erythema from 1% dichloroethyl sulfide in blacks compared with whites. A subsequent study by Weigand et al.[49] reported that after removal of the stratum corneum, there were no differences in irritation as assessed by the induction of erythema. Recent clinical studies report an increase in irritant reactions in darker racial ethnic groups when treated with retinoids.[50,51] However, an exhaustive review of this subject found little evidence supporting differences in the irritant response between Caucasians, blacks, and Asians.[52]

Differences in barrier function assume increasing importance when assessing irritant dermatitis, contact dermatitis, and tolerance to cosmetic formulations. Aggressive anti-aging regimens incorporating the use of retinoids, retinols, and alpha hydroxy acids can induce irritant dermatitis in some darker-skinned patients. Hence, gradual titration to more aggressive formulations is always prudent. Barrier integrity and differences in barrier function are also important considerations when performing chemical peels, microdermabrasion, cosmetic laser resurfacing, and hair removal procedures.

Lipid content

Several studies, albeit with small sample sizes, have measured stratum corneum lipids and ceramide levels in darker racial ethnic groups. Reinertson and Wheatley in 1959 measured lipids and sterols in living and cadaver skin of black and white men. Lipid content and sterols were higher in black skin compared with white.[53] Since then, two other studies have assessed lipids. In contrast to the later studies, Sugino et al. reported 50% lower levels of ceramides in blacks compared with Hispanics and Caucasians.[54] However a study of stratum corneum lipid content in 41 subjects from the United Kingdom and 62 subjects from Thailand showed no differences in scalp lipid levels.[55]

Lipid levels may significantly influence and/or determine epidermal water content, an important variable in evaluating or considering the response to topical cosmeceutical and pharmaceutical agents.

DERMAL STRUCTURE

Fibroblasts, mast cells, and blood vessels

Very few studies have assessed basic dermal differences in darker racial ethnic groups. Dermal changes associated with chronologic aging and photoaging are discussed in Chapter 3. Black skin has a thick and compact dermis in which the distinction between the papillary and reticular layers is less clear compared with Caucasian skin. The dermis of blacks contains many fiber fragments composed of collagen fibrils and glycoproteins.[56] In addition, there is close stacking of the collagen fiber bundles, which run parallel to the surface of the epidermis. In general, the dermis of blacks shows minimal evidence of photodamage. Table 2-2 compares differences in the dermis of black and white skin.

Table 2-2		
Comparison of dermal structure between black and white skin		
	White	Black
Dermis	Thinner and less compact	Thick and compact
Papillary and reticular layer	More distinct	Less distinct
Collagen fiber bundles	Bigger	Smaller. Close stacking and surrounded by ground substance
Fiber fragments	Sparse	Prominent and numerous
Melanophages (macrophages that phagocytize). Melanosomes that spill into the dermis	Many	Numerous and larger
Lymphatic vessels	Moderate, dilated	Many dilated, empty lymph channels, usually surrounded by masses of elastic fibers
Fibroblasts	Not as numerous. Some binucleated cells	Numerous and large. Many binucleated and multinucleated cells
Elastic fibers	More. In photodamage, only fibers in papillary and reticular dermis stain pink; the others stain lilac or deep blue	Less. All dermal elastic fibers stain pink, as found in sun-protected skin. Elastosis is uncommon
Superficial blood vessels	Sparse to moderate	More numerous, mostly dilated
Glycoprotein molecules	Variable	Numerous in the dermis

From Halder RM. *Dermatology and Dermatological Therapy of Pigmented Skins.* Boca Raton, FL: Publisher; 2006:8. With permission from CRC Press, Taylor & Francis Group.

Fibroblasts are large and numerous on black skin, suggesting active biosynthesis, degradation, and turnover. These cells have been shown to be hypertrophic and contain extensive rough endoplasmic reticulum, Golgi bodies, and vesicles. In blacks, this heightened activity could affect keloid and hypertrophic scar formation, common conditions in individuals of African ancestry. Keloids are also more common in Asians, particularly Chinese people, compared with Caucasians.[56]

Montagna and Carlisle[57] reported an equal number of mast cells in black and white skin and found no differences in the staining properties of mast cell granules. In contrast, Sueki et al.[58] performed biopsies on four black and four white subjects and found that mast cells in black skin contained larger granules. Fusion of granules seemed to account for the larger sizes. Proteases, tryptase, and cathepsin G also differed in mast cells of black and white skin. Mast cell mediators include histamine, fibroblast growth factor, and tryptase. Mast cells also have been implicated in the pathogenesis of keloids and hypertrophic scars.[59,60]

Superficial subepidermal blood vessels are reported to be more numerous in black skin.[61] Compared with white dermis, the dermis of blacks has been reported to have many dilated, empty lymph channels. The significance of these dilated lymph channels is unknown.

Skin thickness/facial tissue thickness

There are few comparative studies assessing skin or tissue thickness in lighter versus darker racial ethnic groups.[62–65] No statistically significant differences in skin thickness were observed in non–sun-exposed forearm skin of white and black women.[65] Facial measurements were not taken.

Measurements of facial soft-tissue thickness have been conducted in men and women in American blacks and whites,[62] Japanese,[63] and a mixed South African racial population.[64] Notable differences exist between men and women, with men having increased thickness of facial tissue. Comparison between the results of facial soft-tissue measurements in American blacks, whites, Japanese, and a mixed South African population show that facial tissues of blacks are thicker in the upper and lower face. Measurements in the aforementioned groups of black, white, and Japanese were conducted on cadaver specimens, whereas measurements in the mixed racial population were taken with computerized tomography. Given the popularity of resurfacing procedures, botulinum toxin injections, and injectable filler substances, these data may be of use to the cosmetic surgeon in defining the choice of resurfacing procedure, depth of treatment, and appropriate dosing of denervating agents.

Appendages

Few definitive differences in eccrine and apocrine glands have been reported among darker racial ethnic groups compared with lighter skin types. However, Montagna and Carlisle[57] reported that apocrine glands are more often found in the facial skin of black women compared with Caucasians.

Results of investigations of sebaceous glands and sebaceous gland activity have shown some differences. Several studies have reported larger sebaceous glands in blacks compared with whites,[66,67] Kligman and Shelly[68] reported an increase in sebum production in blacks, and others have reported no differences among different racial/ethnic groups. Grimes et al.[39] assessed sebum production on the forehead of 18 African American women and 19 white women using a sebumeter. No statistically significant differences in sebum production were found. Sebum production was also measured via a sebumeter and sebutape in 20 blacks, 20 Asians, and 20 whites.[69] No significant differences in sebum production were observed. Sebum production and oily skin are key issues of consideration when selecting the appropriate cosmeceutical and pharmaceutical products. Patients with oily skin necessitate special products to combat oil production. In addition, increased sebum production may be a consideration when selecting appropriate resurfacing procedures for darker skin types.

Hair follicles

The hair features of individuals of African ancestry are indeed different as compared with other racial-ethnic groups. Unprocessed virgin hair is characteristically fragile, tightly curled, dry, and brittle. In contrast to other races, the follicles are flat and elliptical. The hair also has a longer axis. Lindelof et al.[70] assessed the structure of the hair shaft in blacks and reported that the black hair follicle has a helical form. In contrast, the Asian follicle is straight, and the Caucasian follicle is a variation of the two. Compared with other groups, the hair of blacks has the smallest mean cross-sectional area. The cross-sectional area is largest in Asians and smallest in Caucasians; however, hair characteristics are becoming increasingly varied because of miscegenation and genetic diversity. An ultrastructural study of hair differences in blacks and whites found fewer elastic fibers anchoring the hair follicles in the dermis in blacks. In addition, the total hair density and total number of terminal hair follicles appears to be significantly lower in African Americans compared with Caucasians.[71] Because of these inherent structural features, the hair is predisposed to breakage. Special grooming procedures are often necessary to straighten the hair. Pressing the hair and chemical relaxing further aggravate hair fragility (see Chapter 30). In addition, the curved follicle predisposes black men and women to pseudofolliculitis barbae.[72] Hair follicle morphology assumes increasing importance in laser hair removal as well as hair transplantation surgery.

CONCLUSION

Statistical projections suggest continued major growth of darker racial populations globally.[5] The unique structural and physiologic differences of the skin of darker racial ethnic groups are paramount considerations in selecting appropriate aesthetic and cosmetic surgical procedures. Cosmetic surgeons must be cognizant of these differences to provide optimal patient care, patient satisfaction, and enhanced quality of life.

REFERENCES

1. Robins AH. *Biological Perspectives on Human Pigmentation.* New York: Cambridge University Press; 1991.
2. Franklin, JH. *Color and Race.* Boston: Beacon Press; 1968:x.
3. Risch N, Burchard E, Ziv E, et al. Categorization of humans in biomedical research: genes, race and disease. *Genome Biol* 2002;3(7):Comment 2007. http://genomebiology.com/2002/3/7/comment/2007
4. Rees JL. Genetics of hair and skin color. *Annu Rev Genet* 2003;37:67–90.
5. U.S. Census Bureau, Population Division, April 12, 2000.
6. The American Society for Aesthetic Plastic Surgery. *Statistics on Cosmetic Surgery, 2005.* New York: http://www.surgery.org/professionals/index.php.
7. Von Luschan F. *Beiträge zur Völkerkunde der Deutschen Schutzgebieten.* Berlin: Deutsche Buchgemeinschaft; 1897.
8. Fullerton A, Fischer T, Lattice A, et al. Guidelines for measurement of skin colour and erythema. *Contact Dermatitis* 1996;35:1–10.
9. Fitzpatrick TB. The validity and practicality of sun reactive skin type I through VI. *Arch Dermatol* 1988;124:869–871.
10. Lancer HA. Lancer Ethnicity Scale (LES) [correspondence]. *Lasers Surg Med* 1998;22:9.
11. Taylor S, Westerhof W, Im S, et al. Noninvasive techniques for the evaluation of skin color. *J Am Acad Dermatol* 2006;54:S282–290.
12. Grimes PE, Camarena E, Elkadi T. Colorimetric assessment of pigmentation and erythema using the Meximeter MX16: correlation with Fitzpatrick's skin type and race. Poster exhibit presented at: Annual Meeting of the American Academy of Dermatology; March 19–24, 1999; New Orleans, LA.
13. Fitzpatrick TB, Szabo G, Wick MM. Biochemistry and physiology of melanin pigment. In: Goldsmith LA, ed. *Biochemistry and Physiology of the Skin.* New York: Oxford Univ Press; 1983:54.
14. Prota G. Regulatory mechanisms of melanogenesis: beyond the tyrosinase concept. *J Invest Dermatol* 1993;100(2 Suppl):156S–161S.
15. Westerhof W. The discovery of the human melanocyte. *Pigment Cell Res* 2006;19(3):183–193.
16. Fitzpatrick TB, Ortonne JP. Normal skin color and general considerations of pigmentary disorders. In: Freedberg IM, ed. *Fitzpatrick's Dermatology in General Medicine,* vol. I. 6th ed. City: McGraw-Hill; 2003:819–826.
17. Szabo G, Gerald AB, Patnak MA, et al. Racial differences in the fate of melanosomes in human epidermis. *Nature* 1969;222:1081–1082.
18. Olson RL, Gaynor J, Everett MA. Skin color, melanin, and erythema. *Arch Dermatol* 1973;108:541–544.
19. Halder RM, Nootheti PK. Ethnic skin disorders overview. *J Am Acad Dermatol* 2003;48(6 Suppl):S143–148.
20. Toda K, Pathak MA, Parrish JA, et al. Alteration of racial differences in melanosome distribution in human epidermis after exposure to ultraviolet light. *Nat New Biol* 1972;236(66):143–145.
21. Babiarz-Magee L, Chen N, Seiberg M, et al. The expression and activation of protease-activated receptor-2 correlate with skin color. *Pigment Cell Res* 2004;17(3):241–251.
22. Sharlow ER, Paine CS, Babiarz L, et al. The protease-activated receptor-2 upregulates keratinocyte phagocytosis. *J Cell Sci* 2000;113 (Pt 17):3093–3101.
23. Seiberg M, Paine C, Sharlow E, et al. The protease-activated receptor 2 regulates pigmentation via keratinocyte-melanocyte interactions. *Exp Cell Res* 2000;254(1):25–32.
24. Seiberg M, Paine C, Sharlow E, et al. Inhibition of melanosome transfer results in skin lightening. *J Invest Dermatol* 2000;115(2):162–167.
25. Kaidbey KH, Agin PP, Sayre RM, et al. Photoprotection by melanin: a comparison of black and Caucasian skin. *J Am Acad Dermatol* 1979;1:249–260.
26. Rijken F, Bruijnzeel PL, van Weelden H, et al. Responses of black and white skin to solar-simulating radiation: differences in DNA photodamage, infiltrating neutrophils, proteolytic enzymes induced, keratinocyte activation, and IL-10 expression. *J Invest Dermatol* 2004;122(6):1448–1455.
27. Quevedo WC, Fitzpatrick TB, Jimbow K. Human skin color: original variation and significance. *J Hum Evol* 1985;14:43.
28. Washington C, Grimes PE. Incidence and prevention of skin cancer. *J Cosmet Dermatol* 2003;16(S3):46–48.
29. Lee JH, Kim TY. Relationship between constitutive skin color and ultraviolet light sensitivity in Koreans. *Photodermatol Photoimmunol Photomed* 1999;15(6):231–235.
30. Abe T, Arai S, Mimura K, et al. Studies of physiological factors affecting skin susceptibility to ultraviolet light irradiation and irritants. *J Dermatol* 1983;10(6):531–537.
31. Grimes PE, Stockton T. Pigmentary disorders in blacks. *Dermatol Clin* 1988;6(2):271–281.
32. Weigand DA, Haygood C, Gaylor JR. Cell layers and density of Negro and Caucasian stratum corneum. *J Invest Dermatol* 1974;62(6):563–568.
33. Corcuff P, Lotte C, Rougier A, et al. Racial differences in corneocytes: a comparison between black, white and oriental skin. *Acta Derm Venereol* 1991;71(2):146–148.
34. Berardesca E, Rigal J, Leveque JL, et al. In vivo biophysical characterization of skin physiological differences in races. *Dermatologica* 1991;182:89–93.
35. Berardesca E, Maibach H. Ethnic skin: overview of structure and function. *J Am Acad Dermatol* 2003;48(6 Suppl):S139–142.
36. Wilson D, Berardesca E, Maibach HI. In vitro transepidermal water loss: differences between black and white skin. *Br J Dermatol* 1988;119:647–652.
37. Reed JT, Ghadially R, Elias PM. Effect of race, gender, and skin type on epidermal permeability barrier function. *J Invest Dermatol* 1994;102:537.
38. Kompaore F, Marty JP, Dupont C. In vivo evaluation of the stratum corneum barrier function in blacks, Caucasians, and Asians with two noninvasive methods. *Skin Pharmacol* 1993;63:200–207.
39. Grimes P, Edison BL, Green BA, et al. Evaluation of inherent differences between African American and white skin

surface properties using subjective and objective measures. *Cutis* 2004;73(6):392–396.

40. Berardesca E, Maibach HI. Sodium-lauryl-sulphate-induced cutaneous irritation: comparison of white and Hispanic subjects. *Contact Dermatitis* 1988;19(2):136–140.

41. Berardesca E, Maibach HI. Racial differences in sodium lauryl sulphate induced cutaneous irritation: black and white. *Contact Dermatitis* 1988;18(2):65–70.

42. Goh CL, Chia SE. Skin irritability due to sodium lauryl sulfate as measured by skin water vapour loss by sex and race. *Clin Exp Dermatol* 1988;13:16–19.

43. Reed JT, Ghadially R, Elias PM. Skin type, but neither race nor gender, influence epidermal permeability barrier function. *Arch Dermatol* 1995;131(10):1134–1138.

44. Aramaki J, Kawana S, Effendy I, et al. Differences of skin irritation between Japanese and European women. *Br J Dermatol* 2002;146:1052–1056.

45. Gaen CJ, Tur E, Maibach HI. Cutaneous responses to topical methyl nicotinate in black, oriental, and Caucasian subjects. *Arch Dermatol Res* 1989;281(2):95–98.

46. Guy RH, Tur E, Bjerke S, et al. Are there age and racial differences to methyl nicotinate-induced vasodilation in human skin? *J Am Acad Dermatol* 1985;12:1001–1006.

47. Berardesca E, Maibach HI. Cutaneous reactive hyperemia: racial differences induced by corticoid application. *Br J Dermatol* 1989;129:787–794.

48. Marshall EK, Lynch V, Smith HV. Variation in susceptibility of the skin to dichloroethylsulfide. *J Pharmacol Exp Ther* 1919;12:291–301.

49. Weigand DA, Haygood C, Gaylor JR. Cell layers and density of Negro and Caucasian stratum corneum. *J Invest Dermatol* 1974;62:563–568.

50. Halder RM, Richards GM. Topical agents used in the management of hyperpigmentation. *Skin Therapy Lett* 2004; 9(6):1–3.

51. Halder RM. The role of retinoids in the management of cutaneous conditions in blacks. *J Am Acad Dermatol* 1998; 39(2 Pt 3):S98–103.

52. Modjtahedi SP, Maibach HI. Ethnicity as a possible endogenous factor in irritant contact dermatitis: comparing the irritant response among Caucasians, blacks, and Asians. *Contact Dermatitis* 2002;47(5):272–278.

53. Reinertson RP, Wheatley VR. Studies on the chemical composition of human epidermal lipids. *J Invest Dermatol* 1959; 32(1):49–59.

54. Sugino K, Imokawa G, Maibach H. Ethnic difference of stratum corneum lipid in relation to stratum corneum function. *J Invest Dermatol* 1993;100:597.

55. Rawlings AV. Ethnic skin types: are there differences in skin structure and function? *Int J Cos Sci* 2006;28:79.

56. Yosipovitch G, Theng CTS. Asian skin: its architecture, function and differences from Caucasian skin. *Cosmetics & Toiletries* 2002;117(9):104–110.

57. Montagna W, Carlisle K. The architecture of black and white skin. *J Am Acad Dermatol* 1991;24:929–937.

58. Sueki H, Whitaker Menezes D, Kligman AM. Structural diversity of mast cell granules in black and white skin. *Br J Dermatol* 2001;144:85–93.

59. Craig SS, DeBlois G, Schwartz LB. Mast cells in human keloid, small intestine, and lung by immunoperoxidase technique using a murine monoclonal antibody against tryptase. *Am J Pathol* 1986;124:427–435.

60. Kischer CW, Bunce H, Shetla MR. Mast cell analysis in hypertrophic scars treated with pressure and mature scars. *J Invest Dermatol* 1978;70:355–357.

61. Basset A, Liautoud B, Ndiaye B. *Dermatology of Black Skin.* Oxford: Oxford University Press, 1946.

62. Rhine JS, Campbell HR. Thickness of facial tissues in American blacks. *J Forensic Sci* 1980;25(4):847–858.

63. Suzuki K. On the thickness of the soft parts of the Japanese face. *J Anthrop Soc Nippon* 1948;60:7–11.

64. Phillips VM, Smuts NA. Facial reconstruction: utilization of computerized tomography to measure facial tissue thickness in a mixed racial population. *Forensic Sci Int* 1996;83:51–59.

65. Whitmore SE, Sago NJ. Caliper-measured skin thickness is similar in white and black women. *J Am Acad Dermatol* 2000;42:76–79.

66. Pochi PE, Strauss JS. Sebaceous gland activity in black skin. *Dermatol Clin* 1988;6(3):349–351.

67. Taylor SC. Skin of color: biology, structure, function, and implications for dermatologic disease. *J Am Acad Dermatol* 2002(46);S41-S62.

68. Kligman AM, Shelly WB. An investigation of the biology of the human sebaceous gland. *J Invest Dermatol* 1958;30(3): 99–125.

69. Abedeen SK, Gonzalez M, Judodihardjo H, et al. Racial variation in sebum excretion rate: Program and abstracts of the 58th Annual Meeting of the American Academy of Dermatology; March 10–15, 2000; San Francisco, CA.

70. Lindelof B, Forslind B, Hedblad M, et al. Human hair form: morphology revealed by light and scanning electron microscopy and computer-aided three-dimensional reconstruction. *Arch Dermatol* 1988;124:1359–1363.

71. Steggerda M, Serbert HC. Size and shape of head hair from six racial groups. *J Hered* 1942;32:315–318.

72. Richards GM, Oresajo CO, Halder RM. Structure and function of ethnic skin and hair. *Dermatol Clin* 2003;21(4): 595–600.

The Aging Face in Darker Racial Ethnic Groups

Pearl E. Grimes, Doris M. Hexsel and Marcio Rutowitsch

The aging face is an amalgam of many elements of time. It is a canvas of photodamage (extrinsic aging) and the imitable changes of time (intrinsic aging), including volumetric loss (fat atrophy) and gravitational soft-tissue movement. It is characterized by the appearance of coarse and fine wrinkles, skin laxity, jowls, mottled pigmentary changes, textural changes, redundancies, and loose skin. The aforementioned signs are unique to each individual, so that in aging, each person presents a greatly variable number of skin and soft-tissue alterations determined by genetic factors and environmental influences, such as sun exposure, smoking, and lifestyle.

Common signs of aging in fair-skinned patients result from photodamage as evidenced by wrinkles, skin laxity, dyschromia, and textural alterations; these tend to appear as early as the second and third decade of life. Darker racial ethnic groups have a higher content of epidermal melanin (see Chapter 2). In addition, fibroblasts are large and active, often giving rise to a thicker dermis. The photoprotective effects of melanin in darker racial ethnic groups retard many of the early telltale signs of aging, such as crow's feet and periorbital wrinkles. Hence, photoaging changes are often minimized in deeply pigmented skin. Instead, soft tissue and gravitational changes may dominate cutaneous aging in darker skin types.

This chapter will review photodamage, intrinsic aging, and soft-tissue gravitational aspects of the intrinsic aging process in darker racial ethnic groups.

PHOTODAMAGE

Photodamage results from the long-term deleterious effects of sun exposure. Clinically, photodamaged skin is characterized by coarse and fine wrinkling, mottled pigmentary changes, sallowness, textural roughness, and telangiectasias (Table 3-1). Histopathological features of photodamaged skin include significant epidermal and dermal alterations.[1] The epidermal thickness may be increased or decreased, corresponding to areas of hyperplasia or atrophy. There is loss of polarity of epidermal cells and keratinocyte atypia. Dermal features include elas-

tosis, degeneration of collagen, and anchoring fibrils. Blood vessels become dilated and twisted. Ultraviolet light exposure activates matrix-degrading metalloproteinase enzymes, including collagenase. Cytokines are released from keratinocytes. The cumulative effect is chronic dermal inflammation.[2-4]

Photoaging affects all races and skin types. Signs of photoaging may begin at an early age, as evidenced by freckles following ultraviolet light exposure. However, the clinical manifestations of photodamage may differ in lighter compared with darker skin types. In individuals with Fitzpatrick's skin types I to III, or lighter-complexioned races, the clinical signs of photoaging—including wrinkles, laxity, dyschromia, and sallowness—may also be accompanied by an increased occurrence of premalignant and malignant skin lesions, including actinic keratoses, basal cell carcinoma, squamous cell carcinoma, and melanoma.

Glogau classified the severity of photodamage based on the extent of epidermal and dermal degenerative changes. Severity of photodamage is categorized from I through IV, ranging from mild to moderate to advanced or severely photodamaged skin (Table 3-2). The Glogau classification often facilitates the selection of appropriate treatment options in the aging Caucasian face.[5] For instance, patients with mild photodamage often respond to topical anti-aging regimens and superficial resurfacing procedures, whereas patients who have moderate to severe photodamage require more aggressive resurfacing procedures or rhytidectomies.

In deeply pigmented skin, photodamage may be characterized by mottled facial pigmentation, texturally rough skin, and fine wrinkles. In contrast to Glogau's scale, advanced and severe photodamage are uncommon in deeply pigmented skin, in particular in African Americans (Fig. 3-2A–D). In a study by Grimes,[6] 100 women of color were surveyed regarding their concern about wrinkles, and the resulting data were compared with results from an age-matched population of 143 white women. Mean age of the white comparison group was 43 years. Sixty-five percent of the women of color—compared with only 20% of the white women—reported that their skin was not wrinkled. Only 2% of the women of color—compared with

Table 3-1

Clinical and histological features of intrinsic and extrinsic aging

Feature	Intrinsic aging (chronological)	Extrinsic aging (photoaging)
Clinical	Smooth, atrophic	Fine and coarse wrinkles
	Finely wrinkled Laxity, unblemished	Sallowness, laxity, mottled pigmentation, textural roughness, telangiectasias
Epidermis	Stratum corneum normal thickness (basket weave pattern), epidermis thinned, atrophic, flattened rete ridges	Basket weave or compact stratum corneum, acanthosis and/or atrophy, keratinocyte atypia, flattened rete ridges
Dermis	Absent Grenz zone, loss of elastic fibers, elastogenesis, decreased thickness, microvasculature normal, no evidence of inflammation	Grenz zone prominent, elastogenesis, elastosis, collagen degeneration, loss of anchoring fibrils
		Microvasculature abnormal:
		Blood vessels dilated, twisted;
		Later stages: Sparse, perivenular lymphohistiocytic infiltrates

Modified from Gilchrest BA. A review of skin aging and its medical therapy. *Br J Dermatol* 1996;135:867–875; and Lavker RM. Cutaneous aging: chronologic versus photoaging. In: Gilchrest BA, ed. *Photodamage*. Cambridge, MA: Blackwell Science;1995:123–135 (34).

20% of the white women—considered their skin moderately wrinkled. These results show a marked difference in perceived photoaging between women of color and white women. Montagna and Carlisle[7] compared the morphology of facial skin of 19 black and 19 white women between the ages of 22 and 50 who had lived in Tucson, Arizona, for 2 or more years. Four-mm punch biopsies were taken from the malar eminence of each subject and processed for light and electron microscopy. These investigators reported that the stratum lucidum of black skin was not altered by ultraviolet light exposure. Black skin rarely showed areas of epidermal atrophy, and there was minimal evidence of elastosis. Overall, compared with white skin, black skin showed minimal evidence of photodamage. Two-mm punch biopsies of six women ages 45 to 50 with skin types V to VI from the Vitiligo and Pigmentation Institute corroborated Montagna's findings.[8] Biopsies were taken from the lateral periorbital region of each subject. There was no evidence of elastosis or epidermal atrophy. These women did, however, manifest mottled facial pigmentation and texturally rough skin, and in some instances, enlarged pores, which had worsened over time (Fig. 3-3A,B).

In contrast to the Montagna and Carlisle study, Whitmore and Sago[9] measured the thickness of the epidermis and dermis on the non–sun-exposed forearm in 86 white women and 40 black women. They reported no statistically significant difference in skin thickness. Controlling for confounding variables—such as age, menopause, oral contraceptive use, hormone replacement therapy, cigarette smoking, and exercise—there was no relationship between race and skin thickness of black (1.39 ± 0.02 mm) and white (1.41 ± 0.01 mm) women. These findings suggest that the sun-exposed skin of whites is far more susceptible to the deleterious effects of ultraviolet light than is black skin.

The clinical features of photoaging in Asian skin differ from Caucasian skin. Asians tend to develop mottled pigmentation, solar lentigo, and seborrheic keratoses. In addition, Asians develop thicker, deeper wrinkles on the forehead, periorbital, and crow's feet area compared with finer wrinkles in the aforementioned areas in Caucasians.[10] Mild solar elastosis has been observed at 20 years of age in sun-exposed facial skin of Korean patients. Severe accumulation of elastotic material was evident in the dermis of Koreans older than 40 years of age. However, in sun-protected skin, solar elastosis was not present.[11]

Goh assessed photoaging in 1,500 Asians of skin types III and IV.[12] The study included subjects of Indonesian,

Table 3-2

Glogau classification of the aging face

Group	Clinical features
I (Mild)	Age: 20s–30s
	Early photoaging
	Mild dyschromia
	No keratoses
	Minimal wrinkling
	Minimal/no makeup
	Minimal/no scarring
II (Moderate)	Age: Late 30s–40s
	Early senile lentigines
	Dyschromia
	Early actinic keratoses
	Parallel smile lines
	Early wrinkling
	Some foundation worn
	Mild acne scarring
III (Advanced)	Age: Usually 50–65
	Dyschromia, telangiectasias
	Visible keratoses
	Wrinkling at rest
	Always wears makeup
	Moderate acne scarring
IV (Severe)	Age: 60–75
	Actinic keratoses
	Prior skin cancers
	Wrinkling throughout
	Makeup cakes and cracks
	Severe acne scarring

Modified from Glogau RG. Chemical peeling and aging skin. *J Geriatr Dermatol* 1994;2:30–35.

Malaysian, and Chinese ancestry. Clinical manifestations of photodamage in this study included hypopigmentation, coarse and fine wrinkles, and tactile roughness.

In a study of photodamage in 407 Koreans, standardized facial photographs were taken and evaluated by independent investigators to assess the severity of wrinkles and dyspigmentation.[13] Wrinkling and pigmentation changes were a major feature of photoaging in Koreans. Women tended to have more severe wrinkles; seborrheic keratoses were the major pigmentary lesions in men, whereas hyperpigmented macules were prominent features in women. The number of hyperpigmented lesions and seborrheic keratoses increased with each decade of age. Cigarette smoking was an independent risk factor for wrinkles, but not for dyspigmentation, and caused additive detrimental effects to wrinkles induced by aging and sun exposure.

Toyoda and Morohashi[14] assessed morphological alterations of epidermal melanocytes in photoaging in 15 Japanese women between the ages of 58 and 81. The investigators compared skin taken from the exposed crow's feet area with the sun protected postauricular regions. Compared with sun-protected skin, the sun-exposed sites showed a statistically significant increase in melanocyte number, marked nuclear heterogeneity, and signs of cell activation. In addition, melanocytes were in close opposition to photodamaged, degenerated keratinocytes. Melanocytes in the sun-exposed areas also contained large intracytoplasmic vacuolar structures.

Photodamage was assessed in 61 Thai patients. Eighty percent of the Thai subjects were women. Biopsies were taken from the cheek. The majority of subjects were classified as Fitzpatrick skin type IV. All subjects were older than 60 years. Baseline biopsies of these subjects revealed significant evidence of photodamage, including atrophy of the epidermis, atypical epidermal cells, hyperpigmentation, elastosis, and collagen degeneration.[15] Many of these patients had a long-term history of intense sun exposure without photo protection.

There is a dearth of information regarding photoaging in Hispanics. Sanchez[16] reported photoaging as the third most common dermatologic concern in 1,000 Hispanics, accounting for 16.8% of visits in a private practice. Given the diverse background of Hispanic populations, fair-skinned Hispanics may have substantial photodamage similar to Caucasians, whereas deeply pigmented Hispanics may have minimal photodamage, as evidenced in African Americans and darker-skinned Asians.

In light of the above findings, there is a spectrum of photodamage in individuals with skin types IV through VI. Clinical manifestations of photodamage in deeply pigmented skin includes mild wrinkling, dyschromias, textural alterations, seborrheic keratoses, and even dermatosis papulosa nigra. Histologic changes may be minimal, as evidenced by biopsies in African Americans; however, more significant photodamage is reported in Asian skin.[6] The biological basis for these observations correlates with many of the well-documented morphological and physiological skin differences in dark as opposed to white skin.[17]

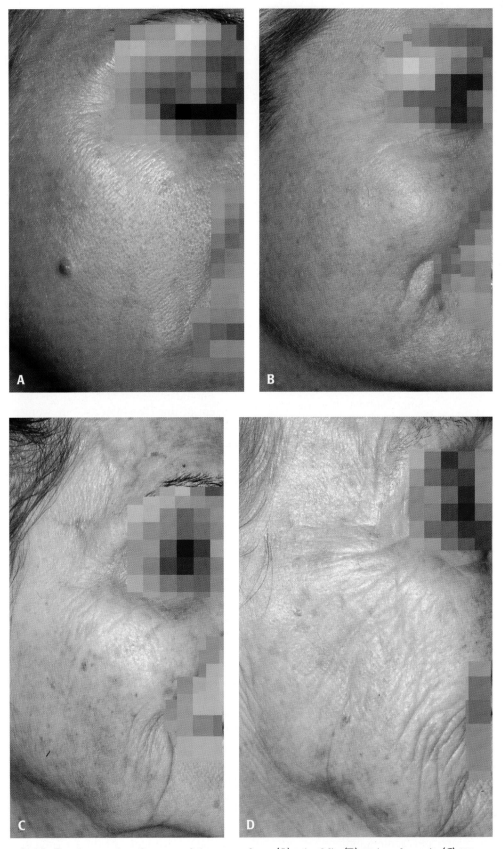

Figure 3-1A–D Glogau classification of the aging face: **(A)** I (mild); **(B)** II (moderate); **(C)** III (advanced); **(D)** IV (severe).

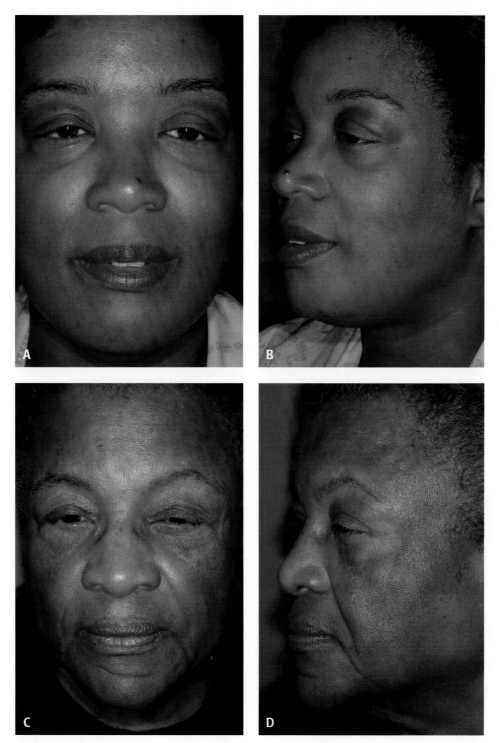

Figure 3-2 A and **B:** A 52-year-old African American woman shows no clinical evidence of photodamage. **C** and **D:** The 82-year-old mother of the patient shown in A and B shows hyperpigmentation, fine wrinkles, laxity, textural changes, and intrinsic aging.

INTRINSIC AGING

All humans experience intrinsic aging. Typically, it is characterized by smooth, relatively atrophic, finely wrinkled or lax skin. Histologically, the stratum corneum is normal. However, the epidermis is atrophic and there is flattening of the dermoepidermal function. Dermal features include decreased thickness, loss of elastic fibers, and a decrease in the biosynthetic capacity of fibroblasts (Table 3-1).

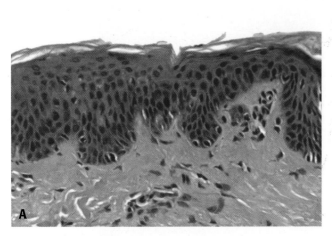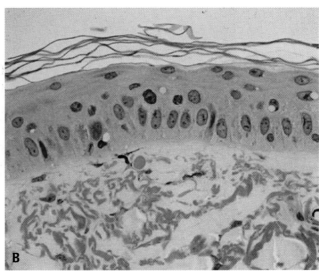

Figure 3-3 Hemotoxylin and eosin stain sections from **(A)** a 50-year-old African American and **(B)** a 50-year-old Caucasian. *Note:* There is minimal histologic evidence of photodamage in the 50-year-old African American. There is severe collagen degeneration in the 50-year-old Caucasian.

There is a scarcity of data regarding the histologic features of chronologic aging in darker racial ethnic groups. Herzberg and Dinehart[18] examined the features of sun-protected skin from six African Americans 6 weeks to 75 years of age with light and electron microscopy.

With aging, the dermoepidermal junction was flattened with multiple zones of basal lamina and anchoring fibril reduplication. Microfibrils in the papillary dermis became irregularly oriented. Compact elastic fibers showed cystic changes and separation of skeleton fibers with age. The area occupied by the superficial vascular plexus in specimens of equal epidermal surface length decreased from the infant to young adult (21–29 years old) to adult (39–52 years old) age groups, then increased in the aged adult (73–75 years old) age groups. With the exception of the vascularity in the aged adult group, the above features were similar to those seen in aging white skin. In addition, there was a decrease in the number of melanocytes with age. Basal keratinocyte melanin granule density increased with age to age 52 and remained dense in the aged adult group, whereas the number of melanocytes decreased. The findings suggest that there are no differences in chronologic aging in black and white skin.

The skin is also a target for various hormones, and sex steroids have a profound influence on the aging process. A decrease in sex steroids thus induces a reduction of those skin functions that are under hormonal control. Sex steroids manifest their effects by two different mechanisms: Genomic and nongenomic effects. Estrogen alone or together with progesterone prevents or reverses skin atrophy, dryness, and wrinkles associated with chronological or photoaging.[19] Estrogen and progesterone stimulate proliferation of keratinocytes, whereas estrogen suppresses apoptosis and thus prevents epidermal atrophy. Estrogen also enhances collagen synthesis, and estrogen and progesterone suppress collagenolysis by reducing matrix metalloproteinase activity in fibroblasts, thereby maintaining skin thickness. Estrogen maintains skin moisture by increasing acid mucopolysaccharide or hyaluronic acid levels in the dermis, whereas progesterone increases sebum secretion.[20]

Figure 3-4 Illustration showing intrinsic aging of the upper, mid-, and lower face, including brow furrows, eyelid ptosis and laxity, nasolabial lines, and jowl formation.

Table 3-3

The aging African American face

The aging African American face

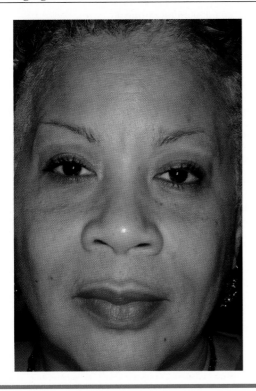

Malar flattening

Prominent nasolabial folds

Nasal lengthening

Recessive chin

Submental skin laxity

Temporal hair loss

Brow ptosis

Furrows: Frontal, glabella

Eyelid:
Upper moderate laxity
Lower minimal laxity
Scleral show

Prominent jowls

Few rhytides

Marionette lines

Modified from Matory WE. Aging in people of color. In: Matory WE, ed. *Ethnic Considerations in Facial Aesthetic Surgery.* Philadelphia: Lippincott-Raven;1998:151–170 (153).

Studies of postmenopausal women reveal that the effects of estrogen deficiency on the skin include wrinkling, dryness, atrophy, laxity, hot flashes, and vulvar atrophy. Subjects using hormone replacement therapy (HRT) demonstrated an improvement in skin moisture, thickness, wound healing, and collagen content.[20–27] However, there is still much debate on the merits of HRT for aging skin. Although a large number of publications have documented the effects of sex hormones on the aging process, it is obvious that HRT should not be administered as an independent treatment for aging skin.

There are few studies available on the influence of testosterone in the male sex. This hormone shows an age-dependent decrease in androgenous tissues like the pubic region, but it remains normal in the regions such as the scrotal and thigh skin.[28] However, there are no studies showing differences in hormonal action between distinct races. Other signs of cutaneous aging are classified as secondary, including reduced sebum production, the number and function of apocrine glands, and slowed hair growth. These signs may represent a reduction in the concentration of androgens in the tissues that occurs with aging.[18,29]

These data suggest that sex steroid hormones also influence the aging process.

Tissue alterations related to intrinsic aging

Facial aging also occurs as a result of loss of hard and soft tissues, including bone remodeling, fat atrophy, and the gravitational redistribution of the skin and subcutaneous tissue. Dark-skinned individuals have a tendency to age prematurely in some areas and late in others because of adipose-tissue atrophy, bone remodeling, and gravitational redistribution of soft tissue.[30] Patients with darker skin, particularly African Americans, tend to manifest signs of aging in the deeper muscular layers of the face, with sagging of the malar fat pads toward the nasolabial folds (Fig. 3-4).

Regarding the upper third of the face, one of the first signs of facial aging in deeply pigmented skin occurs in the periorbital area. Ptosis of the upper eyelid tends to appear around the fourth decade, whereas in fair-skinned individuals, it becomes evident from the third decade.[31] In Hispanics, brows tend to be implanted at a lower level with respect to the supraorbital rim. Nasolabial folds are

Table 3-4
The aging Asian face

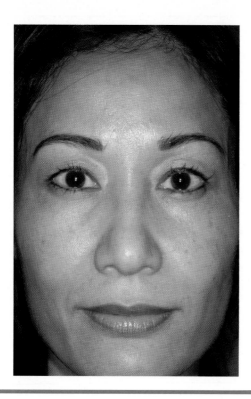

The aging Asian face

Weaker facial skeletal support

Gravitational descent of soft tissues

Malar fat pad ptosis

Tear trough deformity

Descent of thick juxtabrow tissues of the lower orbit

Prominent nasolabial folds

Accretion of submental adipose tissue

Platysmal descent/dehiscence

Few rhytides

Modified from Shirakabe Y, Suzuki Y, Lam SM. A new paradigm for the aging Asian face. *Aesthetic Plast Surg* 2003;27(5):397–402.

common. In addition, there is sagging of the cheeks. However, there are individual variations, such as individuals with hollowed eyes who tend to present drooping upper eyelids later. Some darker-skinned patients have excess skin in the upper eyelids and dark circles. Lower eye bulging and wrinkles are often problems in darker-skinned patients older than 50 years (Tables 3-3, 3-4, and 3-5; Fig. 3-5A-C). As aging progresses, ptosis in black patients is commonly accompanied by the rounding of the outer corner of the eye, with exposure of the sclera.[30] In general, wrinkles in darker ethnic patients are the result of muscular or expression wrinkles, mainly on the upper third of the face, as well as "sleep wrinkles."

In the middle and lower face, the classic signs of aging include tear trough deformity, infraorbital hollowing, ptosis of the subcutaneous adipose tissue in the malar region; increasing nasojugal groove prominence and deepening of the nasolabial fold.[30] Bimaxillary protrusion in the presence of infraorbital hypoplasia is a common feature in individuals of Hispanic, Asian, and African ancestry.[32,33] Given the thicker dermis and subcutaneous tissues of some darker racial ethnic groups, combined with infraorbital hypoplasia, midface aging can occur at an earlier age and can be pronounced.

In the lower face, darker racial ethnic groups experience jowl formation and pronounced melomental lines. Lower face alterations also occur later in dark-skinned patients and are less pronounced than in the white races, with exception of the accumulation of fat in the mentum region. The mentum is an area in which darker-skinned patients present significant facial aging, where an accumulation of fat may occur in the submandibular region as a result of a lower projection of the chin, leading to a slight rounding of the jaw line in African Americans.[34] With age, the lips in general become thinner and flattened. The philtrum, often considered the key element of attractive lips, also diminishes with age. However, the characteristic voluminous lips of blacks prevent the appearance of perioral wrinkles. The loss of lip volume that occurs with aging is not usually a complaint among blacks, and there is little demand for fillers for lip augmentation.

HAIR SENESCENCE

Structural and morphologic differences in hair amongst different racial ethnic groups are described in Chapter 2.

Table 3-5
The aging Hispanic face

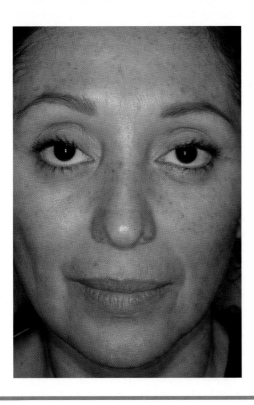

The aging Hispanic face

Minimal facial elastosis

Infraorbital shadowing

Jowl formation

Platysma banding

Few rhytids

Prominent nasolabial folds

Submental fullness

Marionette lines

Modified from Matory WE. The Hispanic patient. In: Matory WE, ed. *Ethnic Considerations in Facial Aesthetic Surgery.* Philadelphia: Lippincott-Raven;1998:303–306.

Whitening of the hair is the most obvious sign of human aging, though its mechanism is, as yet, little understood.[35] Recent studies suggest that the whitening is caused by a defect in the maintenance of the melanocytic stem cells and that this process is dramatically accelerated by deficiency of the Bc12 gene, which causes selective apoptosis in melanocytic stem cells.[35,36] However, there are no studies on the differences in the whitening process between individuals of different skin color.

CONCLUSION

Current concepts regarding facial aging include an interactive relationship between photodamage and intrinsic aging factors, including adipose tissue atrophy, gravitational redistribution of soft tissue, and bone remodeling. However, many facial aging-related alterations are linked to the acquired characteristics and habits of the individual. In darker-skinned patients, the higher content of epidermal melanin and a thicker dermis reduce the appearance of photodamage alterations, including coarse and fine wrinkles, sallowness, and telangiectasias. However, other age-related changes occur because of chronologic aging,

including volumetric loss of fat and gravitational soft-tissue redistribution.

Cosmetic surgery in darker racial ethnic groups continues to grow at a rapid pace. Facial rejuvenation procedures for all skin types have become increasingly popular. As clinicians and cosmetic surgeons, we have much to learn regarding the aging face of darker racial ethnic groups. An expanded knowledge base of the characteristics and alterations of cutaneous aging in such patients will allow us to enhance and grow our armamentarium of appropriate facial rejuvenating procedures. As Francis Bacon said "Knowledge is power." Knowledge is indeed the purveyor of virtue; cosmetic surgical mishaps may arise from ignorance. – Francis Bacon (1561–1626) English Philosopher.

REFERENCES

1. Gilchrest BA. A review of skin aging and its medical therapy. *Br J Dermatol* 1996;135:867–875.
2. Bhawan J, Andersen W, Lee J, et al. Photoaging versus intrinsic aging: a morphologic assessment of facial skin. *J Cutan Pathol* 1995;22:154–159.
3. Grimes PE. Benign manifestations of photodamage: ethnic skin types. In: Goldberg DJ, ed. *Photodamaged Skin*. New York: Marcel Dekker, Inc.;2004: 175–196.

4. Vayalil PK, Mittal A, Hara Y, et al. Green tea polyphenols prevent ultraviolet light-induced oxidative damage and matrix metaloproteinases expression in mouse skin. *J Invest Dermatol* 2004;122:1480–1487.

5. Glogau RG. Chemical peeling and aging skin. *J Geriatr Dermatol* 1994;2:30–35.

6. Grimes PE. Skin and hair issues in women of color. *Dermatol Clin* 2000;18:659–665.

7. Montagna W, Carlisle K. The architecture of black and white skin. *J Am Acad Dermatol* 1991;24:929–937.

8. Grimes, personal database.

9. Whitmore SE, Sago NJ. Caliper-measured skin thickness is similar in white and black women. *J Am Acad Dermatol* 2000;42:76–79.

10. Chung JH. The effects of sunlight on the skin of Asians. In: Giacomoni PU, ed. *Comprehensive Series in Photomedicines, vol 3. Sun Protection in Man.* Amsterdam: Elsevier; 2001: 69–90.

11. Seo JY, Lee SH, Youn CS, et al. Ultraviolet radiation increases tropoelastin mRNA expression in the epidermis of human skin in vivo. *J Invest Dermatol* 2001;116:915–919.

12. Goh SH. The treatment of visible signs of senescence: the Asian experience. *Br J Dermatol* 1990;122(Suppl 35):105–109.

13. Chung JH, Lee SH, Youn CS, et al. Cutaneous photodamage in Koreans. *Arch Dermatol* 2001;137:1043–1051.

14. Toyoda M, Morohashi M. Morphological alterations of epidermal melanocytes in photoaging: an ultrastructural and cytomorphometric study. *Br J Dermatol* 1998;139: 444–452.

15. Kotrajaras R, Kligman AM. The effect of topical tretinoin on photodamaged facial skin: the Thai experience. *Br J Dermatol* 1993;129:302–309.

16. Sanchez MR. Cutaneous disease in Latinos. *Dermatol Clin* 2003;21:689–697.

17. Kaidbey KH, Aging PP, Sayre RM, et al. Photoprotection by melanin: a comparison of black and Caucasian skin. *J Am Acad Dermatol* 1979;1:249–260.

18. Herzberg AJ, Dinehart SM. Chronologic aging in black skin. *Am J Dermatopathol* 1989;11:319–328.

19. Kanda N, Watanabe S. Regulatory roles of sex hormones in cutaneous biology and immunology. *J Dermatol Sci* 2005;38: 1–7.

20. Hall G, Phillips TJ. Estrogen and skin: the effects of estrogen, menopause, and hormone replacement therapy on the skin. *J Am Acad Dermatol* 2005;53:555–568.

21. Brincat M, Versi E, Moniz CF, et al. Skin collagen changes in postmenopausal women receiving different regimens of estrogen therapy. *Obstet Gynecol* 1987;70:123–127.

22. Castelo-Branco C, Duran M, Gonzalez-Merlo J. Skin collagen changes related to age and hormone replacement therapy. *Maturitas* 1992;15:113–119.

23. Varila E, Rantala I, Oikarinen A, et al. The effect of topical oestradiol on skin collagen of postmenopausal women. *BJOG* 1995;102:985–989.

24. Haapasaari KM, Raudaskoski T, Kallioinen M, et al. Systemic therapy with estrogen or estrogen with progestin has no effect on skin collagen in postmenopausal women. *Maturitas* 1997;27:153–162.

25. Sauerbronn AV, Fonseca AM, Bagnoli VR, et al. The effects of systemic hormonal replacement therapy on the skin of postmenopausal women. *Int J Gynaecol Obstet* 2000;68(1): 35–41.

26. Maheux R, Naud F, Rioux M, et al. A randomized, double-blind, placebo-controlled study on the effect of conjugated estrogens on skin thickness. *Am J Obstet Gynecol* 1994; 170:642–649.

27. Callens A, Vaillant L, Lecomte P, et al. Does hormonal skin aging exist? A study of the influence of different hormone therapy regimens on the skin of postmenopausal women using non-invasive measurement techniques. *Dermatology* 1996;193:289–294.

28. Deslypere JP, Vermeulen A. Aging and tissue androgens. *J Clin Endocrinol Metab* 1981;53:430–434.

29. Bolognia JL. Aging skin. *Am J Med* 1995;98(Suppl1A): 1A99S–1A103S.

30. Matory WE. Aging in people of color. In: Matory WE, ed. *Ethnic Considerations in Facial Aesthetic Surgery.* Philadelphia: Lippincott-Raven;1998:151–170.

31. Harris MO. The aging face in patients of color: minimally invasive surgical facial rejuvenation—a targeted approach. *Dermatol Ther* 2004;17:206–211.

32. Shirakabe Y, Suzuki Y, Lam SM. A new paradigm for the aging Asian face. *Aesthetic Plast Surg* 2003;27:397–402.

33. Le TT, Farkas LG, Ngim RC, et al. Proportionality in Asian and North American Caucasian faces using neoclassical facial canons as criteria. *Aesthetic Plast Surg* 2002;26:64–69.

34. Sutter RE, Turley PK. Soft tissue evaluation of contemporary Caucasian and African-American female facial profiles. *Angle Orthod* 1998;68:487–496.

35. Grimes PE. Use of Fillers in Ethnic Skin. Course 101: Soft Tissue Augmentation. Paper presented at: 63rd Annual Meeting of the American Academy of Dermatology; February 18, 2005; New Orleans, LA.

36. Nishimura EK, Granter SR, Fisher DE. Mechanisms of hair graying: incomplete melanocyte stem cell maintenance in the niche. *Science* 2005;307(5710):720–724.

from the camera. Even small changes in the position of the chin can cause distortion of the skin. The camera should have a fixed flash position, F-stop, focal length, and lens. Through-the-lens metering, as used in single-lens-reflex cameras, should be used, as it gives the photographer the ability to compose the image through the same lens with which the picture will be taken. Standardization of image timing is another important factor when performing photography for cosmetic procedures. Posttreatment edema may temporarily reduce wrinkles and improve tone. Images should be taken after edema and erythema has subsided.

Polarized light photography is useful in the assessment of dermal changes, particularly vascular changes and skin surface changes. In studies for disorders of pigmentation, it is primarily used to reduce glare. Ultraviolet (UV) light examination can be used to distinguish between skin color changes that are related to pigmentation and changes that result from other causes, such as collagen deposition, scarring, or vascularity. UV photography is excellent in capturing fine lines as well as pigmentary changes and is 10 times more sensitive than visible light in detecting epidermal melanin. Because most current studies use digital cameras to capture images, it is important to use a resolution of at least 3.0 megapixels to maximize image clarity.[12]

DURATION OF TREATMENT

The duration of any study should be sufficient to allow time for an accurate assessment of efficacy. This may vary depending on the intervention. For example, improvement of telangiectasias with laser surgery can be seen within days, whereas scar therapy with topical agents may require months to demonstrate a difference. Without follow-up, however, it is impossible to assess the overall effect of the intervention. Evaluation of the patient several months or more after treatment establishes the ability of a particular procedure to produce a durable improvement.

COMPLIANCE

The issue of compliance should be addressed in a clinical trial with an assessment made of the amount of study drug used per patient, i.e., number of tubes, weight of drug, and timely attendance of the patients for follow-up visits.

MAINTENANCE TREATMENT

Studies that show improvement of a disorder may need to be prolonged to demonstrate maintenance of improvement. A given therapy may be useless if the effects are not lasting. Good studies usually include follow-up evaluations to document improvement.

Table 5-3

Side effects of therapy from the perspective of the patient and the physician

Patient	Physician
Stinging/burning	Erythema
Pain	Scaling
Tenderness	Erosions
Itching	Crusting
Redness	Inflammation
Scaling/dryness	Irritation
	Hypopigmentation
	Confettilike pigmentation
	Hyperpigmentation
	Postinflammatory hyperpigmentation
	Scarring

SAFETY

The safety of a trial medication should be assessed in terms of local and systemic tolerance, adverse events, and cosmetic appearance. Some examples of safety measures are shown in Table 5-3.

QUALITY OF LIFE

In view of the considerable effect cosmetic disorders have on the health-related quality of life (HRQoL) in affected patients, attempts have been made to assess the benefit of therapy on this important parameter. The existing Dermatology Life Quality Index (DLQI) and SKINDEX-16 are general measures of the impact of skin disease on the HRQoL of patients with various skin disorders; they put equal weight on the physical and psychological effects of a dermatological condition. A new HRQoL instrument for women with melasma, MELASQOL, has been developed.[13] The MELASQOL uses items from the SKINDEX-16 as well as the skin discoloration questionnaire that focus on items that would be more relevant to melasma-specific HRQoL. In the future, cosmetic dermatology studies should include HRQoL measurements to determine the full impact of skin disorders on the patient. To this end, new questionnaires and other QOL instruments that are specifically aimed at cosmetic disorders will need to be developed.

CONCLUSION

Few well-controlled trials have been conducted in patients with cosmetic disorders, and further effort is required to standardize such trials in the future. This will allow clinicians to better compare outcomes of different therapeutic modalities. By using some of the guidelines presented in this chapter, researchers can design well-controlled, randomized trials that will serve the important goal of better care for all patients.

REFERENCES

1. Bigby M. Evidence-based medicine in a nutshell. *Arch Dermatol* 1998;134:1609–1618.
2. Altman DG, Schulz KF, Moher D, et al., for the CONSORT Group. The revised CONSORT statement for reporting randomized trials: explanation and elaboration. *Ann Intern Med* 2001;134:663–694.
3. Moher D, Schultz KF, Altman DG, for the CONSORT Group. The CONSORT statement: revised recommendations for improving the quality of reports of parallel-group randomized trials. *Lancet* 2001;357:1191–1194.
4. Julian DG. What is right and wrong about evidence-based medicine? *J Cardiovasc Electrophysiol* 2003;14(Suppl 9):S2–S5.
5. Guevara IL, Pandya AG. Safety and efficacy of 4% hydroquinone combined with 10% glycolic acid, antioxidants, and sunscreen in the treatment of melasma. *Int J Dermatol* 2003; 42:966–972.
6. Taylor SC, Torok H, Jones T, et al. Efficacy and safety of a new triple combination agent for the treatment of facial melasma. *Cutis* 2003;72:67–72.
7. Hurley ME, Guevara IL, Gonzales RM, et al. Efficacy of glycolic acid peels in the treatment of melasma. *Arch Dermatol* 2002;138:1578–1582.
8. Tse Y, Levine VJ, McClain SA, et al. *J Dermatol Surg Oncol* 1994;20:795–800.
9. White B, Bauer EA, Goldsmith LA, et al. Guidelines for clinical trials in systemic sclerosis (scleroderma). *Arthritis Rheum* 1995;38:351–360.
10. Baryza MJ, Baryza GA. The Vancouver scar scale: an administration tool and its inter-rater reliability. *J Burn Care Rehabil* 1995;16:535–538.
11. Iyer S, Fitzpatrick RE. Long-pulsed dye laser treatment for facial telangiectasias and erythema: evaluation of a single purpuric pass versus multiple subpurpuric passes. *Dermatol Surg* 2005;31:898–902.
12. Shah AR, Dayan SH, Hamilton GS. Pitfalls of photography for facial resurfacing and rejuvenation procedures. *Facial Plast Surg* 2005;21:154–161.
13. Balkrishnan R, McMichael AJ, Camacho FT, et al. Development and validation of a health-related quality of life instrument for women with melasma. *Br J Dermatol* 2003;149: 572–577.

Cosmetic Issues of Concern for Potential Surgical Patients

Chang-Keun Oh, H. Ray Jalian, Stephanie R. Young, and Seong-Jin Kim

Darker-skinned individuals (Fitzpatrick skin type IV through VI) represent 30% of the population, U.S. population and the majority of the global population (see Chapter 2), thus physicians are more likely to encounter such patients in their clinics and practices, and therefore must know how to treat diverse skin types. Until recently, training programs have paid little attention to ethnic skin, focusing instead on procedures and treatments relating to fair-skinned individuals. Today's rapidly increasing population of darker skin types requires that cosmetic surgeons recognize the need for safe, effective treatments for people of color.

Several studies have assessed the incidence of skin diseases in patients of color. Halder et al.[1] assessed the incidence of common dermatoses in 2,000 patients in a pre-dominantly black dermatologic practice. The four most common skin diseases, in order of incidence, were acne vulgaris (27.7% of patients), eczema (23.3.%), pigmentary disorders other than vitiligo (9%), and alopecias (5.3%). Alopecias were predominantly chemical and traction alopecia. Pigmentary disorders were predominantly postin-flammatory hyperpigmentation (PIH) and melasma.

Child et al.,[2] assessing the spectrum of skin disease in a predominantly black population in southeast London, recorded diagnoses in 461 consecutive African, Afro-Caribbean, and mixed-race patients. The most common diagnoses in the 274 adults included in the study were acne vulgaris (13.7%), eczema (9%), psoriasis (4.8%), and keloidal scars (4.1%). Several of the aforementioned conditions are considered "cosmetic."

The cosmetic surgeon should have an in-depth under-standing of the physiological and functional differences that exist between fair-skinned individuals and their dark-skinned counterparts. Data, however, relating to these pri-mary differences remain limited.[3–5] Despite this, surgeons who keep diversity of skin in mind in their practices will do a great benefit to their patients by allowing their postopera-tive experience to be predictable and without complications.

This chapter will provide an introductory overview for cosmetic issues of concern in darker racial ethnic groups. These issues include pigmentation disorders, skin laxity, wrinkles, sensitivity, oily skin and acne, and scar-ring.[6] Many of these disorders will be discussed in depth in other chapters (Table 6-1).

Table 6-1

Cosmetic issues of concern for darker ethnic groups

Pigmentation disorders

Melasma

Postinflammatory hyperpigmentation

Hori's nevus

Solar lentigo

Vitiligo

Irritant contact dermatitis

Wrinkles/photodamage

Oily skin

Acne vulgaris

Hypertophic scars

Pseudofolliculitis barbae

PIGMENTARY DISORDERS

Variation of skin color is believed to have evolved as a result of selective pressures present in particular environments, mainly extremes in light and temperature. The most appar-ent and important morphological difference in darker racial groups involves pigmentation. The reactivity of melanocytes and the profound tendency toward hyperpigmentation are unique characteristics of darker-skinned individuals.

It is well established that there are no racial differ-ences in the number of melanocytes[7] in darker compared with lighter skin types. Differences in melanocytes and melanin production have been discussed in Chapter 2. The increased epidermal melanin content of darker-skinned individuals provides greater intrinsic photopro-tection, perhaps explaining why problems such as photo-damage, actinic keratoses, rhytides, and skin malignancies are less common in deeply pigmented skin. However, the increase in epidermal melanin and the often capricious response of melanocytes to inflammation or injury can lead to distressing dyschromias characterized by hyperpig-mentation or hypopigmentation.

Melasma is a troublesome acquired hypermelanosis, usually occurring symmetrically on the face (Fig. 6-1). Although melasma can affect all people, Asian, Hispanic, and black women are most commonly affected.[8] Although the precise cause of melasma is unknown, multiple factors have been implicated in the etiopathogenesis of this condition. These include genetic influences, sunlight

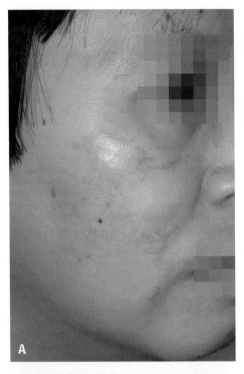

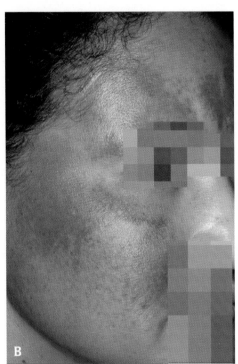

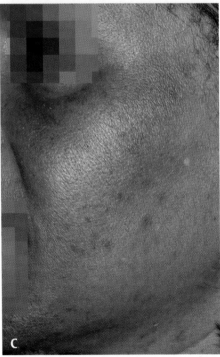

Figure 6-1 A–C Melasma in individuals with skin types IV to VI. **A:** Skin type IV. **B:** Skin type V and **(C)** Skin type VI. Brown hyperpigmented patches of the cheeks and forehead. Note progressive disfigurement in deeply pigmented skin. (Courtesy of Pearl E. Grimes, MD.)

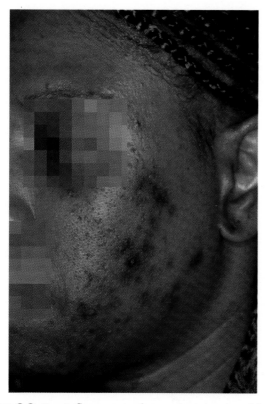

Figure 6-2 Postinflammatory hyperpigmentation. Note hyperpigmented macules and patches of the face. (Courtesy of Pearl E. Grimes, MD.)

exposure, pregnancy, oral contraceptive use, hormone replacement therapy, cosmetics, and medications, such as phototoxic and antiseizure medications. Recently, Grimes et al. reported hyperactive melanocytes and increased epidermal melanin in the affected skin of patients with melasma.[9] Electron microscopy studies showed enlarged melanocytes with increased numbers of melanosomes and prominent dendrites. This study suggested that melasma may be a consequence of hyperactive and hyperfunctional melanocytes causing excessive melanin deposition in the epidermis and dermis.

Another important cosmetic pigmentation issue is PIH (Fig. 6-2). PIH is characterized by an acquired increase in cutaneous pigmentation secondary to an inflammatory process. Excess pigment deposition may occur in the epidermis or in both epidermis and dermis. The condition occurs in all racial and ethnic groups; however, it has a higher incidence in people with darker complexions. Previous studies have suggested that inflammatory reactions that cause a release of arachidonic acid from cell membranes may be a cause of PIH. Mediators implicated in PIH include endothelin 1, prostaglandins, interleukin-1, and stem cell factor.[10,11]

LENTIGINES

Solar lentigo (Fig. 6-3) are common light brown to brown lesions occurring as discrete hyperpigmented macules on

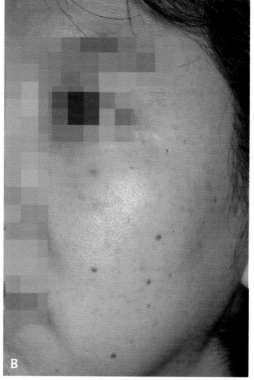

Figure 6-3 Solar lentigo characterized by brown macules of the **(A)** back and **(B)** face. (Courtesy of Pearl E. Grimes, MD.)

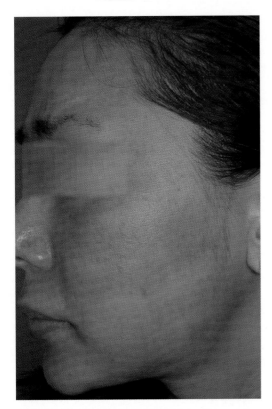

Figure 6-4 Postinflammatory hyperpigmentation after fractional resurfacing.

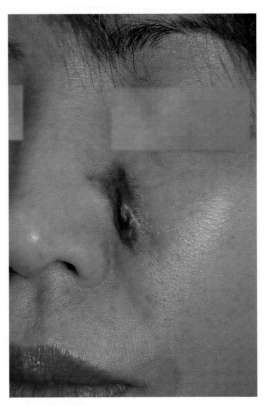

Figure 6-5 Scar after removal of congenital melanocytic nevus with CO_2 laser.

sun-exposed areas of skin, such as the face, arms, chest, and back. Solar lentigo is induced by natural or artificial ultraviolet light sources. Such lesions are common in skin type IV, in particular in Asians and Hispanics. They are less common in blacks. Histologically, they are characterized by elongated rete ridges, club-shaped extensions, and a proliferation of melanocytes, and keratinocytes.[12]

Hori's nevi are acquired bilateral nevus of Ota-like macules symmetrically located on the forehead, temples, eyelids, and malar regions. These often occur in young women with a family history for these lesions. They are also aggravated by sun exposure.[13] Histologically, the overlying epidermis is normal. In the papillary and upper reticular dermis, dendritic melanocytes are present and surrounded by a fibrous sheath.[14]

Treatment with laser light can create unwanted epidermal side effects, such as blistering, dyspigmentation, and scarring, because the higher epidermal melanin content acts as an additional chromophore (Figs. 6-4 and 6-5). A higher level of laser expertise and clinical experience in treating darker skin is mandatory to ensure that patients are treated safely and effectively. Test spots should always be performed as an aid to selecting the safest and most effective parameters of treatment, including determining the appropriate fluence, wavelength, and thermal relaxation time. Efficient cooling devices are essential to prevent the unwanted thermal damage that could potentially cause pigmentary complications. Transient hyperpigmentation can be prevented or relieved by the pre- and postoperative use of hypopigmenting agents.

Vitiligo is a relatively common pigmentary disorder characterized by patches of depigmentation. The disease affects 1% to 2% of the population and shows no racial or ethnic predilection. Vitiligo is indeed a disfiguring and psychologically devastating disease. The disorder may be imperceptible in individuals with skin types I and II. However, the condition is striking in darker racial ethnic groups (Fig. 6-6). Patients with vitiligo experience profound psychological trauma in light of the cosmetic deformity. Psychological profiles document perceived job discrimination, low self-esteem, suicidal ideations, and difficulties in interpersonal relationships.[15,16]. Quality-of-life studies document improvement with treatment of this disorder.[17,18]

Current therapies for dyschromias are reviewed in Chapters 13 through 15.

SKIN LAXITY AND WRINKLES

Darker skin is thought to be more resistant to the deleterious effects of ultraviolet radiation. A physician who has experience in ethnic variations of skin might say that a person with darker skin appears much younger than a fair-skinned person of the same actual age. Higher melanin content and a different pattern of melanosomal dispersion in the epidermis seem to be responsible for this effect.

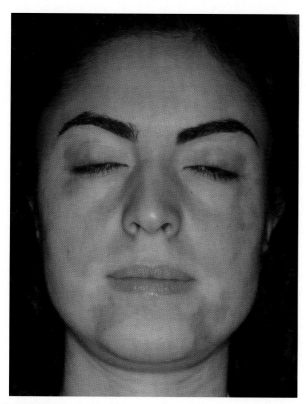

Figure 6-6 Facial vitiligo characterized by areas of depigmentation. (Courtesy of Pearl E. Grimes, MD.)

Recent experimental observations confirmed this hypothesis by measuring cytokines and DNA damage in black and white skin during the skin responses following exposure to solar-simulating radiation.[1,19] It was demonstrated that a dark-skinned individual's epidermis, on average, provided an intrinsic sun protection factor (SPF) of 13.4,[20] which provides the daily protection necessary to maintain "better aging" (see Chapter 3).

Many new products and techniques have arisen that are useful in the rejuvenation of facial skin. Treatment options include topical skin care products, microdermabrasion, chemical peels, and both ablative and nonablative laser/light/radiofrequency skin resurfacing. Surgical intervention, injectable fillers, and neurotoxins are also recommended. In the past, darker-skinned patients were much less likely to undergo facial cosmetic surgery not only because of pervasive cultural attitudes that facial plastic surgery conflicts with a healthy sense of racial identity, but also because of the increased risk of hypertrophic scarring and keloid formation. However, this trend appears to be changing rapidly. Many minimally invasive procedures, such as botulinum toxin injections, soft-tissue augmentation, and resurfacing modalities are well suited for the ethnic patient with midface aging who does not need more drastic lifting procedures. It is recommended to customize treatment plans for the patient, allowing him or her to voice their concerns in the most comprehensive manner possible.

SENSITIVE SKIN

Sensitive skin is generally defined as a reduced tolerance to frequent or prolonged use of cosmetics and toiletries.[21] This intolerance can manifest itself with symptoms that range from objective signs of irritation, such as erythema, dryness, and scaling, to subjective signs of irritation, such as stinging and burning. However, the high variability in the manifestation of sensitive skin makes investigating this issue very complicated. There are a wide variety of test protocols that are employed in an attempt to detect sensitive skin in patients and to assess the irritancy of products. In a recent publication, approximately 50% of women and 40% of men surveyed within a U.K. population regarded themselves as having sensitive skin.[22] Because there is huge variability in the presentation of sensitive skin, subjectively or objectively, some suggest that the perception of "sensitive skin" is possibly influenced by the media, as much published data showed no clear correlation between objective skin findings and patient reports about sensitive skin.[23] Objective findings demonstrating response to irritants, however, suggest that sensitive skin is in fact a real issue. The issue of sensitive skin in darker racial ethnic groups remains controversial.[13]

Jourdain et al.[24] studied ethnic variations in self-assessed sensitive skin by conducting 800 telephone surveys with four different ethnic groups (African Americans, Asians, Euro-Americans, Hispanics). Fifty-two percent of respondents reported sensitive facial skin. No statistically significant differences were identified in the incidence of sensitive skin among different groups, but differences in sensitive skin were identified between ethnic subgroups. African Americans had lower skin reactivity to most environmental factors and lower incidence of recurring facial redness. Euro-Americans had higher skin reactivity to wind and lower reactivity to cosmetics. Asians had higher skin reactivity to spicy food and temperature changes, whereas Hispanics had lower skin reactivity to alcohol. The issue of sensitive skin should be considered when prescribing pharmacologic agents and cosmetic regimens for patients with darker skin types.

Although other studies have suggested an increase in irritation and skin sensitivity in darker racial ethnic groups, a recent detailed review of the subject does not support this occurrence.[1,4,25]

The issue of sensitivity has to be dealt with on an individual basis. Clinical experience suggests that darker-skinned women often experience irritant contact dermatitis (Fig. 6-7) in response to topical products, including cosmetics. However, patch-test results showed a similar incidence of contact dermatitis between blacks and whites in test populations.[26] Studies have shown higher rates of sensitization to formaldehyde-releasing preservatives in whites, whereas African Americans showed higher sensitivity to para-phenylenediamine, cobalt chloride, and thioureas. Overall response rates indicated no significant differences

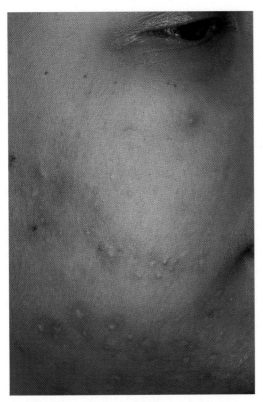

Figure 6-7 Irritant contact dermatitis. Scaly and erythematous patches of the cheeks surrounding hypopigmented acne scars in a patient treated with a benzoyl peroxide product. (Courtesy of Pearl E. Grimes, MD.)

between the two races. Thus, it is more likely related to differences in individual history of allergen exposure.

Commonly used topical irritants include tretinoin, benzoyl peroxide, alpha hydroxy acids, and salicylic acid. These products can be used safely and efficaciously in dark skin; however, they must be cautiously titrated, starting with lower concentrations. Interestingly, it is a consensus of the cosmetic industry in Korea that glycolic acid concentrations higher than 5% are intentionally avoided, because pre-marketing product safety tests showed a marked irritation response. In the United States, in contrast, glycolic acid is available in concentrations up to 8% over the counter.

Whether this difference in tolerability represents true ethnic differences in sensitivity or cultural differences, the therapeutic paradigm may vary to minimize adverse reactions in darker skin. Hypoallergenic cleansers and moisturizers are also recommended to maintain optimal barrier function with postoperative skin care. Maintaining an intact skin barrier is the best protection against irritants, infections, and harmful environmental stimuli.

SCARRING

Hypertrophic scars and keloids are common in darker racial ethnic groups, in particular blacks and Chinese. Keloids are well-demarcated overgrowths of scar tissue that occur in genetically predisposed individuals. Many cutaneous injuries, especially lacerations and surgical trauma, may precipitate keloids. Transforming growth factor beta 1, mast cells, melanocytes, the gli-1 oncogene, and integrins may play a major role in keloid formation. Therapies for keloids and hypertrophic scars are discussed in Chapter 34.

Many individuals avoid surgical procedures for fear of these unwanted scars. Keloids and hypertrophic scarring may indeed complicate surgical procedures in dark skin. Thus, considering whether a darker-skinned patient has a history of keloid or excessive scar formation is an important part of selecting patients for surgery. Also, a careful evaluation of a patient's personal and family history and close physical examination of the patient's skin may reveal any changes secondary to trauma. Even a completely negative evaluation, however, does not guarantee that the patient will be free from these adverse results. However, minimizing scarring and achieving proper wound healing can occur as long as the physician abides by the well-recognized principles of wound healing and care for scar formation in darker skin types (see Chapter 34).

OILY SKIN AND ACNE

Sebum, secreted by the sebaceous glands, is the major component of the lipid film that covers the face. Sebum secretions vary with age, sex, genetics, and topographic variations of the skin.[27–30] The amount of facial sebum secretion is an important consideration in facial skin care. Current studies show no significant differences between African Americans and Caucasians in instrumental measurements of sebum.[25] It is noted that in Asian women, there is a positive correlation between darker pigmentation and the amount of skin surface lipids.[31]

Facial skin types are commonly classified into three types: Oily, normal, or dry (based on the individual's subjective judgment).[32] Excessive skin oiliness can be present in varying degrees in both men and women and may range from being merely a cosmetic burden to a frank disease state, such as severe seborrhea and acne (Fig. 6-8A,B). Excessive seborrhea, characterized by coarse-pored skin, minimal acne, and oily scalp hair, is a well-known clinical entity. It causes considerable concern, has significant social impact, and affects the quality of life in some individuals. Typical treatments include topical tretinoin, glycolic acid, and azelaic acid to improve texture of skin to some degree. Recently, elubiol, a dichlorophenyl imidazoldioxolan, exhibited a clinically significant effect on oily skin.[33] Moreover, superficial chemical peels facilitate and expedite the responses to topical agents. An excellent improvement was observed in rough and oily skin when using a series of salicylic acid chemical peels in patients with skin types V and VI. Salicylic acid peels also improved the appearance of enlarged pores. Although other superficial peels induce similar responses, salicylic

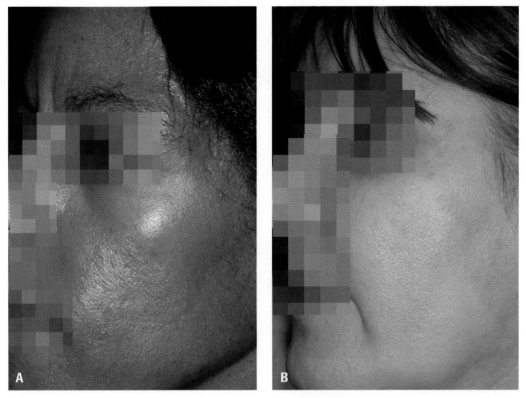

Figure 6-8 Oily and enlarged pores in an **(A)** African American and **(B)** Caucasian. (Courtesy of Pearl E. Grimes, MD.)

acid appears to have maximal efficacy for oily skin because of its lipophilic effects.[34] Recently, Geissler et al. reported that a very low dose of isotretinoin is effective in controlling seborrhea. Daily doses of 2.5 and 5 mg isotretinoin were effective in reducing sebum production.[35] Zileuton, a 5-lipoxygenase inhibitor, also directly inhibits sebum synthesis in a transient manner with the potency similar to low-dose isotretinoin.[36]

Acne vulgaris is common in people of all ethnic skin types (Fig. 6-9A,B,C). Overall, neither race nor ethnicity greatly influence acne prevalence, a disorder that consistently ranks as the top dermatologic diagnosis in populations of all skin types. Similarly, the basic pathophysiology of acne is most likely comparable in all skin phototypes. In dark skin as well as white skin, the well-known quartet of acne pathogenic factors includes excessive sebum production, abnormal follicular keratinization and plugging, proliferation of *Propionibacterium acnes*, and inflammation.[37] Increased sebum production stimulated by androgens is almost always the first listed pathogenic factor promoting acne. A correlation between the severity of acne and facial sebum secretion is generally accepted.

Although this classic pathophysiology is shared, the subsequent evolution of the acne lesion and the degree of inflammation at clinical presentation may vary among individuals according to their skin types. In particular, nodulocystic acne appears to be more common in Caucasians and Hispanics than in African Americans.[38] Patients with darker skin are at an increased risk for developing PIH and keloid scarring subsequent to acne lesions.

The major treatment options for acne itself are also similar for patients across the wide range of skin phototypes. All the approved topical and systemic medications can be considered in patients with ethnic skin. However, the selection, dosing, formulation, timing, and combination of these acne treatments will rely on clinical assessment of each patient's condition—including a careful consideration of the unique acne-related problems of ethnic skin.

The most critical issue related to acne in dark-skinned patients is the development of PIH. PIH can develop in response to the acne itself or to any overly aggressive acne treatment (e.g., thermal, chemical, or trauma) that disturbs the skin. Early and aggressive treatment is always best for avoiding PIH,[39] but the therapy must also be thoughtfully selected to achieve a balance to eliminate the acne without inducing the PIH. Keloid formation is also more common following acne in African American, Hispanic, and Asian patients versus white patients. These keloidal overgrowths of scar tissue are between five and 16 times more frequent in patients with skin of color. Although not as common as PIH, keloidal scarring is more permanent and disfiguring.

Pseudofolliculitis barbae is a common condition observed primarily in men of African descent who shave (Fig. 6-10). However, the condition can occur in other racial

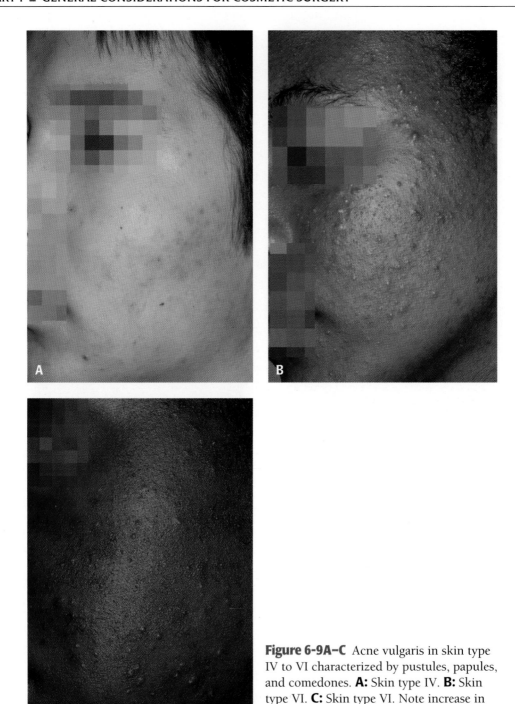

Figure 6-9A–C Acne vulgaris in skin type IV to VI characterized by pustules, papules, and comedones. **A:** Skin type IV. **B:** Skin type VI. **C:** Skin type VI. Note increase in the severity of hyperpigmentation in deeply pigmented skin. (Courtesy of Pearl E. Grimes, MD.)

ethnic groups. It is characterized by inflammatory papules and pustules in the beard region. The condition results from ingrown hairs because of the curved nature of the hair follicle in blacks. Women are also affected by this condition. Treatments include topical antibiotic formulations, benzoyl peroxides, and retinoids. Growing a beard alleviates the condition. Laser hair removal (see Chapter 32) is becoming increasingly popular for facial hair removal in men.

CULTURAL CONCERNS

In spite of the significant influence of the Western world on beauty standards of other countries, there remain tremendous differences between cultures. Culture often dictates beauty standards, as well as choice of cosmetic procedures and surgical outcomes (see Chapter 1). The basic appreciation of these factors is therefore helpful in

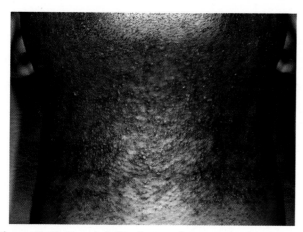

Figure 6-10 Pseudofolliculitis. Inflammatory papules and pustules in the beard area caused by ingrown hairs. (Courtesy of Pearl E. Grimes, MD.)

providing appropriate response to the aesthetic and cosmetic surgery desires and concerns of darker racial ethnic groups.

REFERENCES

1. Halder RM, Grimes PE, McLaurin CI, et al. Incidence of common dermatoses in a predominantly black dermatologic practice. *Cutis* 1983;32(4):388,390.
2. Child FJ, Fuller LC, Higgins EM, et al. A study of the spectrum of skin disease occurring in a black population in south-east London. *Br J Dermatol* 1999;141(3):512–517.
3. Anderson KE, Maibach HI. Black and white human skin differences. *J Am Acad Dermatol* 1979;1:276–282.
4. Taylor SC. Skin of color: biology, structure, function, and implications for dermatologic disease. *J Am Acad Dermatol* 2002;46:S41–46.
5. Berardesca E, Maibach HI. Racial differences in skin pathophysiology. *J Am Acad Dermatol* 1996;34:667–672.
6. Grimes PE. Skin and hair cosmetic issues in women of color. *Dermatol Clin* 2000; 18:659–665.
7. Staricco RJ, Pinkus H. Quantitative and qualitative data on the pigment cells of adult human epidermis. *J Invest Dermatol* 1957;28:33–45.
8. Victor FC, Gelber J, Rao B. Melasma: a review. *J Cutan Med Surg* 2004;8:97–102.
9. Grimes PE, Yamada N, Bhawan J. Light microscopic, immunohistochemical, and ultrastructural alterations in patients with melasma. *Am J Dermatopathol* 2005;27:96–101.
10. Nordlund JJ. Postinflammatory hyperpigmentation. *Dermatol Clin* 1988;6(2):185–192.
11. Imokawa G, Kobayashi T, Miyagishi M, et al. The role of endothelin-1 in epidermal hyperpigmentation and signaling mechanisms of mitogenesis and melanogenesis. *Pigment Cell Res* 1997;10(4):218–228.
12. Okulicz JF, Jozwiak S, Schwartz RA, et al. Lentigo. http://www.emedicine.com/DERM/topic221.htm. Accessed March 13, 2007.
13. Draelos ZD. Sensitive skin: perception, evaluation and treatment. *Am J Contact Dermat* 1997;8:67–78.
14. Lui H, Zhou YZ. Nevi of Ota and Ito. http://www.emedicine.com/DERM/topic290.htm. Accessed March 13, 2007.
15. Picardi A, Pasquini P, Cattaruzza MS, et al. Stressful life events, social support, attachment security and alexithemia in vitiligo: a case report study. *Psychother Psychosom* 2003; 72(3):150–158.
16. Rumpf HJ, Lontz W, Vessler S. A self-administered version of a brief measure of suffering: first aspects of validity. *Psychother Psychosom* 2004;73(1):536.
17. Ongenae K, Van Geel N, De Schepper S, et al. Effect of vitiligo on self-reported health-related quality of life. *Br J Dermatol* 2005;152:1165–1172.
18. Parsad D, Dogra S, Kanwar AJ. Dermatology life quality index score in vitiligo and its impact on the treatment outcome. *Br J Dermatol* 2003;148:373–374.
19. Rijken F, Bruijnzeel PL, van Weelden H, et al. Responses of black and white skin to solar-simulating radiation: differences in DNA photodamage, infiltrating neutrophils, proteolytic enzymes induced, keratinocyte activation, and IL-10 expression. *J Invest Dermatol* 2004;122:1448–1455.
20. Kaidbey KH, Agin PP, Sayre RM, et al. Photoprotection by melanin-a comparison of black and Caucasian skin. *J Am Acad Dermatol* 1979;1:249–260.
21. Chew A, Maibach HI. Sensitive skin. In: Loden M, Maibach HI, eds. *Dry Skin and Moisturizers: Chemistry and Function.* New York: CRC Press;2000:429–440.
22. Willis CM, Shaw S, Lacharriere ODE, et al. Sensitive skin: an epidemiological study. *Br J Dermatol* 2001;145:258–263.
23. Loffler H, Aramaki J, Effendy I, et al. Sensitive skin. In: Zhai H, Maibach HI, eds. *Dermatotoxicology.* New York: CRC Press;2004:123–135.
24. Jourdain R, Lacharriere O, Bastien P, et al. Ethnic variations in self-perceived sensitive skin: epidemiological survey. *Contact Dermatitis* 2002;46(3):162–169.
25. Grimes PE, Edison Bl, Green BA, et al. Evaluation of inherent difference between African American and white skin surface properties using subjective and objective measures. *Cutis* 2004;73(6):392–396.
26. Deleo VA, Taylor SC, Belsito DV, et al. The effect of race and ethnicity on patch test results. *J Am Acad Dermatol* 2002;46:S107–112.
27. Youn SW, Na JI, Choi SY, et al. Regional and seasonal variations in facial sebum secretions: a proposal for the definition of combination skin type. *Skin Res Technol* 2005;11:189–195.
28. Nicolaides N, Rothman S. Studies on the chemical composition of human hair fat. II. The overall composition with regard to age, sex and race. *J Invest Dermatol* 1953;21:9–14.
29. Kligman AM, Shelley WB. An investigation of the biology of the sebaceous gland. *J Invest Dermatol* 1958;30:99–125.
30. Pochi PE, Strauss JS. Sebaceous gland activity in black skin. *Dermatol Clin* 1988;6:349–351.
31. Abe T, Arai S, Mimura K, et al. Studies of physiological factors affecting skin susceptibility to ultraviolet light irradiation and irritants. *J Dermatol* 1983;10:531–537.
32. Youn SW, Kim SJ, Hwang IA, et al. Evaluation of facial skin type by sebum secretion: discrepancies between subjective descriptions and sebum secretion. *Skin Res Technol* 2002;8:168–172.
33. Pierard GE, Ries G, Cauwenbergh G. New insight into the topical management of excessive sebum flow at the skin surface. *Dermatology* 1998;196:126–129.

34. Grimes PE. The safety and efficacy of salicylic acid chemical peels in darker racial-ethnic groups. *Dermatol Surg* 1999;25: 18–22.

35. Geissler SE, Michelsen S, Plewig G. Very low dose isotretinoin is effective in controlling seborrhea [abstract]. *J Dtsch Dermatol Ges* 2003;1:952–958(abst).

36. Zouboulis CC, Saborowski A, Boschnakow A. Zileuton, an oral 5-lipoxygenase inhibitor, directly reduces sebum production. *Dermatology* 2005;210:36–38.

37. Lee DJ, Van Dyke GS, Kim J. Update on pathogenesis and treatment of acne. *Curr Opin Pediatr* 2003;15:405–410.

38. Kelly AP, Sampson DD. Recalcitrant nodulocystic acne in black Americans: treatment with isotretinoin. *J Natl Med Assoc* 1987;79:1266–1270.

39. Callender VD. Acne in ethnic skin: special considerations for therapy. *Dermatol Ther* 2004;17:184–195.

Informed Consent and Treating the Cosmetic Patient

Mathew M. Avram and Daniel E. Kremens

By law, all patients have a right to informed consent before receiving any health-care treatments. This law applies to all procedures and treatments whether they be invasive or noninvasive, oral or topical, medical or cosmetic. Failure to obtain informed consent for a procedure or other treatment constitutes a battery and renders the physician liable for civil damages. This chapter will examine the law of informed consent as it applies to patients undergoing cosmetic procedures, particularly those with darker Fitzpatrick skin phototypes.

BACKGROUND

American jurisprudence has strongly supported the concept of patient autonomy. There is a strong judicial belief that a patient has a right to be free from nonconsensual touching or interference. As stated by Justice Cardozo, "Every human being of adult years and sound mind has a right to determine what shall be done with his own body."[1]

The doctrine of informed consent protects the patient from unwanted contacts. A patient need only demonstrate that he or she was not properly informed of the nature of touching or treatment to prevail in such an action.

Violation of the duty to obtain informed consent from the patient constitutes a battery. The burden of proof is far simpler than that of a negligence action, for which a plaintiff needs to prove a breach of a duty that caused harm. In an action based on battery, physical injury or harm need not be shown to prevail. All that needs to be shown is a nonconsensual touching or treatment. The focus of a battery action is always on whether the touching was consensual. Thus, there is no need for expert witnesses or learned medical treatises in these cases. Indeed, one does not even need to establish a doctor–patient relationship. All that is at issue is whether the patient was informed sufficiently before the physician's treatment.

REQUIREMENTS

There are several factors that must be included in a valid patient consent. The first factor is that the patient must have capacity to make a decision regarding his or her health care.[2] Dermatologists may encounter situations in which capacity is in question. For example, minors lack capacity to consent for many medical procedures. The cosmetic dermatologist therefore should see minors with their parents present, and the physician should determine which, if any, procedures are appropriate for young skin. Similarly, the cosmetic dermatologist may encounter patients with mental illnesses, such as body dysmorphic disorder (BDD), who look to cosmetic procedures as a way to fix their perceived imperfections.[3] Given their underlying pathology, such patients are often not satisfied with even the best results and may sue.[3] The cosmetic dermatologist should have a low threshold to seek appropriate psychiatric consultations before any procedure on a patient suspected of having BDD or other mental illness.

The second factor is that consent must contain adequate information.[2] Most jurisdictions use the "reasonable person" standard to determine what is adequate.[2] The consent must contain the information that a reasonable person requires to make a health care decision.[2] The consent must describe the diagnosis as well as the nature and purpose of the treatment. Furthermore, it must explain the risks and side effects of the procedure, as well as alternatives. For medications, side effects must be described even when there is only a small risk.

In assessing whether to describe each risk, it is important to consider any potentially severe side effects. Thus, even a small risk of serious morbidity or death should be disclosed. One must also consider the particular susceptibilities of the patient. In a patient with a higher Fitzpatrick skin phototype, the risk of pigmentary changes is higher than that of a skin phototype I or II. This should be emphasized both in the patient consultation as well as a proper written consent. For example, there is a higher risk of obvious hypopigmentation in a Fitzpatrick skin phototype VI undergoing laser tattoo removal treatment than in a skin phototype I. The high risk of obvious and cosmetically unappealing hypopigmentation should be emphasized with such a patient. Such practice is not only good from a legal standpoint but also provides a patient with a realistic understanding of potentially troubling side effects. In the event the patient asks more specific questions, the duty expands. Thus, if a patient inquires as to the frequency of side effects such as keloids, the physician would be under a duty to provide more specific information regarding this question than if the patient had not directly asked.

The notion of adequate information also includes alternative treatments. Alternative methods of diagnosis, treatment, and probability of success must all be included in a proper informed consent. Therefore, if a patient is being treated for postinflammatory hyperpigmentation with salicylic acid peels, alternatives such as topical hydroquinone and other bleaching creams should be noted as part of an informed consent. Alternatives should be disclosed even if the procedure entails more side effects or even if the physician has less skill performing those procedures. Alternatives only include those procedures that are within the standard of care. Physicians who practice alternative care are under a duty to discuss traditional medical therapies and procedures as part of an informed consent.

A physician's conflict of interest also comes under the category of adequate information.[4] The physician must disclose all research and economic interests in a particular device or procedure before treatment. Therefore a physician must disclose financial ties to a laser company before treating a patient with that laser.

There are some issues that do not need to be disclosed in a consent form. The risk of poor or unskilled performance need not be disclosed. Moreover, professional training does not need to be included. Thus, if an ophthalmologist performs pulse dye laser for centrofacial rosacea, there is no duty to document lack of dermatology training.

Implicit in the consent for treatment is the option to refuse treatment.[2] In the cosmetic arena, refusal of treatment is typically not a serious concern. However, some jurisdictions require a physician to disclose the consequences of failing to treat as part of an informed consent. A patient refusing intralesional steroid treatment for an incipient keloid has a right to be informed of the consequences of a failure to treat.

The third factor in a valid consent is that the patient must consent freely.[2] Patients must not be coerced by the physician into accepting a cosmetic procedure. Coercion may be as obvious as threatening a patient if he or she does not consent to treatment or as subtle as exaggerating the benefits of accepting the proposed treatment.[2] The dermatologist must be careful not to embellish the expected results of a procedure.

CAUSATION

To establish causation in a battery action, one must demonstrate a link between a failure to disclose and the injury produced. In essence, the patient needs to show that he would have declined treatment in the event he was fully informed. There are two tests for making this determination. The first is the subjective particular patient test in which the determination is made in terms of the jury placing itself in the shoes of the plaintiff. This is the minority rule. The second rule, which is followed in most jurisdictions, is the reasonable person test. This is an objective standard and, accordingly, there is no need for the plaintiff's testimony. Here, the jury places itself in the shoes of the reasonable patient. A determination of whether the risk would be material to a reasonable patient under the circumstances is then made. The medical condition of the patient, patient age, risk of treatment, and risk of alternatives are all considered in making this determination.

DAMAGES

In the event that the duty to obtain an informed consent is breached and a procedure is performed that the patient otherwise would have refused, the physician is liable for all resulting damages.[5]

EXCEPTIONS

True emergency situations almost never arise in cosmetic patients. In the absence of a true emergency, courts are loath to protect a physician claiming this exemption. Courts are equally loath to honor blanket authorizations for medical care.[6] Overbroad waivers are viewed with disfavor and distrust, again because of the basic asymmetric relationship between a patient and a physician. Informed consent requires more specificity. Still, a patient can waive his right to know—i.e., "Doc, just do what you think is best."[7]

A patient who misleads a physician cannot subsequently make a claim based on failure to obtain an informed consent.[8] For example, a tattoo patient who incorrectly denies a history of gold intake cannot sue a physician for failing to discuss the high probability of chrysiasis after Q-switched laser therapy. The patient has a duty to provide the physician with relevant, accurate information as part of an informed consent case. Furthermore, a patient cannot claim miscomprehension in the absence of a showing of incompetence. The courts are skeptical of ex post facto claims of patient incomprehension and mental incompetence.

phenolic thioether amines in melanoma and neuroblastoma cells and the relationship to tyrosinase and tyrosine hydroxylase enzyme activity. *Melanoma Res* 2000;10:9–15.

28. Inoue S, Hasagawa K, Wakamatsu K, et al. Comparison of antimelanoma effects of 4-S-cystaminylphenol and its homologues. *Melanoma Res* 1998;8:105–112.

29. Alena F, Iwashina T, Gili A, et al. Selective in vivo accumulation of N-acetyl-4-S-cystalminylphenol in B16F10 murine melanoma and enhancement of its in vitro and in vivo antimelanoma effect by combination of buthionine sulfoximine. *Cancer Res* 1994;54:2661–2666.

30. Jimbow K. N-acetyl-4-S-cysteaminylphenol as a new type of depigmenting agent for the melanoderma of patients with melasma. *Arch Dermatol* 1991;127;1528–1534.

31. Kimbrough-Green CK, Griffiths CE, Finkel LJ, et al. Topical retinoic acid (tretinoin) for melasma in black patients: a vehicle-controlled clinical trial. *Arch Dermatol* 1994;130:727–733.

32. Griffiths CE, Finkel LJ, Ditre CM, et al. Topical tretinoin (retinoic acid) improves melasma: a vehicle-controlled clinical trial. *Br J Dermatol* 1993;129:415–421.

33. Grimes PE. A microsponge formulation of hydroquinone 4% and retinol 0.15% in the treatment of melasma and postinflammatory hyperpigmentation. *Cutis* 2004;74:362–368.

34. Kligman AM, Willis I. A new formulation for depigmenting human skin. *Arch Dermatol* 1975;111:40–48.

35. Nair X, Parab P, Suhr L, et al. Combination of 4-hydroxisanisol and all-trans retinoic acid produces synergistic skin depigmentation in swine. *J Invest Dermatol* 1993; 145–149.

36. Rendon MI, Benirez AL, Gaviria JI. Treatment of solar lentigines with mequinol/tretinoin in combination with pigment-specific laser: 2 case reports. *Cosmet Dermatol* 2004;17:223–226.

37. Piacquadio D, Farris PK, Downie J, et al. Mequinol 2%/tretinoin 0.01% topical solution monotherapy and combination treatment of solar lentigines and postinflammatory hyperpigmentation. *J Am Acad Dermatol* 2005; 52:145.

38. Tabibian MP. Skin lightening/depigmenting agents. http://www.emedicine.com/derm/topic528.htm. Accessed April 19, 2006.

39. Kollias N, Pote J, Wallo W, et al. Improvements in mottled hyperpigmentation with a soy-based moisturizer. Poster presented at: 61st Annual Meeting of the American Academy of Dermatology; March 21–26, 2003; San Francisco, CA.

40. Fitzpatick RE, Rostan EF. Double-blind, half face study comparing topical vitamin C and vehicle for rejuvenation of photodamage. *Dermatol Surg* 2002;28:231–236.

41. Hakazaki T, Minwalla L, Zhuang J, et al. The effect of niacinamide on reducing cutaneous pigmentation and suppression of melanosome transfer. *Br J Dermatol* 2002;147:20–31.

10

Topical Retinoids in Ethnic Skin

Stefani Takahashi and Julie Iwasaki

Vitamin A (retinol) and its derivatives are known as retinoids.[1] Their topical forms have been used for acne, photoaging, and hyperpigmentation for decades. Throughout the years, many new formulations and vehicles have become available, and continued research can help improve their use. This chapter will discuss all-*trans* retinoic acid, all-*trans* retinol, adapalene, and tazarotene, along with their pharmacology, indications, and side effects. Additional focus will be given to the use of such topical retinoids in ethnic skin.

TOPICAL RETINOIDS

ALL-*TRANS* RETINOIC ACID

All-*trans* retinoic acid (tretinoin), a metabolite of retinol, was developed more than 30 years ago and initially was found to loosen comedones. Thus, it was the first retinoid used for the topical treatment of acne. Ortho Pharmaceuticals introduced this drug as Retin-A in the 1970s. Women using Retin-A for acne coincidentally discovered that it also improved their skin texture, even after their acne was under control. Retin-A was then found to have a new application: to improve photoaging by improving fine lines and enhancing general skin appearance.

As research continued, additional formulations of tretinoin became available. One formulation was Renova, a tretinoin in a new emollient vehicle, which was approved by the FDA to help improve photodamaged skin. Because of the well-known drying properties of Retin-A, Renova was developed to counteract this side effect. Its moisturizing quality was better tolerated in postmenopausal women. Avita is a tretinoin formulation that complexes with polyoprepolymer-2 to slow its absorption into the skin, which decreases irritation. Retin-A Micro uses a microsponge technology to deliver tretinoin in a more controlled manner to similarly reduce irritation.

All-*trans* retinol

All-*trans* retinol is the parent form of vitamin A so it is not considered a drug when it is added to other compounds.

In vitro studies have shown that it is oxidized in the skin to tretinoin; thus, it has similar side effects to this drug. Because it shares tretinoin's irritant qualities, newer formulations were developed to allow for a more controlled delivery. All-*trans* retinol was introduced into cosmetic products by Avon in 1984 to improve photoaging and hyperpigmentation.[2] It is available in formulations of numerous over-the-counter products.

Adapalene

Adapalene, a derivative of naphthoic acid, is commonly available as a 0.1% gel, cream, or lotion to be applied once daily. Adapalene microcrystals penetrate open follicles to the depth of the sebaceous glands within 5 minutes of treatment. Adapalene was found to have a more selective interaction with retinoid receptors than tretinoin; thus, it was developed to improve acne with less skin irritation. In the 1990s, Galderma released this drug as Differin.[2,3]

Tazarotene

Tazarotene, released by Allergan as Tazorac, is a topical retinoid developed to help both acne and psoriasis. The 0.1% tazarotene gel is FDA approved for use in both acne and mild-to-moderate psoriasis; the 0.05% tazarotene gel is only FDA approved for psoriasis. Its side effects include skin irritation and koebnerization. Tazarotene cream 0.1% has also been released by Allergan as Avage to help improve photoaging (facial fine lines, wrinkling, hypopigmentation, hyperpigmentation, and solar lentigines).

PHARMACOLOGY OF TOPICAL RETINOIDS

The first-generation topical retinoids, such as tretinoin, are made by modifying the polar end group and the polyene side chain of vitamin A. Adapalene and tazarotene are both third-generation polyaromatic retinoids that are made by cyclization of the polyene side chain[1] (Fig. 10-1).

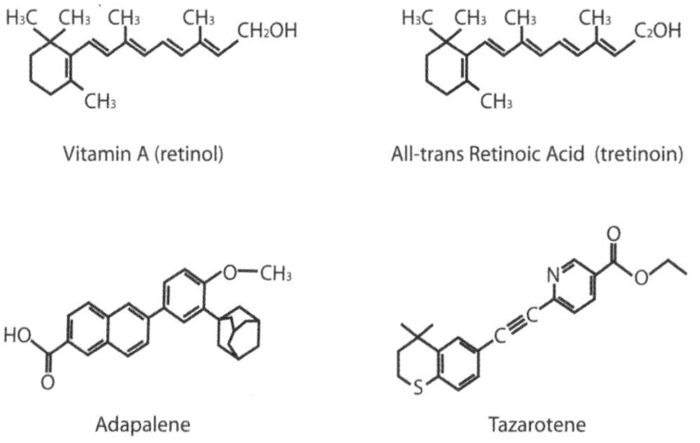

Vitamin A (retinol)

All-trans Retinoic Acid (tretinoin)

Adapalene

Tazarotene

Figure 10-1 Chemical structures of Vitamin A, All-trans Retinoic acid, Adapalene, and Tazarotene.

All-*trans* retinoic acid and all-*trans* retinol

Topical all-*trans* retinol is taken up by epidermal keratinocytes as a fat-soluble drug and binds to cellular or cytosolic retinol-binding protein (CRBP). Inside the keratinocytes, excess all-*trans* retinol is stored as retinyl esters in the form of lipid droplets by acyl CoA:retinol acyl transferase (ARAT). Because topical all-*trans* retinoic acid cannot be reduced to retinol, it increases the amount of intracellular retinoic acid to cause potential side effects. If retinoic acid levels become low in the epidermis, retinol is mobilized from retinyl esters and is oxidized to all-*trans* retinoic acid and its isomers (9-*cis*).

All-*trans* retinoic acid, bound to cellular all-*trans* retinoic acid-binding protein (CRABP), then binds to nuclear retinoic acid receptors (RAR), while the isomers bind to both retinoid X receptors (RXR) and RAR. RAR and RXR belong to the steroid-thyroid hormone family, and each family contains an alpha, beta, and gamma isotype. They form homodimers and heterodimers that bind

to retinoic acid response elements (RAREs) in DNA to directly influence cell differentiation, proliferation, and immune responses (Fig. 10-2).

C-Jun and C-Fos are genes that are involved in photoaging. Levels of C-Jun rise when exposed to ultraviolet (UV) radiation, whereas C-Fos remains the same. C-Jun and C-Fos can then combine to form a heterodimer, activator protein-1 (AP1), which induces collagenase, gelatinase, and stromelysin. Retinoids inhibit the overexpression of C-Jun, which causes an indirect effect from the down-regulation of AP1 by competing for required coactivator proteins. AP1 is normally responsible for proliferative and inflammatory responses; thus retinoids have antiproliferative and anti-inflammatory actions.[1,2,4]

Adapalene

Adapalene is a lipophilic synthetic retinoid with a selective affinity for RAR-beta and RAR-gamma. RAR-gamma is the primary receptor for topically applied adapalene because RAR-beta is not present in epidermal keratinocytes. Only trace amounts of adapalene are absorbed systemically because adapalene's lipophilicity causes selective uptake into the pilosebaceous unit and dissolution within the sebum. The hepatobiliary system removes the systemically absorbed adapalene.[1,2]

Tazarotene

Tazarotene is rapidly hydrolyzed by skin esterases into its active metabolite, tazarotenic acid. Tazarotenic acid binds mostly to RAR-beta and RAR-gamma in the epidermis and has no affinity for RXR. It modulates the expression of retinoid responsive genes to regulate cell proliferation, cell differentiation, and inflammation. Tazarotene down-regulates the expression of keratinocyte transglutaminase I (Tgase I), hyperproliferative keratins (K6 and K16), migration inhibitory factor-related protein (MRP-8), and epidermal

Figure 10-2 Metabolism of topical retinoids. ARAT, acyl CoA:retinol acyl transferase; CRBP, cytosolic retinol-binding protein; CRABP, cellular all-*trans* retinoic acid-binding protein; RA, retinoic acid; RAR, retinoic acid receptors; RAREs, retinoic acid response elements. (Courtesy of Pearl E. Grimes, MD.)

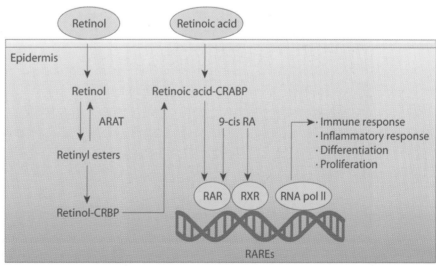

Metabolism of topical retinoids

growth factor receptor, while inducing tazarotene inducible genes (TIGs) 1, 2, and 3.

Although it is rapidly metabolized, a small amount of tazarotene can be absorbed systemically. This is degraded by oxidation to inactive sulfoxine and sulfone derivatives that are excreted in the urine and feces. In normal skin, systemic absorption can be up to 5% of the applied drug, and the maximum blood concentration of tazarotene gel is at 9 hours after the application. The half-life of the drug is less than 20 minutes, and the terminal half-life is about 18 hours.[1,2]

INDICATIONS

The most important aspect of treating a patient with topical retinoids is patient education regarding proper application techniques and expectations. Side effects, such as local skin irritation, and the fact that noticeable results may take months to appear should be discussed. Desquamation corresponds to the hyperproliferative response of RARs to tretinoin, although erythema does not appear to be receptor mediated. Administration of topical retinoids needs to be titrated, depending on the patient's reaction to the medication. A general rule is to start treatment with the lowest strength formulation and then gradually increase it as the patient gains tolerance. Sunscreens and moisturizers should be incorporated as daily regimens.[1]

Acne vulgaris

Topical retinoids are an important, if not essential, component in the treatment of acne vulgaris (Fig. 10-3). Their mechanism of action involves its anti-inflammatory properties and its normalization of the follicular epithelium to loosen comedones and prevent sebum buildup, not sebum production. They are used for mild acne that is nonscarring, has open and closed comedones, and has moderate pustules. For moderate to severe acne, they are used in combination therapy. Topical retinoids need to be maintained to have comedolytic effects. Cystic acne is more severe and does not respond well with monotherapy topical treatment but may be useful in combination therapy or as maintenance therapy once control of the disease has been reached.[2,5]

In treating acne vulgaris with topical retinoids, patients must be aware that onset of improvement may take several weeks. Topical retinoids are usually applied as a thin layer of the retinoid nightly. The disease can worsen in the first month of treatment as the follicular epithelium loosens. After 2 months of sustained treatment, a continued improvement is usually noted. At this point, the main goal of treatment is to prevent development of new comedones. Combination therapy of topical retinoids with mild topical antimicrobial agents is often used.[2]

In a review of acne in African American patients with Fitzpatrick skin types IV through VI, adapalene

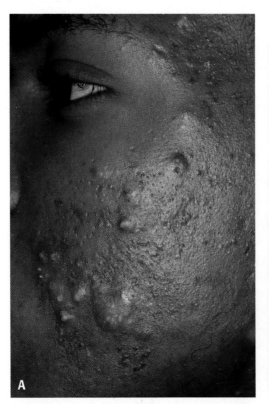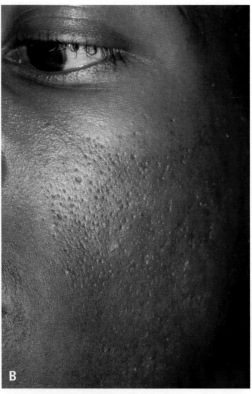

Figure 10-3 Acne treated with tazarotene 0.1% cream in an African American. **A:** Before. **B:** After. (Courtesy of Pearl E. Grimes, MD.)

demonstrated efficacy for the treatment of mild to moderate acne vulgaris. Compared with white patients with acne vulgaris, adapalene significantly reduced the number of inflammatory lesions and caused much less erythema and scaling in black patients. Most of the ethnic patients also had a reduction in number and density of postinflammatory hyperpigmented macules. However, the combined number of inflammatory and noninflammatory lesions was similar in the two patient populations, as well as the dryness that was due to the topical retinoid. Overall, adapalene gel 0.1% can be used to prevent and reduce acne associated hyperpigmentation and decrease the number of both inflammatory and noninflammatory lesions (Fig. 10-4).[5–7]

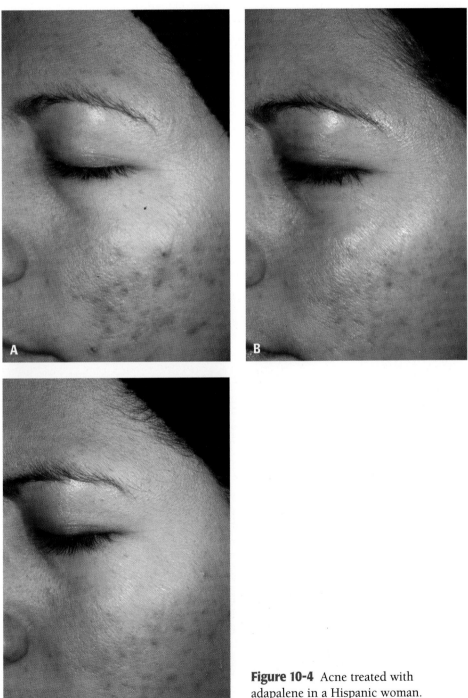

Figure 10-4 Acne treated with adapalene in a Hispanic woman. **A:** Baseline. **B:** 4 weeks. **C:** 8 weeks. (Courtesy of Pearl E. Grimes, MD.)

Acne vulgaris is also a common problem among Asians, who also have a predisposition for postinflammatory hyperpigmentation. Adapalene gel 0.1% was compared with tretinoin gel 0.025% in a randomized study of 150 Chinese patients over an 8-week period. Both adapalene and tretinoin were shown to reduce the number of inflammatory and noninflammatory lesions. Tretinoin caused more irritation than adapalene, although the irritation was mild. In the Chinese population, both adapalene gel 0.1% and tretinoin gel 0.025% are effective treatments for mild to moderate acne vulgaris, but adapalene causes less irritation.[8]

Photodamage

In general, photodamaged skin is characterized by rhytides, telangiectasias, solar comedones, blotchy pigmentation, and actinic keratoses (AKs).[2] The melanin content and melanosomal dispersion pattern in darker skin as compared with lighter skin may provide protection from accelerated aging because of UV radiation. Darkly pigmented skin can still experience photodamage, but this often occurs at a later age. Photoaging in black skin presents as inconsistent pigmentation, such as hypopigmentation or hyperpigmentation. In Asian women, photoaging presents differently as epidermal atrophy, disorderly differentiation, cell atypia, and poor polarity.[9]

All-*trans* retinoic acid has been shown to improve fine wrinkling, increase dermal collagen, and repair elastin fiber formation. Photoaging may be treated with nightly use of tretinoin. Topical alpha-hydroxy acid formulations may be used with topical tretinoin to enhance the penetration in photodamaged skin, but this may cause increased irritation.

Initially, epidermal mucin and temporary compaction of the stratum corneum can improve the texture and fine wrinkles of photodamaged skin. Long-term topical tretinoin treatment can lead to epidermal hyperplasia of atrophic skin, dispersion of melanin granules, removal of dysplastic keratinocytes, new dermal collagen formation, angiogenesis, decreased elastosis, and comedolysis. Clinically, the skin appears smoother, more evenly toned, and has fewer fine lines and wrinkles.[2,10]

Topical tretinoins were found to normalize the differentiation of dysplastic epithelium in AKs. They decrease the amount of AKs on the face by about 50% when used alone for at least 6 months. Topical tretinoin can be used with topical 5-fluorouracil (5-FU) to enhance the penetration of 5-FU in the treatment of actinic keratoses.[2] Retinoids have been used in Thai,[11] Chinese,[12] Japanese,[12] and African American[13] patients with photodamaged skin. The subjects experienced overall improvement in skin texture; the skin surface became less rough and scaly, and small, hyperkeratotic growths tended to disappear (Fig. 10-5).

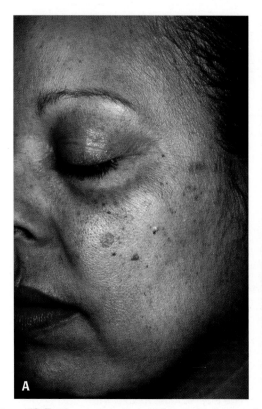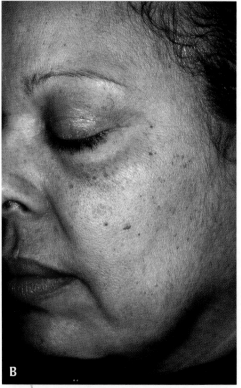

Figure 10-5 Photoaging in an African American characterized by hyperpigmentation and texturally rough skin. **A:** Baseline. **B:** Marked improvement after 12 weeks of treatment. (Courtesy of Pearl E. Grimes, MD and Johnson and Johnson, New Jersey)

Hyperpigmentation

Topical retinoids are also used in the treatment of hyperpigmentation, including that seen in postinflammatory hyperpigmentation (Fig. 10-6), melasma, and solar lentigines. They can be used alone in mild cases, but more severe problems can be treated with combination therapy. Tretinoin has been used with hydroquinone, topical steroids, and/or alpha-hydroxy acids.[2]

In one study, human and murine melanocyte monolayer cultures were studied to evaluate the suppressing effect of tretinoin on melanogenesis. These results showed that tretinoin does not have a direct inhibitory effect on melanogenesis or on cell-cell interactions between melanocytes, keratinocytes, or fibroblasts. Instead, tretinoin may be involved in keratinocyte proliferation, the acceleration of epidermal turnover, and the binding of CRABP-I.[13,14]

In a study of 2,000 black patients who saw a dermatologist, the third most common diagnosis was a pigmentation disorder other than vitiligo. Most of these patients presented with postinflammatory hyperpigmentation.[14] Postinflammatory hyperpigmentation commonly occurs following acne, folliculitis, eczema, or irritation from shaving.[17] It appears to be more severe in darker skin types because of the release of inflammation mediators that trigger melanogenesis and melanocyte proliferation.[5]

In a study by Grimes and Callender,[18] 74 patients from darker racial ethnic groups with acne vulgaris–induced postinflammatory hyperpigmentation were assessed in a double-blind, randomized, vehicle-controlled study. Once-daily application of tazarotene 0.1% cream was shown to be effective against postinflammatory hyperpigmentation, achieving significantly greater reductions compared with vehicle in overall disease severity and in the intensity and area of hyperpigmentation within 18 weeks. Side effects, including erythema, peeling, dryness, and burning, were very minimal.

Tretinoin, 0.1% retinoic acid cream, can also improve postinflammatory hyperpigmentation in black patients. Fifty-four patients were involved in a 40-week-long randomized, double-blind, vehicle-controlled study. After 40 weeks of treatment, the patients who used tretinoin had significantly lighter postinflammatory hyperpigmented lesions on the face than the control patients. The epidermal melanin content of the lesions decreased by 23%, and there was a 40% lightening of the lesions with tretinoin compared with a 3% decrease in epidermal melanin content and 18% lightening of the lesions with the vehicle alone. Tretinoin also lightened the normal skin in black patients. Retinoid dermatitis developed in 50% of tretinoin-treated subjects but diminished as the study progressed.[17]

A triple drug combination of fluocinolone acetonide 0.01%, hydroquinone 4.0%, and tretinoin 0.05% applied once daily at night has been shown to be efficacious in the treatment of postinflammatory hyperpigmentation. The topical corticosteroid suppresses melanocyte secretion of melanin, and the hydroquinone blocks melanin biosynthesis by inhibiting tyrosinase and degrading melanosomes. Tretinoin enhances epidermal turnover, which causes a dispersion of keratinocyte pigment granules. Together, these topical drugs work synergistically to improve postinflammatory hyperpigmentation.[19]

Melasma is an acquired facial hyperpigmentation.[20] It is more prevalent in black, Hispanic, and Asian people and is attributed to hormonal factors, UV radiation, and the liability of melanocytes.[9] Tretinoin was shown to lighten melasma in black patients with minimal side effects. In one study, 28 patients applied 0.1% tretinoin or vehicle cream daily to their faces and were followed over 10 months in a randomized, vehicle-controlled study. Using the Melasma Area and Severity Index Scale to assess improvement, there was a 32% improvement in the tretinoin-treated group compared with a 10% improvement in the vehicle-treated group. Signs of improvement were not significant before week 24. Histologically, tretinoin was observed to cause a decrease in epidermal pigmentation by transferring melanosomes to keratinocytes. Sixty-seven percent of the tretinoin-treated patients did acquire mild retinoid dermatitis. Overall, the use of tretinoin as monotherapy for the treatment of melasma is limited.[20,21] Hence, tretinoin is best used for melasma in combination with other lightening agents.

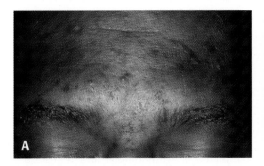 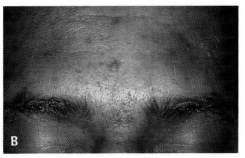

Figure 10-6 Postinflammatory hyperpigmentation and acne treated with tazarotene 0.1% cream. **A:** Baseline. **B:** After 8 weeks. (Courtesy of Pearl E. Grimes, MD.)

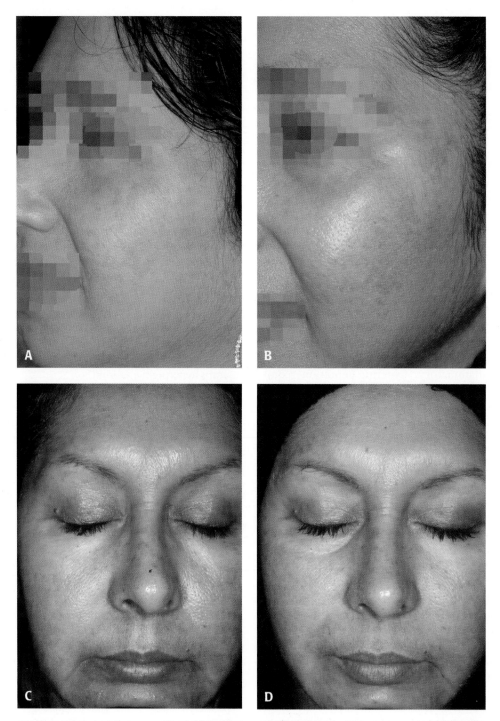

Figure 10-7 Retinoid dermatitis characterized by erythema and irritation of the cheeks **(A)** Baseline and **(B)** 2 weeks after use of retinoid. **C:** Baseline and **(D)** 6 weeks. Note erythema and edema. (Courtesy of Pearl E. Grimes, MD.)

In a community-based trial, a triple combination treatment of fluocinolone acetonide 0.01%, hydroquinone 4.0%, and tretinoin 0.05% in a hydrophilic cream formulation has been shown to improve melasma in all ethnic groups. There were 1,290 patients enrolled from 393 centers in the United States. The treatment signifi-cantly lightened melasma at 4 weeks and had a continued benefit at 8 weeks.[22]

Studies have shown that topical 20% azelaic acid is bet-ter than 2% hydroquinone and is just as effective as 4% hydroquinone for the treatment of melasma and postinflam-matory hyperpigmentation. Tretinoin has been shown to enhance the effect of topical 20% azelaic acid after 3 months of treatment. Azelaic acid may inhibit the energy production, and/or DNA synthesis of hyperactive melanocytes.[23] It may also inhibit tyrosinase activity.

Tretinoin 0.1% cream has also been shown to reduce the hyperpigmentation of lentigines caused by photoaging in the Chinese and Japanese populations. There were 23 Chinese and 22 Japanese patients involved in a double-blind, randomized, vehicle-controlled study conducted over 40 weeks. Ninety percent of the tretinoin-treated patients had significantly lighter lesions compared with 33% of the vehicle-treated patients. According to the histological analysis, the tretinoin-treated patients showed a 41% decrease in epidermal pigmentation compared with a 37% increase in the controls.[12]

SIDE EFFECTS

Side effects of topical retinoids include irritation, erythema, desquamation, pruritus, burning, photosensitivity, dry skin, fissuring, bleeding, and worsening psoriasis (Fig. 10-7). Photoallergy and phototoxicity have not been proven, but patients show photosensitivity by a reduced tolerance to UV radiation. Because of these side effects, noncompliance and discontinuation of the treatment can occur. To reduce the severity of such reactions, the

patients should avoid other products that can cause additional irritation. For example, abrasive soaps and products containing alcohol, salicylic acid, benzoyl peroxide, sulfur, and resorcinol should be avoided.[1] Overall, topical retinoids are safe and effective, as shown by histological examination of skin that was treated up to 4 years. There was no keratinocyte or melanocyte atypia observed that was caused by topical retinoid use.[10]

Because irritation from topical retinoids use can cause postinflammatory hyperpigmentation (Fig. 10-8), newer formulations and synthetic analogues have been used. Cream- and emollient-based preparations are better tolerated, and microsponge vehicles are now used for 0.1% and 0.04% tretinoin gels.[24] Bershad et al. demonstrated that using 0.1% tazarotene gel for up to 5 minutes once or twice daily is a safe and effective method for treating acne while minimizing side effects.[25] Other ways to minimize irritation include applying a small amount of topical retinoid when the skin is completely dry, which slows penetration.

A randomized study by Leyden et al. evaluated tolerability of retinoid concentration, formulation vehicle, skin sensitivity, of individual retinoids in 253 patients. Less irritation and tolerability was seen with lower retinoid concentrations. The researchers found that the irritation induced by a gel or cream formulation depended on the specific retinoid used. Normal skin

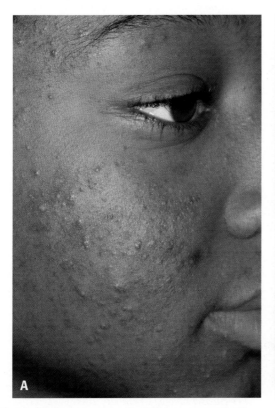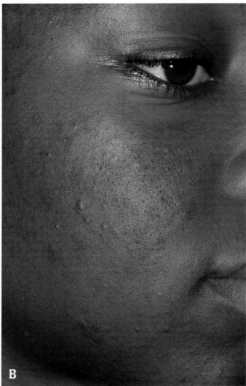

Figure 10-8 Acne treated with tazarotene 0.1% cream. Significant improvement, but patient developed localized and diffuse hyperpigmentation. **A:** Before. **B:** After. (Courtesy of Pearl E. Grimes, MD.)

Table 10-1

FDA pregnancy categories for topical retinoids

Name	Category	Birth defects
Tretinoin	C	Unknown
Adapalene	C	Unknown
Tazarotene	X	Possible

tolerated tazarotene cream better than tretinoin cream, and adapalene and tretinoin microsponge vehicles were tolerated better than tazarotene gel. Sensitive skin tolerated tazarotene and adapalene cream better than tretinoin cream, and adapalene gel was tolerated better than tazarotene gel.[26]

TERATOGENICITY

Vitamin A is required for normal growth and differentiation. The absorption of topical retinoids is usually controlled, but it can become a problem if a large surface area is treated. It is not known whether the drug can affect a developing embryo and fetus, so topical retinoids should be avoided during pregnancy. Also, it is not known whether topical retinoids are present in breast milk, so caution should be taken during this time (Table 10-1).

Tazarotene is contraindicated in women who may become or are pregnant. The patient should be informed of the potential risk to a fetus before the initiation of treatment, and adequate birth control should be used. A negative pregnancy test should be obtained within 2 weeks before treatment, and the treatment should begin during a normal menstrual period. If a patient becomes pregnant while using this drug or if a patient is already pregnant, treatment should immediately be discontinued.[2,27]

CONCLUSION

Topical all-*trans* retinoic acid, all-trans retinol, adapalene, and tazarotene are all used alone or in combination to effectively treat acne vulgaris, photodamaged skin, and hyperpigmentation in ethnic skin. The increased melanin content of darker skin types makes it more prone to pigmentation disorders in response to inflammation, injury, and treatment. With appropriate education on potential side effects and proper medication use, topical retinoids may be used safely and efficiently in darker racial ethnic groups.

REFERENCES

1. Bolognia J. *Dermatology.* Vol. 2. New York: Mosby;2003.
2. Wolverton S. *Comprehensive Dermatologic Drug Therapy.* 7th ed. Philadelphia: W.B. Saunders Company;2001.
3. Katzung B. *Basic and Clinical Pharmacology.* 8th ed. New York: Lange Medical Books/McGraw-Hill;2001.
4. Baumann L. The role of retinoids in photoaging. *Supplement to Skin and Aging.* 2003.
5. Callender VD. Acne in ethnic skin: special considerations for therapy. *Dermatol Ther* 2004;17(2):184–195.
6. Czernielewski J, Poncet M, Mizzi F. Efficacy and cutaneous safety of adapalene in black patients versus white patients with acne vulgaris. *Cutis* 2002;70(4):243–248.
7. Jacyk WK. Adapalene in the treatment of African patients. *J Eur Acad Dermatol Venereol* 2001;15(Suppl 3): 37–42.
8. Tu P, Li GQ, Zhu XJ, et al. A comparison of adapalene gel 0.1% vs. tretinoin gel 0.025% in the treatment of acne vulgaris in China. *J Eur Acad Dermatol Venereol* 2001;15(Suppl 3):31–36.
9. Taylor S. Skin of color: biology, structure, function, and implications for dermatologic disease. *J Am Acad Dermatol (Suppl)* 2002;46(2):S41–S62.
10. Bhawan J. Short- and long-term histologic effects of topical tretinoin on photodamaged skin. *Int J Dermatol* 1998;37(4): 286–292.
11. Kotrajaras R, Kligman AM. The effect of topical tretinoin on photodamaged facial skin: the Thai experience. *Br J of Dermatol* 1993;129:302–309.
12. Griffiths CE, Goldfarb MT, Finkel LJ, et al. Topical tretinoin (retinoic acid) treatment of hyperpigmented lesions associated with photoaging in Chinese and Japanese patients: a vehicle-controlled trial. *J Am Acad Dermatol* 1994;30(1): 76–84.
13. Halder RM. The role of retinoids in the management of cutaneous conditions in blacks. *J Am Acad Dermatol* 1998;39: S98–103.
14. Sanquer S, Reenstra WR, Eller MS, et al. Keratinocytes and dermal factors activate CRABP-I in melanocytes. *Exp Dermatol* 1998;7(6):369–379.
15. Yoshimura K, Tsukamoto K, Okazaki M, et al. Effects of all-trans retinoic acid on melanogenesis in pigmented skin equivalents and monolayer culture of melanocytes. *J Dermatol Sci* 2001;27(Suppl 1):S68–75.
16. Halder RM, Grimes PE, McLaurin EI, et al. Incidence of common dermatoses in a predominantly black dermatologic practice. *Cutis* 1983;32:378–380.
17. Bulengo-Ransby SM, Griffiths CE, Kimbrough-Green CK, et al. Topical tretinoin (retinoic acid) therapy for hyperpigmented lesions caused by inflammation of the skin in black patients. *N Engl J Med* 1993;328(20):1438–1443.
18. Grimes P, Callender V. Tazarotene cream for postinflammatory hyperpigmentation and acne vulgaris in darker skin: a double-blind, randomized, vehicle-controlled study. *Cutis* 2006;77(1):45–50.
19. Nestor M. The use of a triple-drug combination product for the treatment of postinflammatory hyperpigmentation. *Cosmetic Dermatology.* February 2006;19(2):115-118.
20. Kimbrough-Green CK, Griffiths CE, Finkel LJ, et al. Topical retinoic acid (tretinoin) for melasma in black patients. A

vehicle-controlled clinical trial. *Arch Dermatol.* Jun 1994;130(6):727-733.

21. Rendon M. Melasma and Postinflammatory Hyperpigmentation. *Cosmetic Dermatology* 2003;16(S3):9–17.

22. Grimes PE, Kelly AP, Tork H, et al. Community-based trial of a triple-combination agent for the treatment of facial melasma. *Cutis* 2006;77(3):177–189.

23. Breathnach AS. Melanin hyperpigmentation of skin: melasma, topical treatment with azelaic acid, and other therapies. *Cutis* 1996;57(1 Suppl):36–45.

24. Perez A, Sanchez J. Treatment of acne vulgaris in skin of color. *Cosmetic Dermatology* 2003;16(S3):23–28.

25. Bershad S, Kranjac Singer G, et al. Successful treatment of acne vulgaris using a new method: results of a randomized vehicle-controlled trial of short-contact therapy with 0.1% tazarotene gel. *Arch Dermatol* 2002;138(4):481–489.

26. Leyden J, Grove G, Zerweck C. Facial tolerability of topical retinoid therapy. *J Drugs Dermatol* 2004;3(6):641–651.

27. LaGow B. *The PDR Pocket Guide to Prescription Drugs.* New York: Pocket Books;2005.

11

Antioxidants

Fran E. Cook-Bolden and Jocelyne Papacharalambous

Antioxidants have had a key position in the medical and scientific arena since the early 1900s. More recently, they are taking center stage in the dermatologic and aesthetic community, where they are reported to play a critical role in skin health and youthfulness. Another increasingly important role is that they are being used to augment the effects of cosmetic procedures.[1,2] The fuel that has ignited this unquenchable flame for knowledge of antioxidants includes the pursuit of optimal health and well-being, the desire for optimal skin care, the search for longevity and eternal beauty, and the anti-aging movement. Additionally, the increased life span of the population, the desire to align with nature by spending more time outdoors, and the trend toward the use of "natural products" have also contributed to this growing phenomenon.[3] Research has demonstrated a wide range of potential benefits from antioxidants, including improved cognition, improved immune function, prevention of malignancy, overall disease prevention, and anti-aging. Despite the steadily growing popularity of antioxidants and the increase in research in this area, there remains a large gap in detailed information about them, including results demonstrating their direct benefit in the general population.[4] There is an even greater deficit of specific benefits in skin of color (worldwide the majority of the population), as most studies of this nature are performed on skin types I through III.[5]

ANTIOXIDANTS

Antioxidants have been touted as the premier anti-aging substances for scavenging of free oxygen radicals and other harmful agents that have deleterious effects in the body and to the skin. They are defined as oral, topical, or intrinsic substances that protect and possibly correct oxidative injury to the body and the skin caused by free radicals.[6] It has been reported that antioxidants have the ability to actually reverse these and other damaging environmental assaults from sunlight, air pollution, alcohol, cigarette smoke, and stress. Some of these substances not only restrict blood flow to our skin and organs, but also generate potent, destructive free radicals. These free radicals ultimately cause massive internal destruction beyond the cellular layer in every organ system of our body, rapidly increasing the aging and disease process overall, both inside and out. Nonetheless, although there has been a preponderance of speculation and growing clinical investigation supporting the benefits of antioxidants, firm evidence is lacking as to the direct link or cause-and-effect relationship and consistent, reproducible scientific data to guide their usage.[7]

UNDERSTANDING FREE RADICALS AND OXYGEN REACTIVE SPECIES

The molecules that make up the cells of our bodies and skin are held intact and made stable by the bonding of paired electrons. When oxygen molecules are involved in reactions in the body and the skin, these electron pairs are disrupted and lose their partner (the bonds are split), and unstable free radicals are formed. Free radicals (e.g., superoxide, nitric oxide, hydroxyl radicals) and other reactive species (e.g., hydrogen peroxide, peroxynitrite, hypochlorous acid) are produced in the body, primarily as a result of aerobic metabolism. Antioxidants (e.g., glutathione, arginine, citrulline, taurine, creatine, selenium, zinc, vitamin E, vitamin C, vitamin A, and tea polyphenols) and antioxidant enzymes (e.g., superoxide dismutase, catalase, glutathione reductase, and glutathione peroxidases) exert synergistic actions in scavenging free radicals.[8]

As part of an internal process that occurs naturally in the body to repair this state and regain stability, a reaction begins that can affect every cell in the body. These very unstable free radicals quickly react with other compounds in efforts to regain their stability. They do this by attacking the nearest stable molecule to "steal" a partner; this regains stability, but results in the formation of another free radical. The process continues, ultimately ending up with a "chain" of rapid free radical formation and cascading damage to the body and skin. In summary, free radicals

Table 11-1

Antioxidants and their functions   (*continued*)

Antioxidant	Characteristics and functions	
Selenium	Photoprotective properties Decreased intake is associated with increased incidence of some cancers	Role in the formation and function of the selenium dependent glutathione peroxidases, which detoxify hydroperoxides
Soy isoflavone	General skin anti-aging effects Photoprotective properties Osteoporosis prevention	Weak estrogenic activity Used in the treatment of heart disease, cancer, and menopausal symptoms
Zinc	General skin anti-aging	Maintains the integrity of biological membranes resulting in protection against oxidative injury
	Beneficial in wound healing	Vital for proper functioning of the immune system, digestion, reproduction, vision, taste, and smell
	Used to in the treatment of seasonal conjunctivitis	

Vitamin E

Evidence has been obtained showing dietary vitamin E to protect against oxidative damage to DNA in human lymphocytes and white blood cells. Studies on mice have reported reductions in UV-induced skin cancer. Other clear evidence of vitamin E's protective effect has been seen in its suppressive action of low-density lipoprotein (LDL) oxidation both in vitro and in vivo. New evidence on the physiological roles of antioxidants, in addition to their well-known role as free radical scavengers, is emerging from recent research. Early findings suggesting a beneficial effect of vitamin E in improving glucose transport and insulin sensitivity and a possible putative role as a regulator of cell proliferation should open new research dimensions.[37] Vitamin E may be more effective if combined with other antioxidants, such as coenzyme Q_{10} and vitamin C.

Coenzyme Q_{10}

Discovered in 1957 by Frederick Crane, a plant physiologist at the University of Wisconsin Enzyme Institute, coenzyme Q_{10} (CoQ_{10}), or ubiquinone, is the only lipid-soluble antioxidant (in its reduced form, ubiquinol) that is synthesized in the body and present in cellular membranes and in lipoproteins. In 1958, D. E. Wolf and Karl Folkers first described the chemical structure of CoQ_{10}. From 1957 through 1988, there were some 2,300 medical studies on CoQ_{10}. Since then, there have been countless others.[38]

The exceptional antioxidant properties of CoQ_{10} effectively counteract free radical damage and provide significant protection against UVA-induced depletion of cell membrane components, preventing damage to collagen and elastin.[39–41]

CoQ_{10}, an antioxidant that is structurally similar to vitamin E, plays a crucial role in the generation of cellular energy. It is a significant immunologic stimulant, increases circulation, is beneficial for the cardiovascular system, and has anti-aging effects. It appears to qualify as a highly beneficial anti-aging nutrient based on its multiple mechanisms of action, its broad range of effects on a number of life-threatening or debilitating clinical conditions, its life-span–extending properties in more than one species, and its absence of adverse effects. Beneficial effects have been demonstrated in some conditions with as little as 30 to 60 mg per day.[39]

Multiple animal studies have shown an increased life span related to CoQ_{10}.[39–41] As research continues to accumulate, it appears that the higher the dosage, the greater the benefit (as evidenced by supplementation with 390-mg in breast cancer and 1,200-mg in Parkinson disease patients), and that the primary limiting factor on CoQ_{10} dosage is the cost.[39–41]

There are a number of conditions in which CoQ_{10} tissue concentrations are altered with functional consequences. Oxidative stress generated by, for example, physical exercise increases tissue ubiquinone levels by increasing biosynthesis, as does administration of drugs like clofibrate. In contrast, aging is generally associated with decreases in tissue CoQ_{10} levels. For example, levels of CoQ_{10} in the skin are low in childhood, reach a maximum at around 20 to 30 years of age, and then decrease steadily with increasing age. It has been postulated that topically applied CoQ_{10} can penetrate the skin and attenuate

Table 11-2

Miscellaneous antioxidants and their functions

Antioxidants	Purported uses	Function
Acetyl L-carnitine	General skin anti-aging effects, symptomatic diabetic neuropathy	Transport of long-chain fatty acids across the mitochondrial membrane and transport of small and medium chain fatty acids out of the mitochondria
EUK-134	Improvement in skin erythema caused by Ultraviolet (UV) exposure, reduction in adverse developmental outcome due to ethanol exposure in utero, renal dysfunction	A synthetic superoxide dismutase and catalase mimetic with similar actions on the skin
Ferulic acid	General skin anti-aging effects, photoprotection, diabetes, Alzheimer's, macular degeneration, menopause, enhances athletic performance	Arises from the metabolism of phenylalanine and tyrosine
Glutathione	General skin anti-aging, skin lightening, heart disease, osteoarthritis, memory loss, kidney dysfunction, and pulmonary disease	Reduces disulfide bonds formed within cytoplasmic proteins to cysteines by acting as an electron donor Immune system booster and detoxifier Antimelanogenic effects
Grape seed extract	Improvement in skin erythema and wound contraction; used as a laxative and antacid Small human trials have shown possible efficacy in decreasing LDL and increasing total antioxidant activity	Scavenging of hydroxyl and peroxyl radicals; inhibition of the oxidation of LDL
Methionine	General skin anti-aging effects; ingredient in most hair, skin, and nail supplemental vitamins; lowers blood cholesterol; maintains normal body weight	Neutralizes hydroxyl radicals, essential for the production of nucleic acid, collagen, and proteins
Melatonin	Suppresses UV-induced skin damage, modulates the immune system, protects against degenerative diseases, promotes sleep and prevents jet lag	Inhibits metal ion-catalyzed oxidation processes Antiapoptotic activity
Nicotinamide adenine dinucleotide (NADH) (also known as coenzyme 1)	Reduces wrinkles, skin erythema, and hyperpigmentation; improves skin texture; memory enhancer, decreases blood cholesterol, lowers blood pressure	Production of cellular energy
Oligomeric proanthocyanidins (OPCs) (also known as flavonoids)	Photoprotection, reduction in fine lines and wrinkles, protects the liver from damage, repairs connective tissue, slows aging	Moderates allergic and inflammatory responses

both the depth of deep wrinkles characteristic of photoaging, as well as increasing the turnover of epidermal cells. CoQ_{10} is also highly effective in protecting keratinocytes from oxidative DNA damage induced by UV light.

Alpha hydroxy acids

Alpha hydroxy acids (AHAs) are a group of organic carboxylic acids that are naturally occurring and nontoxic and have been used to promote a more youthful complexion by people in many civilizations. In ancient Egypt, Cleopatra used AHAs in the form of milk baths to soften her much-admired skin. AHAs are found in fruit, sour milk, sugarcane, and other products processed through biofermentation.

In low concentrations, AHAs cause a decrease in corneocyte cohesion and facilitate the shedding of corneocytes. In higher concentrations, they result in epidermolysis, upper dermal changes, and may even stimulate the production of collagen and elastin, producing vibrant, less-wrinkled, and more uniformly colored skin.[42] Nonetheless, the specific mechanism of action of AHAs has not been fully determined. It is hypothesized that AHAs act as chelating agents, decreasing local calcium ion concentrations from cation-dependent cell adhesion molecules. Another proposed mechanism for AHA-induced exfoliation is an increase in apoptosis.

The simplest molecule of AHAs and the most widely used in skin care is glycolic acid, made from sugarcane, which is used extensively for photoaging and wrinkles. Studies done by Moy et al. demonstrated that glycolic acid may stimulate collagen production in skin fibroblasts.[43] Another commonly used AHA is lactic acid that is derived from milk. It is widely used as a milder or slightly less irritating alternative to glycolic acid and like glycolic acid is primarily used for anti-aging to soften lines, reduce photodamage from the sun, improve skin texture and tone, and improve overall appearance. Other AHAs include tartaric acid (derived from grapes), malic acid (derived from apples and pears), and citric acid (derived from citrus fruits). All have similar benefits.

Major side effects of alpha hydroxy acids are irritation and sun sensitivity. People with darker skin tones are at a higher risk of long-term pigment changes with aggressive use of AHAs. Their use can increase sun sensitivity by 50%.[42,44,45] Hence, it appears that although AHAs may reverse some of the damage caused by photoaging, they can make the skin more susceptible to photoaging at the same time. Larger cohort studies need to be done to fully evaluate efficacy as well as the specific mechanism of action.

Silymarin

Silymarin, *Silybum marianum* (L.),[46] a flavonoid isolated from milk thistle (present in artichokes), is used clinically in Europe and Asia as an antihepatotoxic agent,[47,48] largely because of its strong antioxidant activity. Because most antioxidants afford protection against tumor promotion, a detailed study was done that assessed the protective effect of silymarin on tumor promotion in a mouse-skin model. It was concluded that silymarin possesses exceptionally high protective effects against tumor promotion (protection against tumor incidence, tumor multiplicity, and tumor volume), and that the mechanism of such effects may involve inhibition of promoter-induced edema, hyperplasia, proliferation index, and the oxidant state.

As a therapeutic agent, silymarin is very well tolerated and largely free of adverse effects.[49,50] It has been marketed recently in the United States for its potential antioxidant benefits. Recent studies show that it may inhibit UVB-promoted cancers in animals. Mechanistic studies have shown that silymarin is a strong antioxidant that is capable of scavenging both free radicals and reactive oxygen species in rodents and in cell cultures, and that it results in a significant increase in cellular antioxidant defense machinery by ameliorating the deleterious effects of free radical reactions.[51–55]

Green tea (tea polyphenols)

Recent scientific studies have indicated that green tea could protect against cancer, heart disease, and osteoporosis; aid in weight loss; and help ward off skin cancer and signs of aging. Green tea is consumed mostly in Asian countries—including India, Japan, Korea, and China—although it is not quite as popular as its cousin, black tea, which is consumed by more than 75% of tea drinkers. Like black tea and oolong tea, green tea comes from the *Camellia sinensis* plant, but its leaves are not fermented before steaming and drying; they remain fresh.

These teas contain large quantities of polyphenols (a class of bioflavonoids) and have been shown to have antioxidant, anticancer, antibacterial, and antiviral properties. Most of the polyphenols in green tea are catechins. Catechins are antioxidants that have also been shown to function as anti-inflammatory and anticancer agents. One of the major catechins in green tea has been shown to be the most effective agent against skin inflammation and cancerous changes in the skin.

There is evidence that the compounds in green tea protected mouse skin from cancer caused by sunlight. Initial experimental studies on human skin by Katyar et al. found that the polyphenols in green tea also had anti-inflammatory and anticancer properties.[56]

Studies by Conney, et al. have been done to determine how green tea protects against cancer.[57] In their initial studies, caffeine was removed from the tea, and the decaffeinated tea was fed to mice at a moderate dose. Results revealed that when the caffeine was removed from green tea, the tea lost most of its effectiveness at inhibiting skin cancer. Reproducible evidence is still scarce to show the benefit in humans.[57]

Superoxide dismutase

Superoxide dismutase is an enzyme that is also a potent antioxidant. It revitalizes cells and reduces the rate of cell destruction by neutralizing superoxide. It converts the reactive oxygen species by converting superoxide radicals into hydrogen peroxide, which is then changed into molecular oxygen and water. Superoxide dismutase levels tend to decline with age, whereas free radical production increases. Its potential as an anti-aging treatment has been suggested. Compounds that mimic superoxide dismutase have been shown to extend the life span of experimental worms by near 50%.[58]

ANTIOXIDANTS AND SURGERY

Cosmetic surgery has increased in popularity, not only as a way to maintain youthfulness, but also to approve general appearance. A 2004 report of the American Society of Plastic Surgeons noted that Botox injections increased by 184% from 2002; chemical peel by 26%; laser skin resurfacing by 13%; and soft-tissue fillers, such as collagen, by 14% and fat by 22%.[59] Total cosmetic minimally invasive procedures increased by 81%. In the past, cosmetic surgery was frowned upon in the black community, but in 2004, African Americans accounted for nearly 5% of the 8.7 million cosmetic-surgery procedures. The basis of the past stigma was multifactorial and included religious factors, lack of trust, economic factors, and ethnic pride in maintaining unique ethnic features. These factors are not unique to African Americans but have been observed across numerous cultures and ethnic groups to varying degrees. Similar results demonstrating the growth of cosmetic procedures were observed in a survey by the American Society for Dermatologic Surgery in 2005. There was an overall 32% increase in minimally invasive cosmetic procedures from 2003 to 2005, with a 58% increase observed from 2001. There was no information on ethnic breakdown of the growth of these procedures.[60]

THE BENEFITS OF ANTIOXIDANTS IN COSMETIC SURGERY OF THE SKIN IN THE ETHNIC POPULATION

Despite the flooding of the media and academic literature of information on antioxidants, there are significant deficits in our understanding of the nuances of antioxidant therapy. Similarly, there is a definite lack of information on racial and ethnic differences in skin structure, physiology, and function stemming from a significant lack of ethnic diversity in currently available clinical investigations. Consequently, few definitive conclusions can be made on skin diseases in ethnic skin, especially in the areas of antioxidants and cosmetic surgery and a relationship between the two. The literature does support a racial differential in epidermal melanin (pigment) content and melanosome dispersion in people of color com-

pared with fair-skinned persons. These differences appear to, at least in part, account for the lower incidence of skin cancer in darker-skinned individuals compared with those with white skin and a lower incidence and different presentation of photoaging in people with skin of color. Regardless of age, all skin types and age ranges need sun protection and can benefit from antioxidants with ingredients that mimic the structure of skin and have cell-communicating ingredients. There is virtually no existing information on the benefits of antioxidants in specific ethnic groups; any conclusions drawn result from extrapolation of the results from studies on fairer skin tones.

Much work remains in efforts to gain a detailed and precise understanding of the specific mechanisms of action, methodology that includes evaluation tools in all skin types, optimum formulation and delivery modes, dosage, and firm evidence of the direct link or cause-and-effect relationship between usage and results. We are, however, well on the way to an improved and more accurate understanding of the varied benefits of antioxidant therapy in disease and cancer prevention, anti-aging, and overall health maintenance. As we continue to achieve this knowledge, we will be able to apply it to more diverse and broader applications, such as specific disease processes, disease prevention, unique benefits that will meet the needs of the various ethnic groups, and many cosmetic procedures.

REFERENCES

1. Brown SA, Coimbra M, Coberly DM, et al. Oral nutritional supplementation accelerates skin wound healing: a randomized, placebo-controlled, double-arm, crossover study. *Plast Reconstr Surg* 2004;114(1):237–244.
2. Baines M, Shenkin A. Use of antioxidants in surgery: a measure to reduce postoperative complications. *Curr Opin Clin Nutr Metab Care* 2002;5(6):665–670.
3. Johnson AW, Nettesheim S. The care of normal skin. In Wintroub B, ed. *Cutaneous Medicine and Surgery: An Integrated Program in Dermatology*. Philadelphia: W.B. Saunders; 1996:75.
4. Podhaisky HP. Skin Antioxidants: assessment of therapeutic value. *Expert Opin Ther Patents* 2003;13(7):969–977.
5. Halder RM, Nootheti PK. Ethnic skin disorders overview. *J Am Acad Dermatol* 2003;48(6 Suppl):S143–148.
6. Di Mambro VM, Fonseca MJ. Assays of physical stability and antioxidant activity of topical formulation added with different plant extracts. *J Pharm Biomed Anal* 2005;37(2):287–295.
7. Gutteridge JMC, Halliwell B. *Antioxidants in Nutrition, Health and Disease*. New York: Oxford University Press;1994: 24–39.
8. Fang YZ, Yang S, Wu G. Free radicals, antioxidants, and nutrition. *Nutrition* 2002;18(10): 872–879.
9. *Understanding Free Radicals and Antioxidants*. February 2006. HealthCheck Systems. February 2006. http://www. healthchecksystems.com/antioxid.htm. Accessed October 2006.

10. *What You Need to Know About Anti-Oxidants.* Product-Watch.net. February 26, 2006. http://www.productwatch.net/catalog/PW/consumer_products/anti_oxidants/index.html. Accessed November 13, 2005.

11. Fernandes D. Beautiful skin. *Elixir News* 2005. http://www.elixirnews.com/newsView.php?id=395&cat10=20. Accessed November 2006.

12. *Theories of Aging.* International Antiaging Systems. November 2005. http://www.antiaging-systems.com/agetheory.htm. Accessed November 2005.

13. Harman D. Aging: a theory based on free radical and radiation chemistry. University of California Rad. Lab. Report No. 3078. July 14, 1955.

14. Harman D. Free radical theory of aging. In: Emerit I, Chance B, eds. *Free Radicals and Aging.* Basel: Birkhauser Verlag, 1992:109–123.

15. Cerami A. Hypothesis: glucose as a mediator of aging. *J Am Geriatr Soc* 1985;33:626.

16. Dilman V, Dean W. *The Neuroendocrine Theory of Aging and Degenerative Disease.* Pensacola, FL: The Center for Bio-Gerontology, 1992.

17. Beguin A. A novel micronutrient supplement in skin aging: a randomized placebo-controlled double-blind study. *Journal of Cosmetic Dermatology* 2005;4:277–284.

18. Kohen R. Skin antioxidants: their role in aging and in oxidative stress—new approaches for their evaluation. *Biomed Pharmacother* 1999;53(4):181–192.

19. Thiele JJ, Schroeter C, Hsieh SN, et al. The antioxidant network of the stratum corneum. *Curr Probl Dermatol* 2003;29:26–42.

20. Kwyer T. The role of glutathione in cell defense with references to clinical deficiencies and treatment. www.fda.gov/ohrms/dockets/ac/00/slides/3652s1_05/index.htm. Accessed November 2006.

21. Sariahmetoglu M, Wheatley RA, Cakycy Y, et al. Evaluation of the antioxidant effect of melatonin by flow injection analysis-luminol chemiluminescence. *Pharmacol Res* 2003; 48:361–367.

22. Balch PA. Prescription for Nutritional Healing, A Practical A-To_Z Reference to Drug-Free Remedies Using Vitamins, Minerals, Herbs & Food Supplements. 4th ed. Garden City Park, NY: Avery Publishing Group; 2006.

23. Uhoda E, Pierard-Franchimont C, Pierard GE. Comedolysis by a lipohydroxyacid formulation in acne-prone subjects. *Eur J Dermatol* 2003;13:65–68.

24. Ling ZQ, Xie BJ, Yang EL. Isolation, characterization, and determination of antioxidative activity of oligomeric procyanidins from the seedpod of Nelumbo nucifera Gaertn. *J Agric Food Chem* 2005;53:2441–2445.

25. Bilska A, Wlodek L. Lipoic acid-the drug of the future? *Pharmacol Rep* 2005;57:570–577.

26. Lin F, Lin JY, Gupta RD, et al. Ferulic acid stabilizes a solution of vitamin C and E and doubles its photoprotection of skin. *J Invets Dermatol* 2005;125:826–832.

27. Villarma CD, Maibach H. Glutathione as a depigmenting agent: an overview. *Int J Cosmetic Sci* 2005;27:147–153.

28. Serwin AB, Chodynicka B. The role of selenium in skin. *Wiad Lek* 2001;54:202–207.

29. Slominski A, Fischer TW, Zmijewski MA, et al. On the role of melatonin in skin physiology and pathology. *Endocrine* 2005;27:137–148.

30. Bissett DL, Miyamoto K, Sun P, et al. Topical niacinamide reduces yellowing, wrinkling, red blotchiness, and hyperpigmented spots in aging facial skin. *Int J Cosmetic Sci* 2004; 26:231–238.

31. Dreher F, Denig N, Gabard B, et al. Effect of topical antioxidants on UV-induced erythema formation when administered after exposure. *Dermatology* 1999;198(1): 52–55.

32. Elmore AR. Final report of the safety assessment of L-ascorbic acid, calcium ascorbate, magnesium ascorbate, magnesium ascorbyl phosphate, sodium ascorbate, and sodium ascorbyl phosphate as used in cosmetics. *Int J Toxicol* 2005;24(Suppl 2):51–111.

33. Farris PK.Topical vitamin C: a useful agent for treating photoaging and other dermatologic conditions. *Dermatol Surg* 2005;31(7 Pt 2):814–817.

34. Fahn S. A pilot trial of high-dose alpha tocopherol and ascorbate in early Parkinson's disease. *Ann Neurol* 1992;32:S128–S132.

35. Christen WG, Ajani UA, Glynn RJ, et al. Prospective cohort study of antioxidant vitamin supplement use and the risk of age-related maculopathy. *Am J Epidemiol* 1999;149(5):476–484.

36. Seddon JM, Ajani UA, Sperduto RD, et al. Dietary carotenoids, vitamins A, C, and E, and advanced age-related macular degeneration. *JAMA* 1994;272:1413–1420.

37. Yu BP, Kang CM, Han JS, et al. Can antioxidant supplementation slow the aging process? *BioFactors* 1998;7(1–2): 93–101.

38. National Cancer Institute. U.S. National Institutes of Health. *Coenzyme Q10.* January 2006. http://www.cancer.gov/cancertopics/pdq/cam/coenzymeQ10. Accessed January 23, 2006.

39. Bliznakov EG. Coenzyme Q10, the immune system, and aging. In: Folkers K, Yamamura Y, eds. Biomedical and Clinical Aspects of Coenzyme Q. Vol. 3 by Amsterdam: Elsevier-North Holland;1981:311–323.

40. Fahy GM. Life extension benefits of CoQ10. *Anti-Aging News* 1983;3:7,73–78.

41. Coles LS, Harris SB. Co Q-10 and life span extension. In: Klatz R, ed. *Advances in Anti-Aging Medicine.* Vol. 1. Larchmont, NY: Mary Ann Liebert, Inc.;1996:205–215.

42. Slavin JW. Considerations in alpha hydroxyl acid peels. *Clin Plast Surg* 1998;25(1):45–52.

43. Moy LS, Howe I, Moy RL. Glycolic acid modulation of collagen production in human skin fibroblast cultures in vitro. *Dermatol Surg* 1996;22(5):439–441.

44. Gilchrest BA. A review of skin ageing and its medical therapy. *Br J Dermatol* 1996;135(6):867–875.

45. *Alpha Hydroxy Acids for Skin Care.* April 1998. Kurtzweil P. http://www.fda.gov/fdac/featurs/1998/298_ahas.html. Accessed September 2006.

46. Mereish KA, Bunner DL, Ragland DR, et al. Protection against microcystin-LR-induced hepatotoxicity by silymarin: biochemistry, histopathology, and lethality. *Pharm Res* 1991;8:273–277.

47. Letteron P, Labbe G, Degott C, et al. Mechanism for the protective effects of silymarin against carbon tetrachloride-induced lipid peroxidation and hepatotoxicity in mice. *Biochem Pharmacol* 1990;39:2027–2034.

48. Ferenci P, Dragosics B, Dittrich H, et al. Randomized controlled trial of silymarin treatment in patients with cirrhosis of the liver. *J Hepatol* 1989;9:105–113.

49. Mourelle M, Muriel P, Favari L, et al. Prevention of CCl$_4$-induced liver cirrhosis by silymarin. Fund Clin Pharmacol 1989;3:183–191.

50. Vogel G, Trost W, Braatz R. Studies on the pharmacodynamics, including site and mode of action, of silymarin: the anti-hepatotoxic principle from *Silybum marianum* (L) Gaertn. *Arzneim-Forsch* 1975;25:82–89.

51. Racz K, Feher J, Csomos G, et al. An antioxidant drug, silibinin, modulates steroid secretion in human pathological adrenocortical cells. *J Endocrinol* 1990;124:341–345.

52. Valenzuela A, Guerra R, Videla LA. Antioxidant properties of the flavonoids silybin and (+)-cyanidanol-3: comparison with butylated hydroxyanisole and butylated hydroxytoluene. *Planta Med* 1986;5:438–440.

53. Comoglio A, Leonarduzzi G, Carini R, et al. Studies on the antioxidant and free radical scavenging properties of IdB1016: a new flavanolignan complex. *Free Radic Res Commun* 1990;11:109–115.

54. Muzes G, Deak G, Lang I, et al. Effect of the bioflavonoid silymarin on the *in vitro* activity and expression of superoxide dismutase (SOD) enzyme. *Acta Physiol Hung* 1991;78: 3–9.

55. Lahiri-Chatterjee M, Katiyar SK, Mohan RR, et al. A flavonoid antioxidant, silymarin, affords exceptionally high protection against tumor promotion in the SENCAR mouse skin tumorigenesis model. *Cancer Res* 1999;59: 622–632.

56. Katiyar SK, Ahmad N, Mukhtar H. Green tea and skin. *Arch Dermatol* 2000;136(8):989–994.

57. Conney AH, Zhou S, Lee MJ, et al. Stimulatory effect of oral administration of tea, coffee, or caffeine on UVB-induced apoptosis in the epidermis of SKH-1 mice. *Toxicol Appl Pharmacol.* 2006 [in press]

58. Lam M, Sulindro M. Anti-Aging Research Brief No. 1 The Academy of Anti-Aging Research. {www.a3r.org}.

59. American Society of Plastic Surgeons Reports 2003 Statistics. http://www.plasticsurgery.org/media/press_releases/DEMAND-JUMPED-IN-2003-FOR-MINIMALLY-INVASIVE-PLASTIC-SURGERY. cfm. Accessed October 2006.

60. 2005 Procedure survey dermasurgery trends and statistics. American Society for Dermatologic Surgery 2005. http://www.asds-net.org/media/Archives/ASDS2005statsReport.pdf. Accessed October 2006.

12

Photoprotection

Vermén M. Verallo-Rowell

The deleterious effects of ultraviolet and visible light on human skin include sunburn, suntan, phototoxic and photoallergic reactions, aggravation of hyperpigmentary disorders, photoaging, immunosuppression, solar keratoses, and the induction of skin cancers. For more than 70 years, commercial sunscreens have been used to mollify these detrimental cutaneous effects of light. The first, containing benzyl salicylate and benzyl cinnamate, was developed and marketed in the United States in 1928.[1]

Since the development of the early formulations to prevent sunburn, sunscreens have evolved as the gold standard for skin protection from ultraviolet light. In general, sunscreens are used to prevent sunburn, limit photodamage, and decrease the risk of skin cancers, including basal cell carcinomas, squamous cell carcinomas, and malignant melanoma. The International Agency for Research on Cancer reported that although the data on sunscreen prevention of actinic keratoses and squamous cell carcinomas is adequate, that on basal cell carcinomas and melanomas is inadequate.[2] Despite this finding, most clinicians and researchers agree that an overall sun protection program should include limited sun exposure, protective clothing, sun visors, hats, and daily use of sunscreen.

INDICATIONS FOR SUNSCREEN USE IN DARKER RACIAL ETHNIC GROUPS

Individuals encompassing Fitzpatrick's skin types III/IV through VI generally have olive, brown, or black skin (see Chapter 2). Such individuals have a substantially lower incidence of skin cancers and photoaging. Photoimmunosuppression has been reported to be milder, and photosensitivity is less common.[3] Why, then, do people with darker skin need sunscreens?

Disorders of hyperpigmentation have emerged as a key indication for sunscreen use in darker skin types. These include melasma, postinflammatory hyperpigmentation (PIH), ephelides, lentigines, Hori's nevus, post-

laser, and phototherapy hyperpigmentation. Albeit less life threatening than cancers and melanomas, these skin problems seriously affect quality of life (see Chapter 6). Skin cancers are another indication. Although still relatively rare among those with darker skin, the incidence is growing. The Cancer Registry in Singapore in 1988 noted increasing incidence of skin cancers, excluding melanoma.[4] By 2002, skin cancer, including melanoma, reached the top-ten cancers list.[5] This higher ranking for skin cancer may be attributed to more affluence, a favoring of increased outdoor leisure activities, longer life spans, and exposure to more solar ultraviolet rays brought on by the factors that promote stratospheric ozone depletion.[6]

Sociological/cultural issues further influence the use of sunscreens in darker skin. A unique irony regarding skin color is that those with lighter skin cherish being darker (i.e., acquiring a tan), whereas many of those with olive or darker skin prefer to have lighter-colored skin. Toward this goal, sun avoidance is a popular practice. Unless demanded by work or for play, when outdoors, those with darker skin who prefer light skin color look for deep shades, use parasols, wear wide-brimmed hats, and cover up with clothing.[7] They also frequently use skin lighteners.[8] Both practices are common among those who are generally of mixed heritage: African Americans;[9] Africans;[10] Asians;[11] Hispanics;[12] Middle Easterners;[13] and Caribbean Islanders.[14] This is true even among some of the more ethnically homogenous Asians from Japan,[15] China,[16] or Korea, who, despite being fairer than other Asians, consider themselves "brown."[17]

Use of sunscreens is not a common practice because darker skin phototypes III/IV to VI do not burn readily and have a baseline color that darkens easily and is perceived to be protective.

Because sun-induced/aggravated hyperpigmentations are common in those with darker skin, their customary sun behavioral practices are obviously not enough to avoid these conditions. What follows is a review of the light wavelengths that sunscreens protect against to understand which to use for the specific indications needed by those with darker skin.

ELECTROMAGNETIC RADIATION WAVELENGTH EFFECTS AND PROTECTION

Sunlight is divided into three components, including ultraviolet (UV) light, visible light (VL), and infrared light (IRL), with UV representing the most important component (Fig. 12-1). UV is divided into three groups based on the wavelength of light: (i) UVC (100–280 nm), which minimally affects the earth's surface because it is blocked by the ozone layer, (ii) UVB (290–320 nm), which causes erythema, sunburn, DNA damage, solar elastosis, hyperpigmentation, and skin cancer, and (iii) UVA (320–400 nm), which requires a higher dose to induce erythema but easily elicits two pigment-darkening responses, both produced by the photo-oxidation of melanin.[18] Immediate pigment darkening (IPD) starts in seconds after UVA exposure and disappears within 2 hours. At higher doses of 8 to 25 J/cm^2 from 2 to 24 hours after exposure, IPD is followed by more pigmentation, the PPD or persistent pigment darkening. In those with lighter skin, this lasts about 24 hours.[19] In those with darker skin, it lasts much longer, often continuing into the delayed tanning effect of both UVB and UVA.[20] UVB does not produce IPD nor PPD, but produces, with UVA, a delayed tanning response that peaks at 72 hours. This is brought on by an increase in the number of active melanocytes and tyrosinase, which together produce new melanosomes, melanin, and transfer to keratinocytes.[21]

IPD and PPD are not photoprotective,[21] an important point to remind those with darker skin who may think that their immediate darkening protects them from the sun. The UVB-induced delayed tanning after erythema has a sun protection factor (SPF) of 3, which is a few points higher in darker skin.[21]

Erythema reactions

Both UVB and UVA produce acute erythema, but UVA is much less efficient than UVB. Approximately 1,000 times more UVA than UVB is needed to elicit the same erythema response.[22]

Solar UVB-induced acute erythema starts after about 4 hours of exposure, peaks at 8 to 24 hours, and fades after a day or so. However, among the very fair or very old, this may last for weeks.[23] The acute erythema induced by UVA for both light and darker skin color is milder than the UVB erythema and biphasic. The first phase appears immediately after exposure and fades in several hours. The second phase starts at about 6 hours and peaks at 24 hours.[24]

After a single erythema response, both UVB and UVA increase epidermal and dermal mitotic activity. That of UVB persists for days to weeks, with much more thickening of the epidermis and dermis.[24] Only after repeated exposures does UVA produce thickening of the epidermis, but this is much less than that from UVB.[24]

Chronic erythema produces P^{53} gene mutation, which is found in 90% of squamous cell carcinomas, 60% of actinic keratosis, and 50% of basal cell carcinomas.[25] Even nonerythemal sun exposure induces reactive oxygen species-mediated DNA change and pyrimidine dimer formation leading to skin cancer in animal models.[26]

Repeated UVA radiation has in recent years been shown to produce even more immunosuppression than UVB.[27] Animal models develop skin alterations of the Langerhans cells—their number, functions and morphology—resulting in photoimmunosupression. This is medi-

Figure 12-1 Schema of the electromagnetic spectrum of light and the wavelengths of its three components discussed in the text in regard to their specific effects on darker skin.

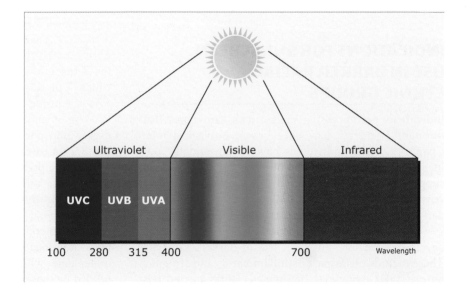

ated in part through the generation of cis-urocanic acid, tumor necrosis factor, and interleukin-10.[28]

UVA, much more than UVB, elicits the photosensitivity reactions to cosmetics, drugs, and environmental chemicals, often resulting in the appearance of PIH in darker skin types.[29]

Visible light

Verallo-Rowell, in a cross-sectional photopatch testing of 20 patients with melasma, compared with 20 without, used VL to irradiate photoallergens.[30] In the melasma group, 29 photopatch tests to 11 fragrances, 11 North American Contact Dermatitis Group (NACDG), and 7 plant allergens were (+), relevant, and significant (*p* = 0.005, CI: 1.54–4.49). A follow-up open study of 20 melasma patients examined the exposed parts of the body. All showed irregular *subtle* pigmentation in a classic pattern of photosensitivity. The subtlety of the dyschromia was attributed to the "sun-shy" behavior of the all Asian patients. Patch tests with the same photoallergens as the previous study, irradiated with UVA at slightly less than the predetermined Minimal Erythema Dose (MED) elicited (+) to (+++), relevant reactions.[31]

Melasma cases that worsened instead of improving as expected following intense pulsed light (IPL) therapy prompted a study by Negishi et al. on very subtle epidermal melasma (VSEM).[32] Best seen under UV photography, VSEM was described as otherwise "invisible to the naked eye," although photographs "under normal light" appear similar to the subtle melasma and photosensitivity among the sun-shy Asians reported by Verallo-Rowell.[31]

The importance of these initial observations is relevant to the VL and IRL-emitting lasers and light devices used to treat melasma. We have just started a multicenter, prospective controlled study on the relationship of melasma and photosensitivity. The results of this study may continue to improve our understanding on the specific sunscreens and light devices to use in the prevention and treatment of melasma patients. In this respect, among Negishi et al.'s 223 IPL-treated melasma patients, 63 (28.3%) had VSEM. Of the 45/63 nonusers of sunscreens, 50.6% had VSEM. Of the rest—18/63 who were sunscreen users—only 13.4% had VSEM.[32]

To summarize, despite outdoor sun avoidance practices, people with darker skin are prone to hyperpigmentations. UVA and VL (much more than UVB) aggravate and elicit photosensitivity, PIH, and melasma. Anti-UVA and anti-VL sunscreens are thus indicated in normal skin to help prevent hyperpigmentations; in the treatment of melasma and other pigmentation problems to inhibit formation, retard proliferation of melanocytes, and protect lightened skin; and overall to facilitate therapeutic effects during and postmelasma treatment. Postlaser and light therapy sunscreens help prevent pigmentations and help avoid the stimulation by light of viable melanocytes. All these also help to avoid potentially more serious sun-related cancers and immunosuppression.[33,34]

SUNSCREENS AGAINST LIGHTS EMITTED BY OUTDOOR/INDOOR LIGHT SOURCES

Outdoors

On the earth's surface, the amounts of solar UVB and UVA, at a ratio of 20:1, are strongest between 10 A.M. and 4 P.M.[22] and vary depending on latitude, altitude, season, time of day, clouds, and ozone layer. Compared with UVB, UVA is of longer wavelength, is less affected by these factors, and can penetrate deeper into the skin.[22] Solar VL and IRL are much more abundant, but have longer, thus weaker, wavelengths, which therefore are considered harmless to the skin.[22]

Indoors

In cars and through windows, clear glass absorbs and acts as a protective shield against the shorter wavelengths (below 320 nm) of UVB.[35] Untinted glass allows UVA through. Ordinary tint can block a large portion of UVA up to about 370 to 380 nm, whereas dark-tinted glass containing metals provides significant protection against UVA and VL. This is limited by the U.S. Federal Motor Vehicle Safety Standard,[36] which requires that side window glass allow the transmission of at least 70% VL radiation. It has been estimated that approximately 50% of outdoor UVR also occurs indoors, from scatter and reflection on bright surfaces or rippling water.[21]

In short, for the hyperpigmentation problems of darker skin types who generally avoid the sun but do not use sunscreens: Indoors, where UVA and VL are ubiquitous, daily anti-UVA and anti-VL sunscreens are needed, especially after cosmetic surgery with laser and lights. Outdoors, in addition to the anti UVA and VL, anti-UVB sunscreens are needed. Sun avoidance,[37] sunglasses,[38] and hats and clothing[39] extend skin photoprotection.

SUNSCREEN INGREDIENTS

Active sunscreen ingredients are best called organic (chemical), or inorganic (physical, chemical-free). Table 12-1 lists the names, light wavelength absorption maximum or range, and their known safety and stability profiles. The U.S.-approved ingredients include 14 organic filters (9 anti-UVB; 5 anti-UVB and A) and 2 inorganic filters.[40] Table 12-1 also lists the European-approved sunscreen ingredients.[41–45] Two, called the Mexoryls, are made by L'Oreal (Clichy, France): Mexoryl SX[41–44] (terephthalydene dicamphor sulphonic acid) and Mexoryl XL (drometrizole trisiloxane). Both are UVA absorbers at

Table 12-1

Absorption, safety, and photostability of some sunscreen ingredients approved by the United States and European Regulatory Boards[40]

Names	Maximum absorption peak/range in nanometers	Safety, photostability
UVB Filters: PABA Derivatives		
Padimate O: (Octyldimethyl PABA)	311: good filter	Photolabile but, less than the other PABAs
Cinnamates		
Octinoxate: (Parsol MCX,OMC: octylmethoxycinnamate, Escalol 557, Eusolex 2292)	311: < potent filter than Padimate O To ↑ SPF, add other UVB filters	Unstable. Encapsulated form: ↓ photodegradation by 53%–35%
Cinoxate: (ethoxy-ethyl-p-methoxycinnamate, Uvinul N-539 Neo HeliopanE1000)	289: less often used filter	
Salicylates (Weaker UVB Filters)		
Octisalate: Octyl salicylate Homosalate: Homomenthyl salicylate Trolamine salicylate	307 308 260–305	↑ effect of other UVB filters, ↓ photodegradation of avobenzone, oxybenzone, others. In water-soluble sunscreens and hair products
Others: Octocrylene Ensulizole (PBZole sulfonic acid)	303: Photostable 310: Water soluble, skin light	Improves product stability; enhances SPF of sunscreen
Benzophenones Bp (Broad-spectrum UVA Filter)		
Oxybenzone (benzo'none-3, Bp3, Eusolex4360,UvinulM40) Sulisobenzone (Bp4,benzophenone-4) Dioxybenzone (benzophenone-8)	Two absorption peaks 288, 325 UVB to UVA strong filter 366 352	Bp group (92) photolabile Inactivates antioxidant systems; stabilized by octocrylene, salicylates, camphor, methylbenzyliden, micronized, ZnO, TiO_2
UVA Filters		
Butyl methoxydibenzoyl methane (avobenzone, Parsol 1789)	380: strong filter BUT: Photolabile: ↓ 50%–60% after 1-hour exposure	Strongly ↑ degrades OMC (99); See Bp on how to ↑ photostability
Anthralinates		
Meradimate (menthyl anthralinate, Ensulizole)	340: weak filter, mainly UVA2	
Inorganic: Favored Name for Nonchemical or Physical[46–50]		
Titanium dioxide: Pigmentary Nonmicronized 200–500 nm Micronized 10–50 nm	>UVB, UVA2, <UVA1 filter. ↑ photoreactive than ZnO Photoexcited, micronized cause cell death	Refractive index = 2.6, thus whiter than 1.9 of zinc oxide, though particle size smaller, more difficult to formulate
Zinc oxide (Z-cote) Microfine	UVA 2 and UVA 1 up to 380 nm; better protection than TiO_2	Photostable

---

Table 12-1

Absorption, safety, and photostability of some sunscreen ingredients approved by the United States and European Regulatory Boards[40] *(continued)*

Mexoryls by L'Oreal[41–44]

Mexoryl SX (terephthalylidene trisiloxane, silatriazole)	345 UVB broad spectrum filter Humans: Prevent UVA-induced pigmentation, epidermal hyperplasia ↓ skin hydration, elasticity photostable	Animals: ↓ UVR-induced cancers, photoaging ↓ formation cis-urocanic acid, epidermal Langerhans cells: role in immunosuppression
Mexoryl XL (drometriazole trisiloxane, silatriazole)	303 and 344; UVB/UVA broad spectrum	Liposoluble Photostable

Tinosorbs by CIBA[45]

Tinosorb M (methylene-bisbenzotriazolyl tetramethylbutylphenol	303 and 358 broad spectrum Microfine organic particles in aqueous phase of emulsion	Both are photostable Stabilize OMC and avobenzone No hormonal activity
Tinosorb S (bis-ethylhexyloxyphenol methoxyphenyl triazine (anisotriazine)	348 nm Broad-spectrum oil soluble	

344- and 345-nm maximum wavelengths. In addition, Mexoryl XL absorbs at UVB with 303 as its maximum wavelength.

In animals, Mexoryl SX studies prevented UVA-induced histochemical alterations associated with photoaging.[41–44] An anti-UVB sunscreen, with (compared with without) the Mexoryl SX significantly suppressed UV ray–induced carcinogenesis,[42] reduced cis-urocanic acid formation, and prevented the decrease in the number of epidermal Langerhans cells, the changes known to play a role in immunosuppression.[43] In humans, Mexoryl SX applied before UVA exposure reduced UV-induced pigmentation, epidermal hyperplasia, skin hydration, and elasticity.[44]

Two new European filters developed by Ciba Specialty Chemicals (Basel, Switzerland) are the Tinosorbs: *M* (methylene-bis-benzotriazolyl tetra-methylbutylphenol and *S* (bis-ethylhexyloxyphenol methoxyphenyl triazine (anisotriazine). Both have been shown to be broad-spectrum filters: Tinosorb M at UVB:303 and UVA:358 nm; Tinosorb S at UVA:348 nm maximum wavelength absorption. Tinosorb M has microfine organic particles, dispersed in the aqueous phase of the sunscreen emulsion, whereas Tinosorb S is oil soluble. Both are photostable and without hormonal activities.[45]

Titanium dioxide (TiO_2) and zinc oxide (ZnO) provide Anti-UVB, UVA, and Anti-VL protection. They are now available in more cosmetically acceptable formulations.[46] The addition of iron oxide pigment to opaque photoprotective agents enhances VL photoprotection and cosmetic acceptability.[47] A broad-spectrum sunscreen with a wide anti-UVB, UVA, and VL range from combining TiO_2 with bisoctrizole is also on the horizon.[48]

The basic formula of colored cosmetic products usually has TiO_2, ZnO, and pigment-inorganic sun filters that make the products, such as a lipstick, inherently photoprotective. A powder makeup may have a baseline SPF of 3 or 4, whereas a foundation makeup, with its higher amounts of TiO_2 and ZnO, may have full-spectrum UVA and VL protection.[49] The actual amount of cosmetics a person applies on the face, however, is less than the 2 mg/cm² amount used in the testing for protection factors. One study showed that by layering—or applying one on top of the other—thin amounts of a sunscreen cream base, powder, and foundation, a protection factor against UVA (PFA) of 14 and protection factor against visible light (PFV) of 1.4 were achieved.[50]

ANTIOXIDANTS

The natural antioxidants are enzymatic (GSH peroxidase, catalase, and superoxide dismutase) or nonenzymatic (GSH, alpha tocopherol, and beta carotene). Plants are a rich source of antioxidants, because unlike man, plants are not able to walk away from the sun.[51–62] Antioxidants neutralize the free radicals formed by the normal oxidative processes in the body. With more oxidative stress, including that from sun exposure, the natural antioxidants may not be able to cope with the increased number of free radicals. Oxidative cell damage can lead to photoaging, immunosuppression, and photocarcinogenesis.[40]

Antioxidants have very weak sunscreen effects, but they are increasingly found in sunscreens, primarily to help deal with UV-induced oxidative stress. In sunscreens, antioxidants need to be present in adequate amounts to be effective. But they are inherently unstable, do not diffuse well enough to cover a wide skin area, and are easily removed by washing, perspiration, or rubbing. The ideal delivery of antioxidants is therefore, ingested as food supplement. Table 12-2 lists some antioxidants, their sources, and their possible effects taken internally or in sunscreens. Among those antioxidants that have been shown to be protective against UVA and/or immunosuppression are vitamins C and E,[51,52] polypodium leucotomos,[53,54] zinc,[55,56] green tea,[57] and N-acetylcysteine.[58,59]

SUNSCREEN PROTECTION FACTORS

Protection factors to look for in anti-UVA and -VL broad-spectrum sunscreens, in order, are the following:

PFA

PFA is assessed by many in vivo and vitro methods, but there is still no universally accepted procedure from either the U.S. FDA or European regulatory bodies.[60] In vivo determinations use the two end points that are visible in the skin after exposure to UVA. These are the IPD[61] and the PPD.[62] Between the two, PPD is more commonly used, as it remains stable between 2 and 24 hours, and is easily read in white skin. In brown skin, the IPD is readily visible, and the dose to elicit both IPD and PPD is virtually the same.[20]

The critical wavelength and UVA:UVB ratio (boots star rating)

The critical wavelength (CW)[60] and UVA:UVB ratio (Boots Star Rating)[63] are derived from similar in vitro methods. A spectrophotometric method is used to determine a sunscreen's transmission/absorption of light at a range of 290 to 400 nm. The sunscreen's CW is calculated as the point at which 90% of the light is absorbed, whereas the Boots Star Rating calculates the data as a ratio of the UVA to the UVB. The German DGK Sun Protection Task Force, from the results of a six intra- and interlaboratories comparative study, concluded that the reproducibility of the CW and the UVA/UVB ratio was superior to any in vivo end point.[64] Hence, they favor the in vitro method, using specific changes to older methods.

The photosensitivity protection factor or protection factor for visible light

Photosensitivity protection factor (PPF) was developed to predict the VL protection factor of sunscreens containing ZnO and pigmentary grade TiO$_2$.[46] For patients sensitive in the visible light range,[47] two SPF-25 sunscreens in vitro achieved a PPF of 4.1 to 9.6. In vivo PPF determination

using blue VL[46] at 430 +/− 30 nm was higher at a range of 3 to >10, (median 8). For consistency with the FDA-recommended name, PFA for UVA protection, PFV for visible light is proposed. The PFV for consumer acceptable cosmetics containing ultrafine dispersions of TiO$_2$ and ZnO ranged from 1 to 4.[50]

Immune protection factor

The immune protection factor (IPF) is assessed using reactions from solar-simulating radiation (SSR), a light source that contains both UVA and UVB. This is based on the ability of sunscreens to inhibit suppression of the induction arm of local contact hypersensitivity response, such as to nickel sulfate, or the elicitation phase of delayed hypersensitivity response to recall antigens. UVA is known to play a significant role in immunosuppression. IPF is rarely used in sunscreen labels, although studies now show that IPF has a better correlation with the UVA than the UVB's SPF.[65]

The *SPF* is the oldest and most popularly recognized factor for outdoor sun protection. It is defined as the ratio of the least amount of ultraviolet exposure required to induce minimal erythema in sunscreen protected skin versus that required for unprotected skin. Against sunburn mainly from UVB and its chronic effects, there is 94% protection with an SPF of 15 and 97% with an SPF of 30.[66]

Summary

Those with darker ethnic skin have commendable sun avoidance behavior, but additionally need protection from UVA and VL, which are present indoors. Based on the American Academy of Dermatology's UVA Consensus Conference,[60] the author recommends: Daily use of sunscreens with organic, inorganic, possibly antioxidant ingredients, and broad-spectrum anti-UVA, -VL, and -UVB claims, with these values:

- CW >370 nm
- UVA:UVB ratio of 0.6 to <0.8 (*** or superior) or ≥0.8 (**** maximum);
- PPF or PFV of at least 4, layered if less
- SPF of 30+ for outdoor use.

HOW MUCH TO APPLY?

Apply about 2 mg/cm^2 of sunscreen, the same amount used in testing for the SPF that is claimed on the sunscreen package. Overall, the median application thickness among mostly Fitzpatrick phototypes I through III[67] and for those who are photosensitive, has been shown to be an average of about 0.5 to 1.0 mg/cm^2. Most inorganic products appear white, so users of inorganic sunscreens apply less: Two-thirds that of the organic ones. Fortunately, more cosmetically acceptable organic sunscreens are now

Table 12-2

Some antioxidants and their action by topical/oral route[40]

Name/source	Topical	Oral
Carotenoids From plants Not a UV filter		Beta carotene:120–180 mg/d ↓ EPP photosensitivity, 4–5 year study ↓ SCC
Vitamin C In fruits, vegetables Not a UV filter	L-ascorbic acid, unstable, but absorbed >20-fold. Other forms more stable, but not converted to L-ascorbic acid	
Antioxidant combinations Work best	Animals: Topical individually effective, but C and E increased protection	L-ascorbic acid 3g/d + alpha tocopherol 2g/d ↑ MED to SSR Animals: Vitamins C and E, ↓ acute effects of SSR, ↓ nickel sensitivity
Polypodium leucotomos Plant extract	↑ UV for IPD, MED ↑ Minimal melanogenic dose ↑ Minimal phototoxic dose	Phototoxic, pigmentary protection, anti- inflammatory
Zinc trace mineral Divalent zinc ion	Protect against free radicals ↓ UVA- and UVB-induced sunburn cell formation	↓ UVA-1 induced apoptosis, protects against UVA- induced DNA damage
Green tea polyphenols Best studied topical/oral: Animals/humans	Protect against UVB-ROS inflammation, photoaging, contact hypersensitivity, ↓ photocarcinogenesis	↓ sunburn cells; ↓ UVR erythema, carcinogenesis, immunosuppression, anti-inflammatory
Isoflavones Soybean—Genistein Equol—Red Clover	After UV exposure protect against inflammation/immunosuppression in a dose-dependent manner	
Plant oligosaccharides Xyloglucans tamarind seeds Aloe barbadensis	Reduction of IL-10. Prevention of UVB-induced systemic immunosuppression	Aloe gel effects decays rapidly, but suppression of DTH is stable over time
N-acetylcysteine:NAC ↑ levels of endogenous antioxidant glutathione	In mice, applied before UVB exposure, can protect against immunosuppression	In cultured human fibroblasts Protects against UVA cytotoxicity
Hydroxycinnamic acids Caffeic Acid: plants Ferrulic Acid: Olives Potent antioxidant	Protects UVB induced erythema in vitro. In vivo (100) prevents photodamage of lotions/sunscreens	In food inhibits lipid peroxidation and oxidative spoilage

DTH, dietary butylated hydroxytoluene; EPP, erythropoietic protoporphyria patients; IPD, immediate pigment darkening; MED, minimal erythema dosing; ROS, reactive oxygen species; SCC, squamous cell carcinoma; SSR, solar-stimulating radiation; UV, ultraviolet; UVA, ultraviolet A; UVB, ultraviolet B; UVR, ultraviolet ray.

available, with more to come, and layering can be used to boost these protection factors.[50]

HOW OFTEN?

For outdoors and beach use, the general recommendations are that sunscreens be applied 15 to 30 minutes before sun exposure, then reapplied after 15 to 30 minutes to compensate for improper initial application, then every 2 to 3 hours, especially after swimming or sweating.[68] For multiday sun exposures, higher SPFs are needed, because the skin is more sensitive on the second day from the UVB-induced erythema peak at 24 hours.[68]

One study found daily use as more protective against UV-induced skin changes than intermittent use of the same product in white skin.[69] For darker skin, daily-use protects not just from outdoor sun, but also indoors from reflected solar UVA and VL, from artificial light sources, as well as from cosmetic surgical light and laser devices.

Lawsuits against sunscreen manufacturers have questioned the accuracy of sunscreen protection factor claims. At the American Academy of Dermatology's Melanoma/ Skin Cancer Detection and Prevention Month 2006 news conference, Draelos clarified this perceived inconsistent performance. Sunscreens are rated under ideal conditions that actual usage often does not mimic. Therefore, follow these guidelines on how to use sunscreens properly: Use at least 1 ounce (about one shot glass full) to ensure a thick enough layer for the whole body, apply 30 minutes before going out, reapply every 2 hours, and don't wipe the sunscreen off.[70]

ADVERSE REACTIONS TO SUNSCREENS

Contact dermatitis

Irritant, allergic, photoallergic, and phototoxic contact dermatitis have been reported,[71] although considering the widespread use of sunscreens, they are relatively uncommon.[72] Among the organic sunscreen filters, BP-3—commonly used as a UVA filter—is the most common photoallergen. Avobenzone, oxybenzone, sulisobenzone, PABA, padimate O, methylbenzylidene camphor, octinoxate, and ensulizole have also been reported to induce reactions.

A Singapore study[73] gave similar results, plus allergic reactions to fragrance mix and/or Balsam of Peru. Worth watching out for are reactions to the organic anti-UVA filters: 4-tert-butyl-4′-methoxy-dibenzoylmethane (Parsol A), 2-(2-hydroxy-5-methylphenyl)-benzotriazole (Tinuvin P), and benzophenone derivatives, which in a Japanese study gave positive results.[74]

Once a reaction occurs, patch and photopatch testing of active ingredients, inactive ingredients, and even the test product itself are valuable, so sunscreens without the specific allergen can be chosen. A general rule to follow is that because fragrance is among the top allergens that cause contact dermatitis and is also a photoallergen, particularly for sensitive patients, the use of totally unscented sunscreens is ideal.

Hypovitaminosis D

A recent review of current nutrition data strongly indicates that vitamin D sufficiency is needed not just for calcemic but also noncalcemic health at all stages of life.[75] This review cites optimum serum levels of 25-hydroxy vitamin D: 25(OH)D to be approximately or higher than 30 to 50 ng/mL (75–125 nmol/L). These serum levels can be maintained by 500 to 1000 IU of vitamin D per day (0.06 ng/mL/IU/day). The best source for vitamin D is sun exposure and secondarily from food and supplements. For darker skin, the MED in the summer noonday sun in the southern United States is about 60 to 80 minutes.[75] From this it has been computed, and we can further extrapolate, that sun exposure to suberythemal doses (25%–50% MED) of about 20% to 40% of the body surface would produce about 1,000 IU of vitamin D.

However, compared with apparently normal Caucasian women of the same age on similar diets, in Boston, African American women 20 to 40 years old were found to have half as much 25(OH)D. In the summer/fall, this was a low 16.5±6.6, down to 12.1±7.9 ng/mL in winter/ spring. It was therefore suggested that sunlight stimulates the skin to make vitamin D, but pigmented skin makes less.[75] The same observation was made of Norwegians living at 60°N, compared with Africans who, despite living at 10°N, had a high rate of vitamin D deficiency.[76] Veiled women have also been found to be vitamin D deficient.[77]

Thus, children and adults with darker skin, in the absence of adequate sun exposure because of strict sun-avoidance practice and daily sunscreen use greater than about 20% to 40% of the body, even if living in the tropics, may need 1,000 IU vitamin D daily supplementation to achieve the 30 to 50 ng/mL blood levels.

Estrogenicity

Bp-3, homosalate, methylbenzylidene camphor, OMC, and octyl dimethyl PABA are among the UVB and UVA filters reported to have estrogenic effects. These studies, all done in animals, are still controversial for many reasons, including the unrealistically high exposure test amounts used in comparison with potential human exposure.[78] So far, there appears to be no biologic relevance or application of the results of these studies to the aesthetics of human skin.

HOW DO DARKER SKIN TYPES DEVELOP THE HABIT OF DAILY SUNSCREEN USE?

Giving people with darker skin types the answers to questions about sunscreens specific to their problems will help them develop the habit of daily use. Doctors need to learn from past failures in trying to change behavior patterns that are ingrained cultural habits. Since the 1980s, dermatologists have established skin cancer prevention and detection programs to educate the public about the sun[79] by the *use* of sunscreens and by sun-avoidance practices. The reasons: to avoid skin cancers, photoimmunosuppresion, and photoaging.

In August 2005, Naylor and Robinson's editorial in the Archives of Dermatology recognized that these campaigns have failed on many fronts.[80] They conclude that a "significant percentage of the population will continue to ignore . . . worse, a substantial number will continue to intentionally seek UV exposure for the purpose of cosmetic tanning."[80]

The immediate gratification provided by the sex appeal of a visually well-tanned body decidedly is more important than the future effects that photoprotection can offer. This mind-set, applied to those with darker skin, suggests that emphasis should be made on the evident attractiveness now of the even-colored nonhyperpigmented skin, and further, that the daily use of sunscreens can keep it looking that way. Sex appeal, sophistication, and good looks are crucial, hence sunscreens/products should be cosmetically desirable, using terms such as ultrasheer, cool, and elegant, and be marketed with a "must-have" look for the daily handbag. Once the daily use of sunscreens is in place, optimal improvements following cosmetic surgery and the prevention of future hyperpigmentations becomes the bonus.

One last lesson learned from Hillhouse and Turrisi[81] concerns the delivery of the sunscreen message. They call it "inconsistent, . . . leading consumers to make purchasing decisions based primarily on price, convenience, and marketing." The message to those with darker ethnic skin should therefore be simple: *"To keep your skin looking great, use your broad-spectrum sunscreen daily."*

Acknowledgement to Drs. Henry Lim and Prisana Kullavanijaya for their article on photoprotection[40], which I used, in part, as a template for comparison with that of darker skin. Kullavanijaya P, Lim H. Photoprotection. J Am Acad Dermatol 2005;52;66:937–958.

REFERENCES

1. Shaath NA. Evolution of modern sunscreen chemicals. In: Lowe NJ, Shaath NA, Pathak MA, eds. *Sunscreens: Development, Evaluation, Regulatory Aspects.* 2nd ed. New York: Marcel Dekker Inc., 1997:3–10.

2. World Health Organization International Agency for Research on Cancer IARC Monographs on the Evaluation of Carcinogenic Risks to Humans. Volume 55 Solar and Ultraviolet Radiation Summary of Data Reported and Evaluation Solar and Ultraviolet Radiation. Volume 55:1–9. http://monographs.iarc.fr/ENG/Monographs/vol55/volume55.pdf. Accessed March 11, 2007.

3. Taylor SC. Skin of color: biology, structure, function, and implications for dermatologic disease. *J Am Acad Dermatol* 2002;46(2 Suppl):S41–62.

4. Lee HP, Duffy SW, Day NE, et al. Recent trends in cancer incidence among Singapore Chinese. *Int J Cancer* 1988;42(2): 159–166.

5. Seow A, Koh WP, Chia KS, et al. *Trends in Cancer Incidence in Singapore 1968–2002 Singapore Cancer Registry-2004, Report No. 6. ISBN:981-05-0868-9. www.nccs.com.sg/cedu/pt_04-3.htm.* Accessed March 10, 2007.

6. de Gruijl FR, Longstreth J, Norval M, et al. Health effects from stratospheric ozone depletion and interactions with climate change. *Photochem Photobiol Sci* 2003;2:16–28.

7. Noel Coward. Mad Dogs and Englishmen. www.sabrizain.demon.co.uk/malaya/coward.htm. Accessed March 10, 2007.

8. Del Guidice P, Yves P. The widespread use of skin lightening creams in Senegal: a persistent public problem in West Africa. *Int J Dermatol* 2002;41(2):69–72.

9. Alfiee MB. A model for differential perceptions of competence based on skin tone among African Americans. *Journal Multicultural Counselling and Development* 1998;26(4):294–322.

10. Schuler C. Africans look for beauty in a Western mirror. The Christian Science Monitor. December 23, 1999. http://www.csmonitor.com/1999/1223/p1s4.html. Accessed March 7, 2007.

11. Sahay S, Piran N. Skin-color preferences and body satisfaction among South Asian-Canadian and European-Canadian female university students. *J Soc Psychol* 1997;137(2):161–171.

12. Jones VE, Pride or prejudice? A formally taboo topic among Asian-Americans and Latinos comes out into the open as skin tone consciousness sparks a backlash. *Puerto Rico Herald.* August 19, 2004. http://www.puertorico-herald.org/issues/2004/vol8n49/PridePreju.shtml. Accessed March 7, 2007.

13. Al-Saleh I, Al-Doush I. Mercury content in skin lightening creams and potential health hazards to the health of Saudi women. *J Toxicol Environ Health* 1997;51:123.

14. Christopher A. Skin bleaching, self-hate, and black identity in Jamaica. *Journal of Black Studies* 2003;33(6):711–718.

15. Ashikari M. Urban middle-class Japanese women and their white faces: gender, ideology, and representation. *Ethos* 2003;31(1):3–25.

16. Altman K. China's frightening beauty industry. http://newsweek.washingtonpost.com/postglobal/kyoko_altman/2007/03/overly_sexualized_china.html. Accessed March 12, 2007.

17. Youn JI, Oh JK, Kim BK, et al. Relationship between skin phototype and MED in Korean brown skin. *Photodermatol Photoimmunol Photomed* 1997;13(5–6):208–211.

18. Parrish JA, Jaenicke KF, Anderson RR. Erythema and melanogenesis action spectrum of normal human skin. *Photochem Photobiol* 1982;36:187.

19. Moyal D, Wichrowski K, Tricaud C. In vivo persistent pigment darkening method: a demonstration of the

reproducibility of the UVA protection factors results at several testing laboratories. *Photodermatol Photoimmunol Photomed* 2006; 22(3):124–128.

20. Verallo-Rowell VMV, Paz LMR. Indoor clinical laboratory study to determine differences between the IPD and PPD, used as end-point in the determination for the PFA of multi-heritage Asian-Filipinos with skin phototypes IV and V. In: Eds. *Skin in the Tropics: Sunscreens and Hyperpigmentations.* Pasig City: Anvil Press; 2002:187–190.

21. Honigsmann H. Erythema and pigmentation. *Photodermatol Photoimmunol Photomed* 2002;18:75–81.

22. NIH Consensus Statement. Sunlight, ultraviolet radiation and the skin. *NIH Consensus Statement* 1989;7:1–29.

23. Guarrera M. Age and skin response to ultraviolet radiation. *J Cutan Ageing Cosmetic Dermatol* 1988;1:135.

24. Pearse AD, Gaskell SA, Marks Rl. Epidermal changes in human skin following irradiation with either UVB or UVA. *J Invest Dermatol* 1987;88:83–87.

25. Verma AK, Lowe NJ, Boutwell RK. Induction of mouse epidermal ornithine decarboxylase activity and DNA synthesis by ultraviolet light. *Cancer Res* 1979;9:1035–1040.

26. Gallagher CH, Canfield PJ, Greenoak GE, et al. Characterization and histogenesis of tumors in the hairless mouse produced by low-dosage incremental ultraviolet radiation. *J Invest Dermatol* 1984;83:169–174.

27. Nghiem DX, Kazimi N, Cldesdale G, et al. Ultraviolet A radiation suppresses an established immune response: implications for sunscreen design. *J Invest Dermatol* 2001;117: 1193–1199.

28. Serre I, Cano JP, Picot MC, et al. Immunosuppression induced by acute solar-simulated ultraviolet exposure in humans: prevention by a sunscreen with a sun protection factor of 15 and high UVA protection. *J Am Acad Dermatol* 1997;37:187–194.

29. Schaefer H, Moyal D, Fourtanier A. Recent advances in sun protection. *Semin Cutan Med Surg* 1998;17:266–275.

30. Verallo-Rowell VM, Villacarlos-Bautista D, Oropeza NS, et al. Indoor lights used in the photopatch testing of a case-controlled group of melasma and non-melasma patients. In: Eds. *Skin in the Tropics: Sunscreens and Hyperpigmentations.* Pasig City: Anvil Press;2002:102–131.

31. Verallo-Rowell VM. Photopatch test positive melasma with subtle photosensitivity among sun shy Asians. Paper presented at: 7th Asian Congress of Dermatology; September 29, 2005; Kuala Lumpur, Malaysia; and Occupational and Contact Dermatitis Conference; October 26, 2005; Manila, Philippines.

32. Negishi K, Kushikata N, Tezuka Y, et al. Study of the incidence and nature of "very subtle epidermal melasma" in relation to intense pulsed light treatment. *Dermatol Surg* 30(6):881–886.

33. Pandya AG, Guevara IL. Disorders of hyperpigmentation. *Dermatol Clin* 2000;18(1):91–98.

34. Grimes PE. Melasma. Etiologic and therapeutic considerations. *Arch Dermatol* 1995;131:1453–1457.

35. Johnson JA, Fusaro RM. Broad-spectrum photoprotection: the roles of tinted auto windows, sunscreens and browning agents in the diagnosis and treatment of photosensitivity. *Dermatology* 1992;185:237–241.

36. Federal register: rules and regulations. *Fed Reg* 1999;64:27687.

37. Carolyn B, Lyde R, Bergstresser PR. Ultraviolet protection from sun avoidance. *Dermatol Ther* 1997;4:72–78.

38. Davis JK. The sunglass standard and its rationale. *Optom Vis Sci* 1990;67:414–430.

39. Georgouras KE, Stanford DG, Pailthorpe MT. Sun protective clothing in Australia and the Australian/New Zealand standard: an overview. *Australas J Dermatol* 1997;38(Suppl): S79–82.

40. Kullavanijaya P, Lim H. Photoprotection. *J Am Acad Dermatol* 2005;52;66: 937–958.

41. Fourtanier A, Labat-Robert J, Kern P, et al. In vivo evaluation of photoprotection against chronic ultraviolet-A irradiation by a new sunscreen Mexoryl SX. *Photochem Photobiol* 1992;55:549–560.

42. Fourtanier A. Mexoryl SX protects against solar-simulated UVR-induced photocarcinogenesis in mice. *Photochem Photobiol* 1996;64:688–693.

43. Krien PM, Moyal D. Sunscreens with broad-spectrum absorption decrease the trans to cis photoisomerization of urocanic acid in the human stratum corneum after multiple UV light exposures. *Photochem Photobiol* 1994;60:280–287.

44. Seite S, Moyal D, Richard S, et al. Mexoryl SX: a broad absorption UVA filter protects human skin from the effects of repeated suberythemal doses of UVA. *J Photochem Photobiol B* 1998;44:69–76.

45. Learn DB, Sambuco CP, Forbes PD, et al. Twelve month topical study to determine the influence of bemotrizinol and bisoctrizole on photocarcinogenesis in hairless mice. European Society for Photobiology. 2005 Poster Session I: 157–158.

46. Moseley H, Cameron H, MacLeod T, et al. New sunscreens confer improved protection for photosensitive patients in the blue light region. *Br J Dermatol* 2001;145:789–794.

47. Kaye ET, Levin JA, Blank IH, et al. Efficiency of opaque photoprotective agents in the visible light range. *Arch Dermatol* 1991;127(3):351–355.

48. European Medicines Agency. Titanium dioxide and bisoctrizole for the treatment of UV-A and visible light-induced photosensitivity disorders (chronic actinic dermatitis, cutaneous porphyrias, actinic prurigo and solar urticaria). Orphan designation (EU/3/05/262) granted by the European Commission, application for Pre-authorisation Evaluation of Medicines for Human Use, London, 1 July 2005.

49. Kollias N. The absorption properties of "physical sunscreens." *Arch Dermatol* 1999;135:209–210.

50. Verallo-Rowell VM, Belicena H, Paz LMR, et al. SPF and PFA of colored cosmetics. In: Eds. Skin in the Tropics: Sunscreens and Hyperpigmentations. Pasig City: Anvil Press;2002:209–241.

51. Darr D, Dunston S, Faust H, et al. Effectiveness of antioxidants (vitamin C and E) with and without sunscreens as topical photoprotectants. *Acta Derm Venereol* 1996;76:264–268.

52. Fuchs J, Kern H. Modulation of UV-light-induced skin inflammation by D-alpha-tocopherol and L-ascorbic acid: a clinical study using solar simulated radiation. *Free Radic Biol Med* 1998;25:1006–1012.

53. Gonzalez S, Pathak MA, Cuevas J, et al. Topical or oral administration with an extract of Polypodium leucotomos prevents acute sunburn and psoralen-induced phototoxic reactions as well as depletion of Langerhans cells in human skin. *Photodermatol Photoimmunol Photomed* 1997;13:50–60.

54. Gomes AJ, Lunardi CN, Gonzalez S, et al. The antioxidant action of Polypodium leucotomos extract and kojic acid:

reactions with reactive oxygen species. *Braz J Med Biol Res* 2001;34:1487–1494.

55. Rostan EF, DeBuys HV, Madey DL, et al. Evidence supporting zinc as an important antioxidant for skin. *Int J Dermatol* 2002;41:606–611.

56. Record IR, Jannes M, Dreosti IE. Protection by zinc against UVA- and UVB-induced cellular and genomic damage in vivo and in vitro. *Biol Trace Elem Res* 1996;53:19–25.

57. Katiyar SK, Elmets CA. Green tea polyphenolic antioxidants and skin photoprotection. *Int J Oncol* 2001;18:1307–1313.

58. Van den Broeke LT, Beijersbergen vHG. Topically applied N-acetylcysteine as a protector against UVB-induced systemic immunosuppression. *J Photochem Photobiol B* 1995;27:61–65.

59. Steenvoorden DP, Hasselbaink DM, Beijersbergen VHG. Protection against UV-induced reactive intermediates in human cells and mouse skin by glutathione precursors: a comparison of N-acetylcysteine and glutathione ethylester. *Photochem Photobiol* 1998;67:651–656.

60. Lim HW, Naylor M, Honigsmann H, et al. American Academy of Dermatology consensus conference on UVA protection of sunscreens: summary and recommendations. *J Am Acad Dermatol* 2001;(44):505–508.

61. Kaidbey KH, Barnes A. Determination of UVA protection factors by means of immediate pigment darkening in normal skin. *J Am Acad Dermatol* 1991;25:262–266.

62. Moyal D, Chardon A, Kollias N. Determination of UVA protection factors using the persistent pigment darkening (PPD) as the end point (part 1): calibration of the method. *Photodermatol Photoimmunol Photomed* 2000;16:245–249.

63. Kelly DA, Seed PT, Young AR, et al. A commercial sunscreen's protection against ultraviolet radiation-induced immunosupression is more than 50% lower than protection against sunburn in humans. *J. Invest Dermatol* 2003; 120(1): 65–71.

64. Gers-Barlag H, Klette E, Bimczok R, et al. Members of the DGK (German Society for Scientific and Applied Cosmetics) Task Force. Sun protection: In vitro testing to assess the UVA protection performance of sun care products. *Int J Cosmet Sci* 2001;23:3–14.

65. Baron ED, Fourtanier A, Compan D, et al. High ultraviolet A protection affords greater immune protection confirming that ultraviolet A contributes to photoimmunosuppression in humans. *J Invest Dermatol* 2003;121:869–875.

66. Diffey BL, Grice J. The influence of sunscreen type on photoprotection. *Br J Dermatol* 1997;137:103–105.

67. Stenberg C, Larko O. Sunscreen application and its importance for the sun protection factor. *Arch Dermatol* 1985;121:1400–1402.

68. Diffey BL. When should sunscreen be reapplied? *J Am Acad Dermatol* 2001;45:882–885.

69. Phillips TJ, Bhawan J, Yaar M, et al. Effect of daily versus intermittent sunscreen application on solar simulated UV radiation-induced skin response in humans. *J Am Acad Dermatol* 2000;43:610–618.

70. American Academy of Dermatology Public Resource Center. Sunscreen 101: Dermatologist Reveals What Every American Should Know About Good Sun Protection. New York (May 3, 2006).

71. Schauder S, Ippen H. Contact and photocontact sensitivity to sunscreens: review of a 15-year experience and of the literature. *Contact Dermatitis* 1997;37:221–232.

72. Darvay A, White IR, Rycroft RJ, et al. Photoallergic contact dermatitis is uncommon. *Br J Dermatol* 2001;145:597–601.

73. Ang P, Ng SK, Goh CL. Sunscreen allergy in Singapore. *Am J Contact Dermat* 1998;9(1):42–44.

74. Hayakawa R. Contact/photocontact dermatitis due to sunscreen products in Japan: review. *Japan Soc Contact Derm* 1994; 1,2:98–105.

75. Grant WB, Holick MF. Benefits and requirements of vitamin D for optimal health: a review. *Altern Med Rev* 2005;10(2):94–111.

76. Feleke Y, Abdulkadir A, Mshana R, et al. Low levels of serum calcidiol in an African population compared to a North European population. *Eur J Endocrinol* 1999;141:358–360.

77. Grover SR, Morley R. Vitamin D deficiency in veiled or dark-skinned pregnant women. *MJA* 2001;175:251–252.

78. Bolt HM, Guhe C, Degen GH. Comments on "in vitro and in vivo estrogenicity of UV screens." *Environ Health Perspect* 2001;109:A358–361.

79. Dobes WL. Public education: an approach: skin cancer awareness project using the solar meter. *J Am Acad Dermatol* 1986;14:676–679.

80. Naylor M, Robinson JK. Sunscreens, sun protection and our many failures. *Arch Dermatol* 2005;14:1025–1027.

81. Hilhouse J, Turrisi R. Skin cancer risk behaviors. A conceptual framework for complex behavioral change [editorial]. *Arch Dermatol* 2005;141:1028–1031.

PART 3

Therapies for Dyschromias

been considered safe; however the effect of treatment can be inconsistent, as some CALMs may even darken after treatment. Thus, a test spot should be performed using conservative parameters that produce a visible response. The treatment area is re-evaluated 4 to 8 weeks later for clinical response and adverse effects. Hyperpigmentation can occur but usually improves over several months with topical bleaching regimens. Hypopigmentation is a potential risk, particularly with the shorter wavelength lasers. The risk of dyspigmentation is especially higher in darker-skinned individuals and should be taken in consideration when treating CALMs in patients with skin types IV through VI in whom the initial lesion may already be less apparent.

The Q-switched ruby, alexandrite, and Nd:YAG lasers have been shown to treat CALMs with varying degrees of efficacy. Grossman et al. found variable response in treating CALMs with a 694-nm QS ruby laser and a 532-nm frequency doubled Q-switched Nd:YAG laser.[50] Nine lesions were treated, half with each laser. At 6 months, five of the lesions showed lightening, and one resolved. One lesion resolved after the first month, but recurred at the 3-month follow-up, whereas two lesions darkened 1 month after the first treatment. Clinical experience with multiple Q-switched laser treatments has yielded inconsistent results, with 50% of the cases achieving total clearance and repigmentation occurring in the other half.[45] Other reports suggest a single laser treatment may lighten up to 50% of café au lait spots and almost clear 20% to 50% of lesions. However, one third of these showed repigmentation.[51–53]

Longer-pulsed lasers have been used in treating CALMs, but have also yielded inconsistent long-term results. The 510-nm pulsed dye laser has been used to treat café au lait macules. A report described its use to successfully treat a facial café au lait macule in a patient with Fitzpatrick skin type V using the following parameters: 2.5 J/cm^2, 300 nsec, with single, nonoverlapping laser pulses every 2 months for six treatments.[54] In another study using the QS alexandrite laser to treat CALMs, 9 out of 10 patients

had 60% to 100% response after a mean of 6.7 treatments. Three patients had partial or complete recurrence. One patient had PIH, and another had hypertrophic scarring. A preliminary study described a lower risk of recurrence with the normal-mode ruby laser (42% recurrence) in 33 patients with café au lait patches compared with the Q-switched ruby laser (82% recurrence).[41] The data were limited to a 3-month follow-up after a single treatment. The authors proposed that the longer pulse width may reduce the recurrence rate by affecting the follicular melanocytes.

Nevus of Ota

Nevus of Ota is a benign pigmentary disorder that usually manifests as blue-brown or gray patches over facial skin innervated by the first and second trigeminal nerve. Associated lesions include scleral melanocytosis as well as involvement of the nasopharynx, auricular mucosa, tympanic membrane, palate, and dura. It is seen most commonly in Asians and is typically congenital or acquired by adolescence. The use of the Q-switched lasers is the current treatment of choice for the cutaneous component (Fig. 13-3).

Several studies have reported successful clearing after multiple treatments using various Q-switched laser systems. A study of 114 patients with Ota's nevi treated with the QS ruby resulted in good to excellent clearing after three or more treatment sessions.[55] Transient hyperpigmentation after the first treatment was the most common complication. A Japanese study also reported the safe and successful use of the Q-switched ruby laser in treating nevi of Ota in 106 adults and 46 children using the following parameters: 30-ns pulse duration, 4-mm spot size, and 5- to 7-J/cm^2 fluence at 3- to 4-month intervals.[56] They found the average number of sessions to achieve significant clearing was less in the younger age group (3.5 sessions) than the older age group (5.9 sessions).

In a study of 55 Korean patients with Ota's nevi treated with the Q-switched alexandrite laser for three sessions every 3 months, 49% of patients had excellent pigment

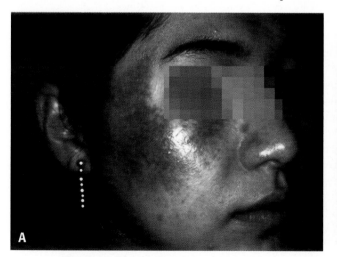
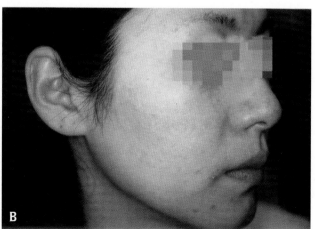

Figure 13-3 Nevus of Ota treatment with Q-switched laser. **A:** Initial treatment with Q-switched laser. **B:** After treatment with Q-switched laser.

clearing, and 31% had good pigment clearing. PIH developed in 55% of patients, which resolved within 4 months.[57] Chan et al. compared the use of the Q-switched alexandrite and the Q-switched Nd:YAG for nevi of Ota in 40 Asian women, noting the Nd:YAG to be more effective as evaluated by two independent clinicians. However, scores by only one clinician was found to be statistically significant.[58]

Although excellent clearing of nevus of Ota can be achieved with multiple laser treatment lesions, patients should be counseled on the potential for incomplete clearing, erythema, postinflammatory hyper- and hypopigmentation, recurrence of condition, and scarring. In a retrospective study of 211 Q-switched alexandrite and Nd:YAG laser-treated sites, Chan et al. noted the following complications: 15.3% had hypopigmentation, 2.9% had hyperpigmentation, 2.9% had textural changes, and 1.9% had scarring.[59] Recurrence after laser clearance of nevi of Ota is approximately 0.6% to 1.2%.[60]

Hori's nevus or acquired bilateral nevus of Ota-like macules

Hori's nevus is an acquired bilateral nevus of Ota-like lesions that usually presents symmetrically on the face. It is seen most commonly in middle-aged women of Asian descent. Unlike nevus of Ota, it does not have mucosal involvement. Histologically, irregular-shaped melanocytes are seen in the middle and upper dermis similar to that seen in nevus of Ota. Electron microscopy demonstrates dermal melanocytes that contain many singly dispersed melanosomes in stages II, III, and IV of melanization.[61]

As in treatment of Ota's nevi, Q-switched lasers have been successfully used to treat Hori's nevi. Multiple treatments are typically required. A study evaluated the Q-switched alexandrite laser for the treatment of Hori's nevi in 32 Chinese women, noting more than 50% clearing in more than 80% of patients after a mean of seven treatment sessions every 4 weeks. Temporary erythema was seen in 41% of patients and transient hypopigmentation in up to 50% of patients. Hyperpigmentation occurred in 12.5% of patients. This was treated with topical bleaching agents.[62] In a study of 66 Asian patients treated up to seven times with the Q-switched Nd:YAG laser, Polnikorn et al. found 50% of patients had good to excellent clearing.[63] Another study using the Q-switched Nd:YAG laser (fluence of 8–10 J/cm[2], spot size 2 or 4 mm) demonstrated 100% clearance of Ota's nevi after two to five sessions in 68 out of 70 patients. Fifty percent of patients had temporary hyperpigmentation. The results persisted at 3 to 4 years follow-up.[64]

Table 13-1

Laser therapies for disorders of hyperpigmentation

Diagnosis	Lasers/light source used	Outcomes
Melasma	CO_2 laser	Poor
	Erbium laser	Poor
	QS lasers	Poor
	Fractional photothermolysis	Variable
Postinflammatory hyperpigmentation	QS lasers	Poor
Medication-induced hyperpigmentation	QS Alexandrite	Variable
	QS Nd:YAG	Variable
Lentigines	QS Alexandrite	Variable
	QS Nd:YAG	Variable
	Long pulsed dye laser	Variable
	Long pulsed Nd: YAG laser	Variable
	Intense pulsed light	Variable
Café au lait macules	QS Alexandrite	Variable
	QS Nd:YAG	Variable
	Long pulsed dye laser	Variable
Nevus of Ota	QS Alexandrite	Positive
	QS Nd:YAG	Positive
Acquired bilateral nevus of Ota-like macules	QS Alexandrite	Positive
	QS Nd:YAG	Positive

Combination treatment with lasers has also been used to treat Hori's nevi. A scanned carbon dioxide laser followed by a Q-switched ruby laser was found to be effective in 13 Thai patients with skin types III to IV. However, all patients had posttreatment erythema at 1 month follow-up, which persisted in two patients at 3-month follow-up.[65] Recently, in a split-face study of 10 Asian women with Hori's nevi, combination treatment using the Q-switched 532-nm Nd:YAG laser followed by the Q-switched 1,064-nm laser showed a greater degree of lightening compared with the 1,064-nm alone at 6 months follow-up. However, this combination had a higher incidence of mild postinflammatory adverse effects, which lasted for 2 months.[66] Laser therapies for disorders of hyperpigmentation are summarized in Table 13-1.

REFERENCES

1. Roberts WE. Chemical peeling in ethnic/dark skin. *Dermatol Ther* 2004;17:196–205.
2. Grimes PE. Melasma: etiologic and therapeutic considerations. *Arch Dermatol* 1995;131:1453–1457.
3. Pathak MA, Fitzpatrick TB, Kraus EW. Usefulness of retinoic acid in the treatment of melasma. *J Am Acad Dermatol* 1986;15:894–899.
4. Nanda S, Grover C, Reddy BS. Efficacy of hydroquinone (2%) versus tretinoin (0.025%) as adjunct topical agents for chemical peeling in patients of melasma. *Dermatol Surg* 2004;30:385–358; discussion 389.
5. Sarkar R, Kaur C, Bhalla M, et al. The combination of glycolic acid peels with a topical regimen in the treatment of melasma in dark-skinned patients: a comparative study. *Dermatol Surg* 2002;28:828–832; discussion 832.
6. Grimes PE. The safety and efficacy of salicylic acid chemical peels in darker racial-ethnic groups. *Dermatol Surg* 1999;25:18–22.
7. Khunger N, Sarkar R, Jain RK. Tretinoin peels versus glycolic acid peels in the treatment of melasma in dark-skinned patients. *Dermatol Surg* 2004;30:756–760; discussion 760.
8. Sharquie KE, Al-Tikreety MM, Al-Mashhadani SA. Lactic acid as a new therapeutic peeling agent in melasma. *Dermatol Surg* 2005;31:149–154; discussion 154.
9. Fitzpatrick RE, Goldman MP, Ruiz-Esparza J. Laser treatment of benign pigmented epidermal lesions using a 300 nsecond pulse and 510 nm wavelength. *J Dermatol Surg Oncol* 1993;19:341–347.
10. Grekin RC, Shelton RM, Geisse JK, et al. 510-nm pigmented lesion dye laser: its characteristics and clinical uses. *J Dermatol Surg Oncol* 1993;19:380–387.
11. Goldberg DJ. Benign pigmented lesions of the skin: treatment with the Q-switched ruby laser. *J Dermatol Surg Oncol* 1993;19:376–379.
12. Taylor CR, Anderson RR. Ineffective treatment of refractory melasma and postinflammatory hyperpigmentation by Q-switched ruby laser. *J Dermatol Surg Oncol* 1994;20:592–597.
13. Manaloto RM, Alster T. Erbium:YAG laser resurfacing for refractory melasma. *Dermatol Surg* 1999;25:121–123.
14. Angsuwarangsee S, Polnikorn N. Combined ultrapulse CO2 laser and Q-switched alexandrite laser compared with Q-

switched alexandrite laser alone for refractory melasma: split-face design. *Dermatol Surg* 2003;29:59–64.
15. Fisher GH, Geronemus RG. Short-term side effects of fractional photothermolysis. *Dermatol Surg* 2005;31:1245–1249; discussion 1249.
16. Manstein D, Herron GS, Sink RK, et al. Fractional photothermolysis: a new concept for cutaneous remodeling using microscopic patterns of thermal injury. *Lasers Surg Med* 2004;34:426–438.
17. Rokhsar CK, Fitzpatrick RE. The treatment of melasma with fractional photothermolysis: a pilot study. *Dermatol Surg* 2005;31:1645–1650.
18. Tannous ZS, Astner S. Utilizing fractional resurfacing in the treatment of therapy-resistant melasma. *J Cosmet Laser Ther* 2005;7:39–43.
19. Halder RM, Grimes PE, McLaurin CI, et al. Incidence of common dermatoses in a predominantly black dermatologic practice. *Cutis* 1983;32:388–390.
20. Pandya AG, Guevara IL. Disorders of hyperpigmentation. *Dermatol Clin* 2000;18:91–98, ix.
21. Epstein JH. Postinflammatory hyperpigmentation. *Clin Dermatol* 1989;7:55–65.
22. McBurney EI. Side effects and complications of laser therapy. *Dermatol Clin* 2002;20:165–176.
23. Bulengo-Ransby SM, Griffiths CE, Kimbrough-Green CK, et al. Topical tretinoin (retinoic acid) therapy for hyperpigmented lesions caused by inflammation of the skin in black patients. *N Engl J Med* 1993;328:1438–1443.
24. Grimes PE, Callender VD. Tazarotene 0.1% cream in the treatment of facial post-inflammatory hyperpigmentation associated with acne vulgaris: a two-center, double-blind, randomized, vehicle-controlled study. Poster presented at: 61st Annual Meeting of the American Academy of Dermatology; March 21–26, 2003; San Francisco, CA.
25. Jacyk WK, Mpofu P. Adapalene gel 0.1% for topical treatment of acne vulgaris in African patients. *Cutis* 2001;68:48–54.
26. Kligman AM, Willis I. A new formula for depigmenting human skin. *Arch Dermatol* 1975;111:40–48.
27. Burns RL, Prevost-Blank PL, Lawry MA, et al. Glycolic acid peels for postinflammatory hyperpigmentation in black patients: a comparative study. *Dermatol Surg* 1997;23:171–174; discussion 175.
28. Yoshimura K, Harii K, Aoyama T, et al. Experience with a strong bleaching treatment for skin hyperpigmentation in Orientals. *Plast Reconstr Surg* 2000;105:1097–1108; discussion 1109–1110.
29. Callender VD. Acne in ethnic skin: special considerations for therapy. *Dermatol Ther* 2004;17:184–195.
30. Tafazzoli A, Rostan EF, Goldman MP. Q-switched ruby laser treatment for postsclerotherapy hyperpigmentation. *Dermatol Surg* 2000;26:653–656.
31. Atkin DH, Fitzpatrick RE. Laser treatment of imipramine-induced hyperpigmentation. *J Am Acad Dermatol* 2000;43:77–80.
32. Karrer S, Hohenleutner U, Szeimies RM, et al. Amiodarone-induced pigmentation resolves after treatment with the Q-switched ruby laser. *Arch Dermatol* 1999;135:251–253.
33. Green D, Friedman KJ. Treatment of minocycline-induced cutaneous pigmentation with the Q-switched alexandrite laser and a review of the literature. *J Am Acad Dermatol* 2001;44:342–347.

34. Becker-Wegerich PM, Kuhn A, Malek L, et al. Treatment of nonmelanotic hyperpigmentation with the Q-switched ruby laser. *J Am Acad Dermatol* 2000;43:272–274.

35. Friedman IS, Shelton RM, Phelps RG. Minocycline-induced hyperpigmentation of the tongue: successful treatment with the Q-switched ruby laser. *Dermatol Surg* 2002;28:205–209.

36. Alster TS, Gupta SN. Minocycline-induced hyperpigmentation treated with a 755-nm Q-switched alexandrite laser. *Dermatol Surg* 2004;30:1201–1204.

37. Ortonne JP, Pandya AG, Lui H, et al. Treatment of solar lentigines. *J Am Acad Dermatol* 2006;54:S262–271.

38. Stern RS, Dover JS, Levin JA, et al. Laser therapy versus cryotherapy of lentigines: a comparative trial. *J Am Acad Dermatol* 1994;30:985–987.

39. Farris PK. Combination therapy for solar lentigines. *J Drugs Dermatol* 2004;3:S23–26.

40. Chan HH. Effective and safe use of lasers, light sources, and radiofrequency devices in the clinical management of Asian patients with selected dermatoses. *Lasers Surg Med* 2005;37:179–185.

41. Chan HH, Kono T. The use of lasers and intense pulsed light sources for the treatment of pigmentary lesions. *Skin Therapy Lett* 2004;9:5–7.

42. Chan H. The use of lasers and intense pulsed light sources for the treatment of acquired pigmentary lesions in Asians. *J Cosmet Laser Ther* 2003;5:198–200.

43. Lee PK, Rosenberg CN, Tsao H, et al. Failure of Q-switched ruby laser to eradicate atypical-appearing solar lentigo: report of two cases. *J Am Acad Dermatol* 1998;38:314–317.

44. Downs AM, Rickard A, Palmer J. Laser treatment of benign pigmented lesions in children: effective long-term benefits of the Q-switched frequency-doubled Nd:YAG and long-pulsed alexandrite lasers. *Pediatr Dermatol* 2004;21:88–90.

45. Shimbashi T, Kamide R, Hashimoto T. Long-term follow-up in treatment of solar lentigo and cafe-au-lait macules with Q-switched ruby laser. *Aesthetic Plast Surg* 1997;21:445–448.

46. Kono T, Manstein D, Chan HH, et al. Q-switched ruby versus long-pulsed dye laser delivered with compression for treatment of facial lentigines in Asians. *Lasers Surg Med* 2005;38:94–97.

47. Chan HH, Fung WK, Ying SY, et al. An in vivo trial comparing the use of different types of 532 nm Nd:YAG lasers in the treatment of facial lentigines in Oriental patients. *Dermatol Surg* 2000;26:743–749.

48. Kawada A, Shiraishi H, Asai M, et al. Clinical improvement of solar lentigines and ephelides with an intense pulsed light source. *Dermatol Surg* 2002;28:504–508.

49. Chun EY, Lee JB, Lee KH. Focal trichloroacetic acid peel method for benign pigmented lesions in dark-skinned patients. *Dermatol Surg* 2004;30:512–516; discussion 516.

50. Cook KK, Cook WR Jr. Chemical peel of nonfacial skin using glycolic acid gel augmented with TCA and neutralized based on visual staging. *Dermatol Surg* 2000;26:994–999.

51. Lugo-Janer A, Lugo-Somolinos A, Sanchez JL. Comparison of trichloroacetic acid solution and cryosurgery in the treatment of solar lentigines. *Int J Dermatol* 2003;42:829–831.

52. Li YT, Yang KC. Comparison of the frequency-doubled Q-switched Nd:YAG laser and 35% trichloroacetic acid for the treatment of face lentigines. *Dermatol Surg* 1999;25:202–204.

53. Grossman MC, Anderson RR, Farinelli W, et al. Treatment of cafe au lait macules with lasers: a clinicopathologic correlation. *Arch Dermatol* 1995;131:1416–1420.

54. Kilmer SL, Garden JM. Laser treatment of pigmented lesions and tattoos. *Semin Cutan Med Surg* 2000;19:232–244.

55. Carpo BG, Grevelink JM, Grevelink SV. Laser treatment of pigmented lesions in children. *Semin Cutan Med Surg* 1999;18:233–243.

56. Acland KM, Barlow RJ. Lasers for the dermatologist. *Br J Dermatol* 2000;143:244–255.

57. Alster TS, Williams CM. Cafe-au-lait macule in type V skin: successful treatment with a 510 nm pulsed dye laser. *J Am Acad Dermatol* 1995;33:1042–1043.

58. Watanabe S, Takahashi H. Treatment of nevus of Ota with the Q-switched ruby laser. *N Engl J Med* 1994;331:1745–1750.

59. Kono T, Chan HH, Ercocen AR, et al. Use of Q-switched ruby laser in the treatment of nevus of Ota in different age groups. *Lasers Surg Med* 2003;32:391–395.

60. Kang W, Lee E, Choi GS. Treatment of Ota's nevus by Q-switched alexandrite laser: therapeutic outcome in relation to clinical and histopathological findings. *Eur J Dermatol* 1999;9:639–643.

61. Chan HH, Ying SY, Ho WS, et al. An in vivo trial comparing the clinical efficacy and complications of Q-switched 755 nm alexandrite and Q-switched 1064 nm Nd:YAG lasers in the treatment of nevus of Ota. *Dermatol Surg* 2000;26:919–922.

62. Chan HH, Leung RS, Ying SY, et al. A retrospective analysis of complications in the treatment of nevus of Ota with the Q-switched alexandrite and Q-switched Nd:YAG lasers. *Dermatol Surg* 2000;26:1000–1006.

63. Chan HH, Leung RS, Ying SY, et al. Recurrence of nevus of Ota after successful treatment with Q-switched lasers. *Arch Dermatol* 2000;136:1175–1176.

64. Hori Y, Takayama O. Circumscribed dermal melanoses: classification and histologic features. *Dermatol Clin* 1988;6:315–326.

65. Lam AY, Wong DS, Lam LK, et al. A retrospective study on the efficacy and complications of Q-switched alexandrite laser in the treatment of acquired bilateral nevus of Ota-like macules. *Dermatol Surg* 2001;27:937–941; discussion 941–942.

66. Polnikorn N, Tanrattanakorn S, Goldberg DJ. Treatment of Hori's nevus with the Q-switched Nd:YAG laser. *Dermatol Surg* 2000;26:477–480.

67. Kunachak S, Leelaudomlipi P. Q-switched Nd:YAG laser treatment for acquired bilateral nevus of Ota-like maculae: a long-term follow-up. *Lasers Surg Med* 2000;26:376–379.

68. Manuskiatti W, Sivayathorn A, Leelaudomlipi P, et al. Treatment of acquired bilateral nevus of Ota-like macules (Hori's nevus) using a combination of scanned carbon dioxide laser followed by Q-switched ruby laser. *J Am Acad Dermatol* 2003;48:584–591.

69. Ee HL, Goh CL, Khoo LS, et al. Treatment of acquired bilateral nevus of Ota-like macules (Hori's nevus) with a combination of the 532 nm Q-switched Nd:YAG laser followed by the 1,064 nm Q-switched Nd:YAG is more effective: prospective study. *Dermatol Surg* 2006;32:34–40.

Cosmetic Leukodermas: Therapeutic Approaches

Pearl E. Grimes

Persistent leukoderms or hypopigmentation caused by a variety of aesthetic procedures are indeed dreaded complications. Hypopigmentation can occur after ablative or nonablative resurfacing procedures, chemical peels, dermabrasion, and laser hair removal. In addition, hypopigmented and/or depigmented splayed facelift scars are particularly distressing for many patients. Of these conditions, pigmentary alterations are most often associated with laser resurfacing procedures. Such complications have been reported in all skin types. However, it is most distressing in darker racial ethnic groups. Hyperpigmentation and hypopigmentation are relatively common side effects of ablative laser resurfacing.[1–5] The frequency of hyperpigmentation varies from 2% to 37%. It is primarily observed in darker skin types and in some instances is amendable to topical bleaching agents. In contrast, hypopigmentation is more often a late sequela, usually occurring after 6 or 7 months. Published studies report frequencies ranging from 1% to 20%.[1–5] Many physicians have considered cosmetic leukoderma a permanent sequela of resurfacing procedures; however, in my experience, these conditions are amenable to therapeutic intervention.

PATHOGENESIS OF HYPOPIGMENTATION

The precise mechanism of pigment loss is unknown. It has been reported that after every resurfacing procedure, there is some loss of melanocytes.[6] Hypopigmentation is a common occurrence after phenol peeling, which causes a deep dermal wound. In addition to the induction of dermal fibrosis, phenol and thymol are toxic to melanocytes[7,8]. Liew et al.[9] described the histologic changes of hypopigmentation in nine patients treated for hair removal using the ruby laser. S-100 positive melanocytes remained constant, whereas DOPA oxidase activity appeared to decrease. These findings suggested that the ruby laser caused hypopigmentation by blocking melanin synthesis rather than destroying melanocytes. Laws et al.[10] assessed the histologic features of

hypopigmentation after CO_2 resurfacing in a 62-year-old woman. There was no decrease in the number of melanocytes compared with a pretreatment biopsy. However, there was a decrease in the content of epidermal melanin as assessed with Fontana-Masson staining.

Grimes et al.[11] assessed the histopathological features of hypopigmentation caused by laser resurfacing. Biopsies were taken from the affected areas of pigment loss and normal skin for comparison in four patients. All biopsy specimens demonstrated varying quantities of epidermal melanin as well as residual epidermal melanocytes. Mild perivascular inflammation was evident in two specimens (Fig. 14-1). There was superficial dermal fibrosis in all specimens. These findings suggested that laser resurfacing pigment loss was due to a suppression of melanogenesis rather than loss of melanocytes. In addition, dermal fibrosis is also a contributing factor.

THERAPEUTIC APPROACHES

Albeit challenging, there are several therapeutic regimens that have proven beneficial for patients with hypopigmentation caused by aesthetic procedures.

Topical photochemotherapy

The use of psoralens as repigmenting agents for vitiligo was described as early as 1400 B.C.E.[12] In the Indian sacred book *Atharva Veda,* there is discussion of a plant that produced even skin color. Psoralens are furocoumarin compounds: Photodynamically active drugs that are capable of absorbing radiant energy. They are also found in limes, lemons, celery, figs, and parsnips.[12]

Psoralens were introduced into the field of modern dermatology by El Mofty in 1947. El Mofty observed repigmentation of vitiliginous lesions after the use of powdered seeds prescribed by native herbalists in Egypt. Early clinical studies in Egypt further documented the effectiveness of the *Ammi majus* plant extract 8-methoxypsoralen (8-MOP) taken orally or applied topically in combination with

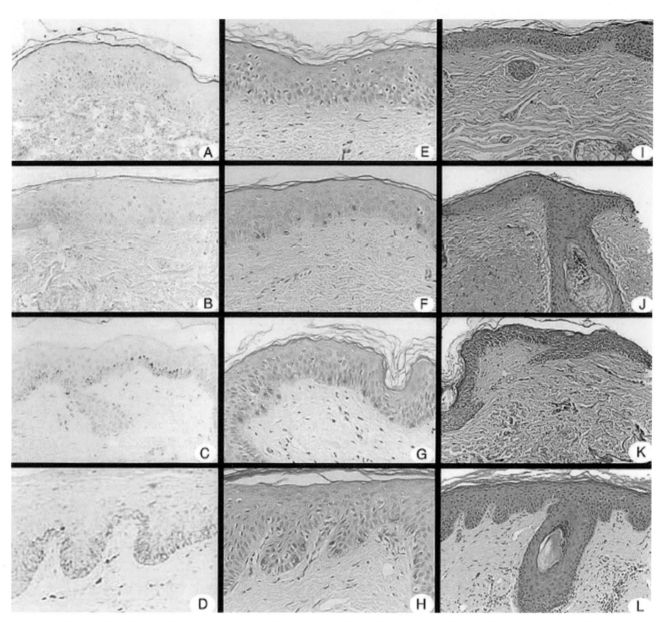

Figure 14-1 Histopathological features of laser-induced hypopigmentation. Composite photomicrographs showing representative areas of four patients **(A–D)**. Sparse **(A,B)** to moderate **(C,D)** epidermal melanin. Note melanophages in upper dermis **(C,D)** (Fontana-Masson; magnification 40X). Basal melanocytes on immunostaining with Mel-5. Note slightly reduced numbers in **(E)** but normal appearing in **(F,G)** (**H**, magnification 40X). Upper dermal fibrosis is seen in all patients **(I–L)**. Note mild to moderate perivascular lymphoid cell infiltrate and melanophages in **(K)** and **(L)** (hematoxylin and eosin; magnification 20X). From Grimes PE, Bhawan J, Kim J, et al. Laser resurfacing–induced hypopigmentation: histologic alterations and repigmentation with topical photochemotherapy. *Dermatol Surg* 2001;27:515–520.

sunlight or ultraviolet (UV) lamps. The acronym *PUVA* (psoralens + UVA) was introduced in 1974 to describe the use of oral psoralen (8-MOP) with the newly invented high-intensity long-wave (320–400 nm) ultraviolet phototherapy units. More than 30 skin conditions, including vitiligo, have been successfully treated with PUVA therapy.[12]

Although initially used for treatment for vitiligo, topical photochemotherapy has proven efficacious for treatment of cosmetic leukodermas. Grimes et al.[11] reported the efficacy of topical photochemotherapy treatments for treatment of laser resurfacing induced hypopigmentation. Seven patients were treated twice a week using 0.001% and 0.01% methoxsalen followed by exposure to artifical UVA light sources. The treatment induced moderate to excellent repigmentation in 71% of the treated patients. Side effects were minimal.

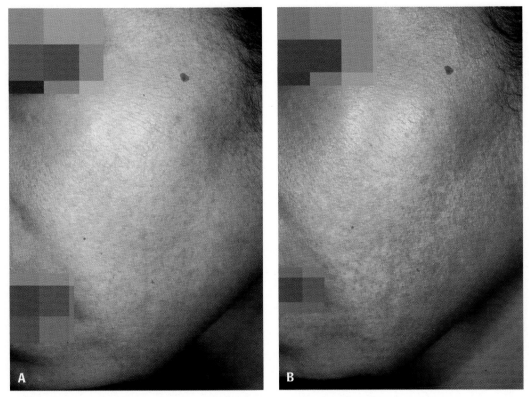

Figure 14-2 Hypopigmentation from a medium depth TCA peel. **A:** Baseline. **B:** After twice-weekly topical photochemotherapy treatments (methoxsalen 0.01%).

The author's standard protocol uses methoxsalen lotion 1% (Oxsoralen, Valiant Pharmaceuticals, Costa Mesa, CA). Methoxsalen stimulates melanocyte proliferation and melanogenesis. The lotion is diluted to a concentration of 0.001% and 0.01% in Aquaphor. A thin coat of 0.001% concentration is applied to hypopigmented areas 30 minutes before UVA exposure. Patients are treated with an initial UVA fluence of 0.20 J/cm². The fluence is then increased by 0.20 to 0.50 J per treatment, according to skin type and sensitivity. Lower initial doses and increments are indicated for skin types I and II. After mild to moderate asymptomatic erythema achieved, UVA fluence is maintained at a level sufficient to retain erythema. Treated areas are then cleansed with Cetaphil and water. A broad-spectrum sunscreen is applied after treatment. Patients are treated twice weekly. After 8 to 10 treatments, the concentration of methoxsalen can be increased to 0.01% if therapeutically indicated. High-intensity UVA light sources, such as the Daavlin Spectra 311/350, are used. However, smaller high-intensity UVA units can be used for small areas. Unaffected areas are protected with sunscreen or clothing (Fig. 14-2A,B and Fig. 14-3A,B).

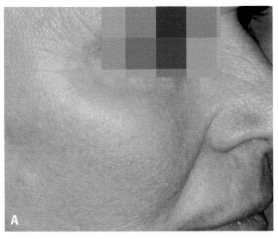

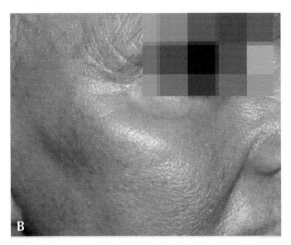

Figure 14-3 Hypopigmentation from CO_2 laser resurfacing in skin type II. Before **(A)** and after **(B)** 28 topical photochemotherapy treatments.

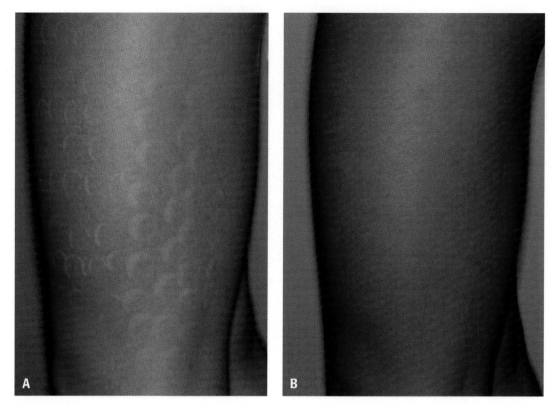

Figure 14-4 Severe hypopigmentation from laser hair removal. Before **(A)** and after **(B)** 17 narrowband UVB treatments.

For some patients who find it difficult to travel to an office for twice-weekly treatments, topical photochemotherapy with daily sunlight exposure is a viable alternative regimen. A thin coat of 0.001% methoxsalen is applied to hypopigmented areas. After an interval of 20 to 30 minutes, the affected areas are exposed to sunlight for 10 to 20 minutes. For lighter skin types (I–II), initial exposure to sunlight is for 5 to 10 minutes. After 2 weeks, exposure time can be increased to 30 minutes if mild erythema has not occurred. Following sun exposure, the treated sites are washed with soap and water. A broad-spectrum sunscreen is applied after treatment.

The author has treated many patients with this regimen. It is efficacious with minimal complications.

Narrowband UVB

Narrowband UVB (NB-UVB) involves the use of TL01 UV lamps with a peak emission around 311 nm.[13] The shorter wavelengths provide high-energy fluences and induce less cutaneous erythema. NB-UVB induces local immunosuppression and stimulation of melanocyte-stimulating hormone, and increases melanocyte proliferation and melanogenesis. NB-UVB has shown substantial efficacy for treatment of vitiligo. Westerhof and Nievweboer-Krobotova[14] were the first investigators to assess the efficacy of NB-UVB for pigment loss. They compared the efficacy of

NB-UVB with topical PUVA in a series of 67 patients with vitiligo. Significantly enhanced repigmentation was achieved in patients with NB-UVB as compared with those treated with topical PUVA. Studies have further confirmed the efficacy of NB-UVB phototherapy for cosmetic leukoderma, such as striae distensae.[15]

Patients with leukodermas induced by cosmetic procedures are treated two or three times weekly with NB-UVB. Normal skin areas are protected with clothing and/or broad-spectrum sunscreen. The initial NB-UVB dose of 150 mJ is usually given with increments of 10% to 15% each visit. Broad-spectrum sunscreens are applied to the affected areas following NB-UVB exposure (Fig. 14-4 A,B). Excellent results have been achieved in patients with extensive pigment loss from laser hair removal.

Targeted light therapy

Targeted phototherapy systems deliver high-intensity light only to the affected areas through a controlled handpiece. Hence, ultraviolet light exposure is avoided on normal skin. Targeted light systems decrease cumulative UV light doses to affected areas. Such units include the excimer laser, broad band UVB units, and combination UVA/UVB systems. These units are commonly used for repigmentation of vitiligo. Friedman and Geronemus[16] treated two patients with the 308-nm excimer laser for postresurfacing

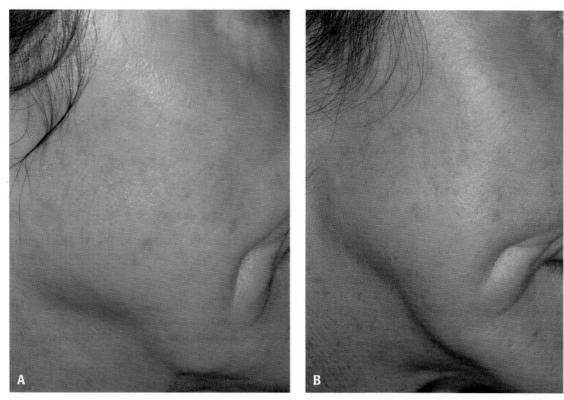

Figure 14-5 Hypopigmentation from ablative resurfacing. Baseline **(A)** and after **(B)** 30 treatments with XeCl excimer laser.

leukoderma. Sites treated included the upper lip and the cheek. The authors reported improvement in both patients. A subsequent study by Alexiades-Armenakas et al.[17] assessed the efficacy of the 308-nm excimer laser for hypopigmented scars and striae alba. The hypopigmented scars are distributed on the face, torso, or extremities. Lesions were randomized to receive treatment or not with site-matched control lesions. Therapy was initiated with a minimal erythema dose minus 50 mJ/cm^2 to affected lesions. Treatments were performed biweekly until 50% to 70% repigmentation was achieved, then every 2 weeks thereafter. The mean percentage pigment correction by visual assessment compared with control skin was 61%. Pigmentation gradually faded during the 6-month follow-up, suggesting that maintenance treatment every 1 to 4 months may be necessary to maintain the cosmetic benefit.

Goldberg et al.[15] treated hypopigmented striae with either the 308 nm excimer laser or a UVB targeted light device (ReLume). After 6 months, all subjects showed clinical evidence of some persistence of clinically significant pigmentation. Analysis of biopsy specimens showed an increase in the number of melanocytes as well as the content of epidermal melanin. Hypertrophy of melanocytes was also evident.

The author has also observed improvement for cosmetic leukoderms treated with the excimer laser (Fig. 14-5A,B). The standard protocol involves an initial excimer

laser dose of 100mJ/cm^2 for skin types I through III and 150 mJ/cm^2 for skin types IV through VI. The fluence is then increased by 50mJ per treatment until mild erythema is achieved. Treatments are given twice weekly.

COMPLICATIONS

Side effects of topical photochemotherapy, narrowband UVB, and targeted light treatment include temporary perilesional hyperpigmentation, blistering reactions, erythema, erosions, and pain.[11–17] The perilesional hyperpigmentation resolves on cessation of treatment. It is never a permanent sequela. It can be minimized by avoiding overlapping treatments with normal skin. Blistering reactions caused by targeted light systems, topical photochemotherapy, or narrowband UVB systems are treated for 2 to 5 days with midpotency to high-potency topical steroids and cool compresses. Patients are usually able to resume treatment in 7 to 10 days. At that time, dosing should be lowered to 50% of the dose at the time of blistering (Fig. 14-6).

SURGICAL INTERVENTION

Autologous grafting procedures have been used extensively in patients with stable, localized areas of vitiligo

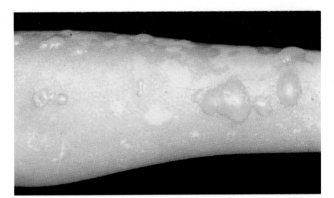

Figure 14-6 Blistering reactions from topical photochemotherapy.

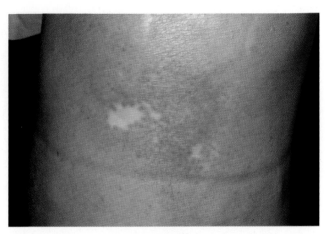

Figure 14-8 Micropigmentation for depigmented patch of the knee area. Note green discoloration of tattooed area.

since the 1980s.[18] For localized areas of hypopigmentation that fail to respond to the aforementioned medical approaches, autologous 1-mm punch grafts are viable. The technique is described in detail in Chapter 15. In brief, the technique involves harvesting 1-mm grafts from the hip, removing 1-mm grafts from the recipient area, and transplanting the graft to recipient areas. Sites are covered with Steri-strips and gauze dressings, which are removed in 7 days. I have had success in using this technique in patients who do not respond to phototherapy regimens (Fig. 14-7; Table 14-1).

MICROPIGMENTATION

Micropigmentation is a process of uniform implantation of minute iron oxide pigment granules into the dermis using a variety of tattoo machines/units. Although not a recommended therapeutic treatment for cosmetic leukoderma, micropigmentation has been used aesthetically to camouflage various medical conditions related to dermatology and plastic surgery. It is not a widely accepted modality for repigmenting hypopigmented skin. Immediate adverse

effects include ecchymosis, crusting, and edema lasting 2 to 3 days, reactivation of herpes simplex virus infection, secondary bacterial infection, and contact allergy to pigments. Micropigmentation should be performed with caution in patients with cosmetic leukoderma given the likelihood of pigment oxidation and further discoloration over time (Fig. 14-8).

In addition, the Tyndall effect—characterized by a bluish discoloration of the treated area—can develop several months later.[19]

CONCLUSION

Cosmetic leukoderma is a dreaded complication of aesthetic resurfacing procedures. Patients are often devastated by this side effect. Although pigmentary disorders are physically benign disorders, the psychosocial aspects of hypopigmentation and depigmentation are often malignant. Self-image, self-esteem, and emotional well-being are affected.[20–22]

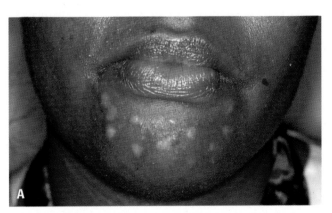

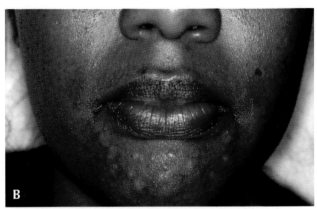

Figure 14-7 A: Hypopigmented scars from CO_2 laser resurfacing for acne scars. **B:** 1-mm autologous grafting.

Table 14-1

Therapeutic approaches for cosmetic leukodermas: mechanisms of action, advantages, and disadvantages

	Mechanism of action	Advantages	Disadvantages
Topical Photochemotherapy	Enhances type IV collagen production Stimulates proliferation and hypertrophy of Follicular border, and residual melanocytes Alters cell-mediated immune response Depletes of expression of epidermal growth factor receptor Inhibits degranulation of mast cells	Efficacious therapeutic option In office or sunlight Minimal practice expense 0.001% methoxalen well tolerated	Repigmentation rates vary considerably Accurate/precise formulations needed Blistering reactions Sometimes unpredictable border hyperpigmentation
Narrowband UVB	Decreases Langerhans cells Increases apoptosis Increases melanocyte proliferation and melanogenesis Increases αMSH Increases βFGF Increases ϵf-1 Increases endothelin 1	Ease and comparable efficacy Lack of systemic side effects No posttreatment ocular protection Excellent safety profile Minimal photoxicity	Requires three treatments per week for maximal efficacy Long-term carcinogenic effects unknown Permanency of repigmentation unknown
Excimer Laser 308 nm	Melanocyte proliferation Melanogenesis Activation of protein kinase C Alteration of cytokine production Stimulation of αMSH Formation of photoproducts	High-intensity light to affected skin areas Increased precision Avoids exposure to normal skin Rapid therapeutic responses Cumulative UV exposure decreased Synergistic effect with topical agents	Temporary hyperpigmentation Blistering similar to a sunburn Erythema Erosions Pain Expense Border hyperpigmentation
Combination UVA/UVB units (Theralight)	Melanocyte proliferation Melanogenesis Activation of protein kinase C Alteration of cytokine production Stimulation of αMSH Formation of photoproducts	High-dose therapy yields rapid result Fewer treatments required No need to fully disrobe Healthy skin not exposed to UV light Minimal side effects Greater convenience	Temporary hyperpigmentation Blistering similar to a sunburn Erythema Erosions Pain Expense Border hyperpigmentation
Surgical Grafting	New reservoir of melanocytes Immature melanocytes express c-kit protein Melanocyte migration Melanocyte proliferation Melanogenesis increased	Transfer of healthy melanocytes to areas of hypopigmentation for migration, proliferation, and repigmentation Adequate repigmentation Available procedures in most anatomic locations	Contraindications are hypertrophic scars and keloids Poor repigmentation in acral areas Infection Scarring Postinflammatory hyperpigmentation Cobblestoning Expense

Data from references 11, 12, [23–34].

FGF, fibroblast growth factor; MSH, melanocyte-stimulating hormone; UV, ultraviolet; UVB, ultraviolet B.

Cosmetic leukodermas are amenable to treatment via topical photochemotherapy, narrowband UVB, excimer laser, targeted UVA/UVB light sources, and surgical grafting. Clinical evidence indicates that substantial improvement can be achieved with minimal side effects. However, for some patients, intermittent retreatment may be required to maintain pigment in the affected areas. Additional studies are necessary to further substantiate the efficacy of these modalities in both the duration of improvement and the mechanism of action.

REFERENCES

1. Weinstein C. Erbium laser resurfacing: current concepts. *Plast Reconstr Surg* 1999;103:602–616.
2. Nanni CA, Alster TS. Complications of carbon dioxide laser resurfacing: an evaluation of 500 patients. *Dermatol Surg* 1998;24:315–320.
3. Ross EV, Grossman MC, Duke D, et al. Long-term results after CO₂ laser skin resurfacing: a comparison of scanned and pulsed systems. *J Am Acad Dermatol* 1997;37:709–718.
4. Bernstein LJ, Kauvar ANB, Grossman M, et al. The short- and long-term side effects of carbon dioxide laser resurfacing. *Dermatol Surg* 1997;23:519–525.
5. Manuskiatti W, Fitzpatrick RE, Goldman MD. Long-term effectiveness and side effects of carbon dioxide laser resurfacing for photo-aged facial skin. *J Am Acad Dermatol* 1999;40:401–411.
6. Stegman SJ, Tromovitch TA. Chemical peel: cosmetic dermatologic surgery. In: Stegman SJ, Tromovitch TA. *Cosmetic Dermatologic Surgery*. Chicago: Yearbook Medical Publishers, 1983:27–46.
7. Kligman AM, Baker TJ, Gordon H. Long-term histologic follow-up of phenol face peels. *Plast Reconstr Surg* 1985;75:652–659.
8. Brown AM, Naplan LM, Brown ME. Phenol-induced histological skin changes: hazards, techniques, and uses. *Br J Plast Surg* 1960;13:158–169.
9. Liew SH, Grobbelaar A, Gault D, et al. Hair removal using the ruby laser: clinical efficacy in Fitzpatrick skin types I–V and histological changes in epidermal melanocytes. *Br J Dermatol* 1999;140:1105–1109.
10. Laws RA, Finley IM, McCollorign ML, et al. Alabaster skin after carbon dioxide laser resurfacing with histological correlation. *Dermatol Surg* 1998;24:633–636.
11. Grimes PE, Bhawan J, Kim J, et al. Laser resurfacing–induced hypopigmentation: histologic alterations and repigmentation with topical photochemotherapy. *Dermatol Surg* 2001;27:515–520.
12. Grimes PE. Psoralen photochemotherapy for vitiligo. *Clin Dermatol* 1997;15:921–926.
13. Parrish JA, Jaenicke KF. Action spectrum for phototherapy of psoriasis. *J Invest Dermatol* 1981;76:359–362.
14. Westerhof W, Nievweboer-Krobotova. Treatment of vitiligo with UV-B radiation vs. topical psoralen plus UVA. *Arch Dermatol* 1997;133:1525–1528.
15. Goldberg DJ, Marmur ES, Schmults C, et al. Histologic and ultrastructural analysis of ultraviolet B laser and light source treatment of leukoderma in striae distensae. *Dermatol Surg* 2005;31:385–387.
16. Friedman PM, Geronemus RG. Use of the 308 nm excimer laser for post-resurfacing leukoderma. *Arch Dermatol* 2001;137(6):824–825.
17. Alexiades-Armenakas MR, Bernstein LJ, Friedman PM, et al. The safety and efficacy of the 308 nm excimer laser for pigment correction of hypopigmented scars and striae alba. *Arch Dermatol* 2004;140(8):955–960.
18. Falabella R. Surgical approaches for stable vitiligo. *Dermatol Surg* 2005;31:1277–1284.
19. Garg G, Thami GP. Micropigmentation: tattooing for medical purposes. *Dermatol Surg* 2005;31:928–931.
20. Porter J, Beuf A, Lerner A, et al. Response to cosmetic disfigurement: a study of patients with vitiligo. *Cutis* 1987;39:493–494.
21. Porter J, Beuf A, Lener A, et al. Psychological reaction to chronic skin disorders: a study of patients with vitiligo. *Gen Hosp Psychiatry* 1979;1:73–77.
22. Balkrishnan R, McMichael AJ, Hu JY, et al. Corrective cosmetics are effective for women with facial pigmentary disorders. *Cutis* 2005;75:181–187.
23. Morelli JG, Yohn JJ, Zekman T, et al. Melanocyte movement in vitro: role of matrix proteins and integrin receptors. *J Invest Dermatol* 1993;101:605–608.
24. Ortonne JP, MacDonald DM, Micoud A, et al. PUVA-induced repigmentation of vitiligo: a histochemical (split DOPA) and ultrastructural study. *Br J Dermatol* 1979;101:1–7.
25. Kao CH, Hsen SY. Comparison of the effect of 8-methoxypsoralen (8-MOP) plus UVA (PUVA) on human melanocytes in vitiligo vulgaris and in vitro. *J Invest Dermatol* 1992;98:734–740.
26. Stern RS, Lange R. Nonmelanoma skin cancer occurring in patients treated with PUVA five to ten years after first treatment. *J Invest Dermatol* 1988;91:120–124.
27. Cooper KD. Cell mediated immunosuppressive mechanisms induced by UV radiation photochemistry and photobiology. *Photchem Photobiol* 1996;63:400–405.
28. Yaron I, Yaron R, Oluwole SF, et al. UVB irradiation of human derived peripheral blood lymphocytes induces apoptosis but not T-cell energy: additive effects with various immunosuppressive agents. *Cell Immunol* 1996;168:258–266.
29. Freeman SE, Gange RW, Sutherland JC, et al. Production of pyrimidine dimers in DNA of human skin exposed in situ to UVA radiation. *J Invest Dermatol* 1987;88:430–433.
30. Funasaka Y, Chakaraborty AK, Hayashi Y, et al. Modulation of melanocyte-stimulating hormonal receptor expression on normal human melanocytes: evidence for a regulatory role of ultraviolet B, interleukin-1-alpha, interleukin-1 beta, endothelin-1 and tumour necrosis factor-alpha. *Br J Dermatol* 1998; 139:216–224.
31. Kondo S, Sauder DN. Keratinocyte-derived cytokine and UVB induced immunosuppresssion. *J Dermatol* 1995;22:888–893.
32. Iwai I, Natao M, Naganuma M, et al. UVA-induced immune suppression through an oxidative pathway. *J Invest Dermatol* 1999;112:19–24.
33. Abdel-Nasser MB, Hann SK, Bystryn JC. Oral psoralen with UVA therapy releases circulating growth factors that stimulate cell proliferation. *Arch Dermatol* 1997;133:1530–1533.
34. Gilchrest BA, Park HY, Eller MS, et al. Mechanisms of ultraviolet light-induced pigmentation. *Photchem Photobiol* 1996; 63:1–10.

information, explaining to health providers that this is not merely a "cosmetic" repair.

EXPERIENCE WITH VITILIGO SURGERY

Vitiligo therapy has changed dramatically with the surgical approach. Since initial attempts for repigmentation of vitiligo and leukoderma with thin Thiersch grafts in 1960,[30] and later on with epidermal grafting in 1971,[31] minigrafting in 1988,[15,32] epidermal suspensions in 1992,[33] and in vitro cultured epidermal sheets in 1989,[34,35] many publications have proven beyond doubt that surgical methods with transplantation of melanocytes have a place in vitiligo therapy in patients with refractory disease.

The highest repigmentation figures have been found for unilateral (segmental, asymmetric) vitiligo, the most stable form of the disease.[36] On the contrary, in bilateral vitiligo (vulgaris, symmetrical), only half the patients so treated have such rates of repigmentation, provided that they are completely stable when surgery is performed;[37] nevertheless, success and quality of repigmentation is dependent on the appropriate selection of cases and technique used.

REIMBURSEMENT IN VITILIGO: AN "INVENTED DISEASE" ARISING FROM A COSMETIC PROBLEM?

Vitiligo is a painless and symptomless condition; at the most, slight pruritus is a symptom in a few patients. However, patients face many difficulties when dealing with their medical plans, because it is frequently claimed that their illness is not covered for reimbursement because they suffer from no disease but just developed a "harmless cosmetic problem."

There are several reasons to disregard vitiligo as a cosmetic problem and consider it as a true disease as any other—with important implications interfering with normal life activities and employment:

- It is an acquired disease, not congenital.
- Patients are frequently segregated and stigmatized because of their unsightly appearance.[2,17]
- As opposed to cosmetic problems that refer mostly to the normal aging process, vitiligo affects profoundly the self-image of patients who suffer it.
- In particular for vitiligo surgery, some patients can be cured definitively if the condition belongs to the group of refractory and stable disease.

Therefore, appropriate selection of patients who are good candidates for surgical interventions with high pos-

sibilities of permanent repigmentation is encouraged. Dermatologists should provide all the necessary information to patients to assure their medical care and reimbursement.

REFRACTORY AREAS TO SURGICAL TREATMENT

For unknown reasons, some areas may become very difficult to repigment with surgical interventions, even though treatment is reasonably indicated. Areas with much mobility or prone to slight or mild daily trauma—such as joints, lips, dorsum of hands and feet, and especially fingers and toes—are the most resistant and "hard" areas for repigmentation. Although no explanation can be given for this difficulty, it is conceivable that a "take" failure may be one of the probable explanations. Other areas such as eyelids, genitalia, and cutaneous folds are not easy to treat because of anatomical difficulties placing the grafts. Regrafting and combination methods are indicated after initial surgical failure, and appropriate immobilization and protection of treated sites may enhance the possibilities of a good graft survival.

SELECTING THE SURGICAL TECHNIQUE

The surgical method is chosen according to the dermatologist's preference, training, and experience. Expertise in a given method may be achieved with any of the available methods, and high repigmentation figures can be obtained if performed appropriately. Comparison among different methods has been done and frequently published in the literature in favor of one method in particular, but this may also reflect the expertise of a given author in such method.

Another basic issue is that the less invasive the method, the better cosmetic results will be achieved. Procedures with much dermal manipulation, in terms of depth and area, have a tendency to originate scarring and unsightly repigmentation.

DONOR AREAS

When performing any transplantation procedure, it is of prime importance to select the appropriate donor site, usually a hidden anatomical area, but also with sufficient donor skin as required. The gluteal region is an excellent donor site for minigrafting and epidermal grafting. The skin folds or gluteal region may be used for in vitro culturing, and flat skin surfaces may be used for thin dermoepidermal grafts harvested with dermatome as well as for skin cultures. In general, the achieved improvement by surgical methods should be far more satisfactory for the patient than the possible damage inflicted to the donor site when harvesting melanocytes for repigmentation.

SURGICAL TECHNIQUES FOR REPIGMENTATION

Although many articles have been published about multiple techniques for melanocyte transplantation, many on them deal with modifications of the five basic surgical techniques that may be used for repigmentation in vitiligo: Noncultured epidermal suspensions, thin dermoepidermal grafts, suction epidermal grafting, punch minigrafting, and in vitro cultured epidermis with melanocytes or cultured melanocyte suspensions.[26]

Noncultured melanocyte suspensions (by trypsin digestion)

This method is performed by grafting noncultured epidermal suspensions with keratinocytes and melanocytes on depigmented skin. A donor skin piece is digested with 0.25% trypsin during 2 hours at 37°C until separation of epidermis from dermis occurs. By vigorous pipetting, keratinocytes and melanocytes separate to constitute a cell suspension, and by centrifugation, a pellet is obtained. The cells are washed with phosphate buffer saline and reconstituted in a cell suspension that is injected into blisters raised by liquid nitrogen freezing[33,38] or "seeded" on a denuded recipient site previously prepared by removal of the depigmented epidermis with superficial dermabrasion. The treated area is covered for 7 days with nonadherent dressings. If a good take occurs, repigmentation will begin 2 to 3 weeks later and continue gradually during the following months. The epidermal cells may be enriched by adding a melanocyte culture medium to the cell suspension, which may enhance the activity of melanocytes; therefore, larger depigmented defects may be treated.[39] The repigmentation yield is approximately a 1:2 ratio or higher according to the dilution used in the cell suspension. Advantages of this method are the evenness of repigmentation and absence of scarring if recipient sites are appropriately manipulated.

Thin dermoepidermal grafts (by dermatome harvesting)

Very thin dermoepidermal grafts harvested with a suitable dermatome from the donor site, not thicker than 0.1 to 0.3 mm, are grafted onto depigmented recipient sites that were prepared by very superficial dermabrasion. To get the best results, only the epidermis and papillary dermis should be removed when harvested, and the thin dermoepidermal sheets are grafted directly onto abraded areas. Grafts are placed close to each other, leaving no space between them; covered with nonadherent dressings; and secured with surgical wrappings during 7 days. Thin grafts and appropriate immobilization are essential for good results in this procedure. Repigmentation is achieved in a few weeks because melanocytes are present within grafts. With this method, refractory areas, as the dorsum of hands and fingers, have been grafted with success.[40] Although simple to perform, the yield is only that of a 1:1 ratio. A similar miniprocedure of this technique has been published as the "flip-top" graft by inserting small 3- to 5-mm, thinly shaved, dermoepidermal fragments under very thin flaps raised on the recipient site. There is a coalescence of pigment spread arising from multiple grafts implanted at a distance similar to the graft diameter. The treated areas should be repigmented within several months postgrafting.[41]

Epidermal grafting (by suction harvesting)

This is a method that has gained popularity, probably because of the excellent results and lack of scarring. In addition, donor sites may be reused for future procedures, allowing treatment of relatively extensive areas.

The technique requires a suction device for harvesting the epidermal grafts. Different publications illustrate several types of custom-made suction devices,[23,28,29,31] some of which are diverse types of syringes successfully used as suction devices.[42,43] The best suction diameter for individual blisters should not be larger than 1 cm to avoid excessive bulging of the skin within the suction device that may interfere with blistering. Blister grafts are obtained in 2 to 4 hours, but timing may be reduced to 30 minutes if heat at 42° to 43°C is provided during suction.[28,44]

Removal of vitiliginous epidermis may be achieved by liquid nitrogen freezing on small 5- to 10-mm spots 2 days before surgical interventions, so that grafting is performed after inflammation subsides; the blistered epidermis is removed just before implanting the epidermal grafts. Similar and faster results for epidermis removal include superficial dermabrasion[40] or ultrapulse CO_2 laser.[45]

When recipient sites are ready, blister grafts are cut with iris scissors; transferred with a thin transparent spatula, glass slide, or acetate films;[46] and grafted onto the recipient site.[29] The grafted surface is dressed with nonadherent gauze and wrapped with elastic bandages for 5 to 7 days. Pigment spread will gradually occur around grafts until repigmentation is complete. By adding PUVA, repigmentation occurs deeply and faster.[28,29] The repigmentation yield is about 1:5 or even higher when grafts are placed at a distance similar to the diameter of grafts. An advantage of this method is the absence of scarring in donor and recipient sites.

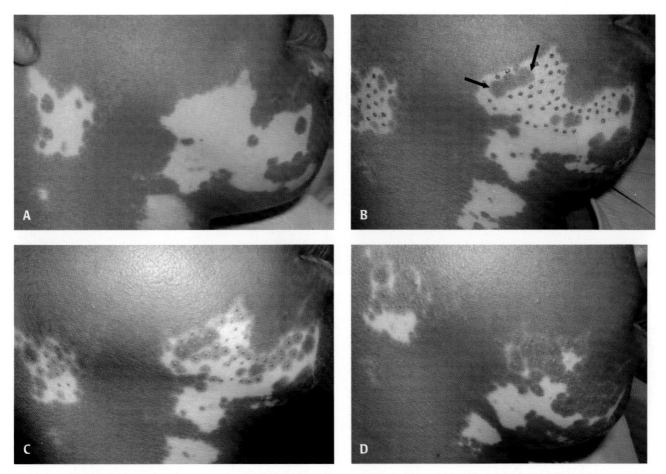

Figure 15-3 *Minigrafting sequence.* A 13-year-old boy of dark ethnic skin with refractory unilateral vitiligo illustrates the results of a single minigrafting session: **A:** Preoperatory aspect. **B:** Minigrafts immediately postgrafting (*arrows* depict minigrafting test done 4 months before). **C:** Partial repigmentation in progress 2½ months postgrafting. **D:** Six months after surgery, 95% repigmentation of treated areas was achieved.

Minigrafting (by small punch grafting)

Among all methods of melanocyte transplantation, minigrafting is the most popular technique used by many dermatologists, probably because of its simplicity.

Initially, after infiltration with 1% lidocaine without epinephrine, multiple perforations on depigmented skin are performed with a small 1- to 1.2-mm punch, separated at a distance of 3 to 5 mm apart from each other; the depigmented skin punches are discarded. The area under treatment is covered with compresses moistened with normal saline solution, allowing protection from contamination and facilitating blood clotting while harvesting minigrafts.

Minigrafts of similar size are then harvested very close to each other from the donor site with iris scissors and a fine-tipped forceps, placed onto a nonadherent dressing moistened with normal saline solution and kept sterile until grafting.

For grafting, minigrafts are transferred to the recipient site with the fine forceps, and when grafting is complete,

Micropore tape is directly applied on the surgical surface to assure adequate immobilization of minigrafts. After 14 days, the dressings are removed carefully to avoid detachment of grafts.[15] Semipermeable or nonadherent dressings may also be used according to the surgeon's experience.

For facial and neck lesions in young patients, a 1.0-mm punch is recommended, leading to good repigmentation and no scarring at all; 1.2-mm minigrafts can be used in the trunk and extremities. Larger-size grafts may provoke an unsightly "cobblestone" appearance.[26] Repigmentation occurs gradually around each minigraft up to 2 mm from the edge of grafts, and by coalescence originated by pigment spread, the total area becomes repigmented (Fig. 15-3A–D and Fig. 15-4A–D).[15,32,47]

Repigmentation rates vary from 1:10 to 1:20. Advantages of this method are its simplicity and the few instruments required: Minipunch, iris scissors, and a fine-tipped forceps. However, expertise should be good enough to avoid "cobblestoning," particularly by using very small punches.

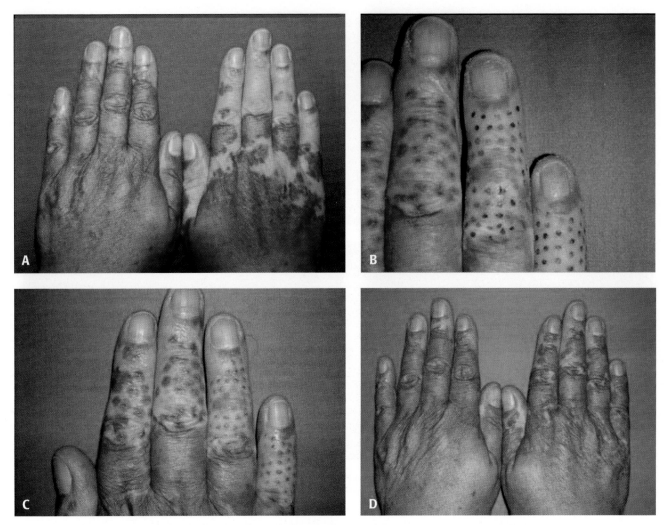

Figure 15-4. *Difficult areas for repigmentation.* **A:** This 50-year-old man had bilateral vitiligo since age 20. Lesions became stable after a few years, and at age 34, he had an in vitro cultured epidermal sheets transplantation on the left hand, with nearly 100% recovery (see reference 22). **B** and **C:** The patient came back 15 years later for additional treatment on his right hand, and after two minigrafting sessions with 1.2-mm grafts, pigment spread began shortly after each procedure. Different stages of repigmentation are observed. **D:** Six months later, 95% repigmentation was achieved. Notice that repigmentation effects are similar with two different techniques.

Cultured epidermis with melanocytes and melanocyte suspensions (by in vitro culture techniques)

A small donor skin sample provides the appropriate number of cells to be cultured in vitro and to be used as pigmented grafts for vitiligo. The skin piece is digested with 0.25% trypsin, and an epidermal suspension is obtained. Next, the cell suspension is seeded in culture flasks with appropriate culture media, and in 3 weeks thin epidermal sheets are achieved. These sheets are removed from the culture vessels using nonadherent polyestirene gauze as a graft carrier and transferred to the recipient site, previously denuded with liquid nitrogen freezing (or superficial dermabrasion, CO_2 lasers, pulsed Erbium-YAG lasers, or diathermosurgery).[48,49]

Pure melanocyte suspensions may be cultured with melanocyte culture media in a similar manner; melanocytes replicate exponentially, and the enriched cultured cell suspension is spread onto the recipient depigmented surface previously prepared by epidermal removal. Next, the area is covered with semipermeable or nonadhering dressings for 5 to 7 days until a good cellular take occurs.[50,51] Repigmentation is followed after surgery in both types of grafts during the next weeks and becomes complete after several months. Other methods providing good results include a hyaluronic artificial matrix for growing keratinocytes and melanocytes,[52] and melanocyte suspensions kept under freezing for several months and recultured after thawing; this latter method speaks in favor of the enormous potential of this technology for vitiligo therapy in the future.[53]

The most important advantage with in vitro culturing techniques is the exponential population of cells obtained from a small donor site, which solves the problem of treating extensive areas in a single session. Cost and infrastructure are the main restrictions at present for a wider use in clinical practice.

POSTSURGICAL CARE AND ADDITIONAL PROCEDURES

Neomelanogenesis depends on the type of technique used. Thin dermoepidermal grafts and epidermal grafts usually provide a full amount of melanocytes, and repigmentation is practically immediate if grafts are placed next to each other. On the contrary, epidermal suspensions, minigrafts, and in vitro cultured grafts or cultured suspensions depend on melanocyte proliferation before reaching full repigmentation. For faster and deeper repigmentation, either natural sunlight, 10 to 15 minutes daily, or PUVA are used; sessions can be initiated 2 weeks after healing takes place and continued until full repigmentation is reached. It is frequently observed that if no UV exposure is additionally administered, repigmentation may be slow, incomplete, or may even fail.

The grafted surface sometimes exhibits a slight hyperpigmented appearance, but this effect usually subsides, matching the surrounding skin aspect in most patients. Additional procedures may be tried with the same or different technique if repigmentation is not complete. Minigrafting is an easy technique for repigmenting small areas not improved in previous interventions.

COMPLICATIONS OF VITILIGO SURGERY

Vitiligo surgery involves invasive methods of donor and recipient sites. When performing such procedures, it is always important to consider to what extent additional defects may be provoked in a patient having a pigmentation disturbance. A careful evaluation of the patient's possibilities for appropriate repigmentation or side effects should be performed before therapy is accomplished. The main difficulties are described.

Postinflammatory hyperpigmentation

Some patients, especially those of darker ethnic skin groups with phototypes III to VI, may develop significant hyperpigmentation with surgery for vitiligo. The cause is not known, but in vitro experiments have demonstrated increased dendricity and edema; higher levels of tyrosinase and immunoreactive b-locus protein in pigment cells cultured with prostaglandin D2 (PGD2); leukotrienes B4, C4, D4, and E4; thromboxane B2; and 12-hydroxy eicosatetraenoic acid (HETE), suggesting a possible role of these arachidonic acid metabolites in the pathogenesis of postinflammatory hyperpigmentation.[54,55] Prostaglandin E2 has also been described having similar effects.[48] Most patients undergo spontaneous resolution, but some of them develop permanent hyperpigmentation; in those patients, it is also conceivable that genetic factors may be implicated. When permanent areas with hyperpigmentation secondary to local trauma are found in a patient, surgery for vitiligo may be contraindicated.

Cobblestoning

Cobblestoning is a complication of minigrafting when large punches are used. Punch grafts of 3 to 4 mm are not recommended, because the cobblestoning aspect may overweight the benefits of repigmentation achieved.[56] The preferred sizes are 1.2 mm for trunk and extremities and 1 mm for facial areas, particularly in young patients.

Scarring

When performing thin dermoepidermal grafts, hypertrophic scars, thick grafts, and irregular surfaces may occur at donor or recipient sites. An adequate dermatome for harvesting thin dermoepidermal sheets is important to avoid this side effect. Surgical blades manipulated by hand for shaving large grafts do not provide thin and even graft thickness, resulting in poor cosmetic results.

Infection

Infection is infrequent in most procedures, but a good aseptic technique must always be carried out.

Keloids

A previous history of keloids, either personal or familial, should be evaluated, and patients under this category should not be treated. This complication can be prevented by a careful evaluation and adequate past history. When still in doubt, a minigrafting test should be tried and evaluated before performing any procedure.

CONCLUSIONS AND FUTURE DIRECTIONS

At present, surgical techniques provide acceptable repigmentation for patients with stable and refractory vitiligo not responding to medical therapy. Results vary from patient to patient, but the most important factor to get a high repigmentation percentage is the appropriate selection of patients.[19] Unilateral vitiligo is the type responding better than any other form of vitiligo, and approximately 50% of those with bilateral disease, after reaching the stage of stability, may also achieve good results. Most areas respond to repigmentation procedures, but acral areas do so poorly. Several cytokines have been identified as having important effects on melanocyte migration *in vitro*, and in time, they may have a future role in clinical practice to enhance repigmentation in combination with medical therapy.[57,58] Surgical interventions could also facilitate repigmentation by selectively providing additional melanocytes implanted within depigmented lesions, which would act as multiple repigmentation foci that could contribute to pigmentation spread and coalescence for complete and faster repigmentation of vitiligo lesions.[59,60] In addition, combination therapy of medical and surgical methods, together with eximer lasers, could enhance the repigmentation rates by stimulating different stages of the repigmentation process. However, it is important that future studies should include control patients to ascertain the validity of findings, as recently demonstrated with epidermal suspensions for treating vitiligo.[61]

REFERENCES

1. Hann SK, Nordlund JJ. Clinical features of generalized vitiligo. In: Hann SK, Nordlund JJ, eds. *Vitiligo.* Oxford: Blackwell Science Ltd.;2000:35–48.

2. Alkhateeb A, Fain PR, Thody A, et al. Epidemiology of vitiligo and associated autoimmune disease in Caucasian probands and their families. *Pigment Cell Res.* 2003;16:208–214.

3. Cui J, Shen LY, Wang GC. Role of hair follicles in the repigmentation of vitiligo. *J Invest Dermatol* 1991;97:410–416.

4. Tobin DJ, Swanson NN, Pittelkow MR, et al. Melanocytes are not absent in lesional skin of long duration vitiligo. *J Pathol* 2000;191:407–416.

5. Grichnik JM, Ali WN, Burch JA, et al. KIT expression reveals a population of precursor melanocytes in human skin. *J Invest Dermatol* 1996;106:967–971.

6. Porter JR, Beuf AH. Racial variation in reaction to physical stigma: a study of degree of disturbance by vitiligo among black and white patients. *J Health Soc Behav* 1991;32:192–204.

7. Bystryn JC. Theories on the pathogenesis of depigmentation: immune hypothesis. In: Hann SK, Nordlund JJ, eds. *Vitiligo.* Oxford: Blackwell Science Ltd.;2000:129–136.

8. Hann SK, Chun WH. Autocytotoxic hypothesis for the destruction of melanocytes as the cause of vitiligo. In: Hann SK, Nordlund JJ, eds. *Vitiligo.* Oxford: Blackwell Science Ltd.;2000:137–141.

9. Schallreuter KU, Beazley WD, Wood JM. Biochemical theory of vitiligo: a role of pteridines in pigmentation. In: Hann SK, Nordlund JJ, eds. *Vitiligo.* Oxford: Blackwell Science Ltd.;2000:151–159.

10. Boissy RE. The intrinsic (genetic) theory for the cause of vitiligo. In: Hann SK, Nordlund JJ, eds. *Vitiligo.* Oxford: Blackwell Science Ltd.;2000:123–128.

11. Orecchia GE. Neural pathogenesis. In: Hann SK, Nordlund JJ, eds. *Vitiligo.* Oxford: Blackwell Science Ltd.;2000: 142–150.

12. Njoo MD, Westerhof W. Vitiligo: pathogenesis and treatment. *Am J Clin Dermatol* 2001;2:167–181.

13. Klisnick A, Schmidt J, Dupond JL, et al. Vitiligo in multiple autoimmune syndrome: a retrospective study of 11 cases and a review of the literature. *Rev Med Interne* 1998;19: 348–352.

14. Hann SK, Nordlund JJ. Definition of vitiligo. In: Hann SK, Nordlund JJ, eds. *Vitiligo.* Oxford: Blackwell Science Ltd.; 2000:3–6.

15. Falabella R. Treatment of localized vitiligo by autologous minigrafting. *Arch Dermatol* 1988;124:1649–1655.

16. Mulekar SV. Melanocyte-keratinocyte cell transplantation for stable vitiligo. *Int J Dermatol* 2003;42:132–136.

17. Gupta S, Kumar B. Epidermal grafting in vitiligo: influence of age, site of lesion, and type of disease on outcome. *J Am Acad Dermatol* 2003;49:99–104.

18. Mulekar SV, Al Issa A, Al Eisa A, et al. Genital vitiligo treated by autologous, noncultured melanocyte-keratinocyte cell transplantation. *Dermatol Surg* 2005;31:1737–1740.

19. Falabella R, Arrunategui A, Barona MI, et al. The minigrafting test for vitiligo: detection of stable lesions for melanocyte transplantation. *J Am Acad Dermatol* 1995;32:228–232.

20. Falabella R. The minigrafting test: validation of a predicting tool. *J Am Acad Dermatol* 2004;51:672–673.

21. Falabella R. Surgical therapies for vitiligo. In: Hann SK, Nordlund JJ, eds. *Vitiligo.* Oxford: Blackwell Science Ltd.; 2000:193–200.

22. Falabella R, Escobar C, Borrero I. Treatment of refractory and stable vitiligo by transplantation of in vitro cultured epidermal autografts bearing melanocytes. *J Am Acad Dermatol* 1992;26:230–236.

23. Falabella R. Surgical techniques for repigmentation. In: Robinson SK, Arndt KA, LeBoit PE, et al., eds. *Atlas of Cutaneous Surgery.* Philadelphia: W.B. Saunders Co.;1996:175–184.

24. Olsson MJ, Juhlin L. Transplantation of melanocytes in vitiligo. *Br J Dermatol* 1995;132:587–911.

25. Falabella R. Grafting and transplantation of melanocytes for repigmenting vitiligo and leukoderma. *Int J Dermatol* 1989; 28:363–369.

26. Falabella R. Surgical therapies for vitiligo. *Clin Dermatol* 1997;15:927–939.

27. Falabella R, Barona M, Escobar C, et al. Surgical combination therapy for vitiligo and piebaldism. *Dermatol Surg* 1995;21: 852–857.

28. Skouge JW, Morison WL. Vitiligo treatment with a combination of PUVA therapy and epidermal autografts. *Arch Dermatol* 1995;131:1257–1258.

29. Hann SK, Im S, Bong HW, et al. Treatment of stable vitiligo with autologous epidermal grafting and PUVA. *J Am Acad Dermatol* 1995;32:943–948.

30. Behl PN. Vitiligo: treatment by dermabrasion and epithelial sheet grafting. *J Am Acad Dermatol* 1994;30:1044.

31. Falabella R. Epidermal grafting: an original technique and its application in achromic and granulating areas. *Arch Dermatol* 1971;104:592–600.

32. Falabella R. Repigmentation of segmental vitiligo by autologous minigrafting. *J Am Acad Dermatol* 1983;9:514–521.

33. Gauthier Y, Surleve-Bazeille JE. Autologous grafting with noncultured melanocytes: a simplified method for treatment of depigmented lesions. *J Am Acad Dermatol* 1992;26: 191–194.

34. Falabella R, Escobar C, Borrero I. Transplantation of in vitro cultured epidermis bearing melanocytes for repigmenting vitiligo. *J Am Acad Dermatol* 1989;21:257–264.

35. Brysk MM, Newton RC, Rajaraman S, et al. Repigmentation of vitiliginous skin by cultured cells. *Pigment Cell Res* 1989;2:202–207.

36. Mulekar SV. Long-term follow-up study of segmental and focal vitiligo treated by autologous, noncultured melanocyte-keratinocyte cell transplantation. *Arch Dermatol* 2004;140:1211–1215.

37. Mulekar SV. Melanocyte-keratinocyte cell transplantation for stable vitiligo. *Int J Dermatol* 2003;42:132–136.

38. Gauthier Y. Les techniques de greffe melanocytaire. *Ann Dermatol Venereol* 1995;122:627–631.

39. Olsson MJ, Juhlin L. Leucoderma treated by transplantation of a basal cell layer enriched suspension. *Br J Dermatol* 1998;138:644–648.

40. Kahn A, Cohen MJ. Vitiligo: treatment by dermabrasion and epithelial sheath grafting. *J Am Acad Dermatol* 1995;33:646–648.

41. McGovern TW, Bolognia J, Leffell DJ. Flip-top pigment transplantation: a novel transplantation procedure for the treatment of depigmentation. *Arch Dermatol* 1999;135:1305–1307.

42. Kim HU, Yun SK. Suction device for epidermal grafting in vitiligo: employing a syringe and a manometer to provide an adequate negative pressure. *Dermatol Surg* 2000;26:702–704.

43. Gupta S, Shroff S, Gupta S. Modified technique of suction blistering for epidermal grafting in vitiligo. *Int J Dermatol* 1999;38:306–309.

44. Peachey RD. Skin temperature and blood flow in relation to the speed of suction blister formation. *Br J Dermatol* 1971;84:447–452.

45. Oh CK, Cha JH, Lim JY, et al. Treatment of vitiligo with suction epidermal grafting by the use of an ultrapulse CO_2 laser with a computerized pattern generator. *Dermatol Surg* 2001;27:565–568.

46. Albert S, Shenoi SD. Acetate sheets in the transfer of epidermal grafts in vitiligo. *J Am Acad Dermatol* 2001;44:719–720.

47. Falabella R. Surgical therapies for vitiligo and other leukodermas, part 1: minigrafting and suction epidermal grafting. *Dermatol Ther* 2001;14:7–14.

48. Kaufmann R, Greiner D, Kippenberger S, et al. Grafting of in vitro cultured melanocytes onto laser-ablated lesions in vitiligo. *Acta Derm Venereol* 1998;78:136–138.

49. Guerra L, Capurro S, Melchi F, et al. Treatment of "stable" vitiligo by timed surgery and transplantation of cultured epidermal autografts. *Arch Dermatol* 2000;136:1380–1389.

50. Lontz W, Olsson MJ, Moellmann G, et al. Pigment cell transplantation for treatment of vitiligo: a progress report. *J Am Acad Dermatol* 1994;30:591–597.

51. Olsson MJ, Juhlin L. Transplantation of melanocytes in vitiligo. *Br J Dermatol* 1995;132:587–591.

52. Andreassi L, Pianigiani E, Andreassi A, et al. A new model of epidermal culture for the surgical treatment of vitiligo. *Int J Dermatol* 1998;37:595–598.

53. Olsson MJ, Moellman G, Lerner A, et al. Vitiligo repigmentation with cultured melanocytes after cryostorage. *Acta Derm Venereol (Stockh)* 1994;74:226–228.

54. Tomita Y, Maeda K, Tagami H. Melanocyte-stimulating properties of arachidonic acid metabolites: possible role in postinflammatory pigmentation. *Pigment Cell Res* 1992;5:357–361.

55. Tomita Y, Iwamoto M, Masuda T, et al. Stimulatory effect of prostaglandin E2 on the configuration of normal human melanocytes in vitro. *J Invest Dermatol* 1987;89:299–301.

56. Malakar S, Dhar S. Treatment of stable and recalcitrant vitiligo by autologous miniature punch grafting: a prospective study of 1,000 patients. *Dermatology* 1999;198:133–139.

57. Morelli JG, Kincannon J, Yohn JJ, et al. Leukotriene C4 and TGF-alpha are stimulators of human melanocyte migration in vitro. *J Invest Dermatol* 1992;98:290–295.

58. Horikawa T, Norris DA, Yohn JJ, et al. Melanocyte mitogens induce both melanocyte chemokinesis and chemotaxis. *J Invest Dermatol* 1995;104:256–259.

59. Falabella R. What's new in the treatment of vitiligo (editorial). *J Eur Acad Dermatol Venereol* 2001;15:287–289.

60. Falabella R. Surgical treatment of vitiligo: why, when and how (editorial). *J Eur Acad Dermatol Venereol* 2003;17:518–520.

61. Van Geel N, Ongenae K, De Mil M, et al.. Modified technique of autologous noncultured epidermal cell transplantation for repigmenting vitiligo: a pilot study. *Dermatol Surg* 2001;27:873–876.

Resurfacing Procedures

16

Microdermabrasion

Joyce Teng Ee Lim

Microdermabrasion is a popular superficial skin resurfacing procedure performed by both physicians and nonphysicians. It is a simple, safe, and easy-to-perform cosmetic procedure with almost no downtime. This procedure is suitable for all ages. It is well tolerated with minimal side effects in darker racial ethnic groups (Fitzpatrick's skin type IV through VI). Microdermabrasion is indicated for various cosmetic skin problems, including photodamage,[1,2] facial rejuvenation,[3] cutaneous hyperpigmentation,[4] acne,[5] striae,[6] and acne scars.[7] Although little is known about the exact mechanism of action, there is evidence of dermal remodeling with minimal epidermal disruption. However, most of the studies involved small groups of patients. Despite the paucity of solid scientific data, most patients and some physicians are happy with microdermabrasion and perceived benefits from it.

MICRODERMABRASION PROCEDURE

The first reported microdermabrasion was performed in Italy in 1985 by Marini and Lo Brutto, who reported both micro- and macroscopic improvement in the skin.[2] They used a closed-loop negative pressure system that used microcrystals to abrade the skin. Since then, there have been many different machines using different types of crystals and different types of suction pressure systems. Initially, aluminum oxide crystals were used, but in later units, sodium chloride, sodium bicarbonate, or magnesium oxide crystals are used to minimize the risks from chronic inhaled aluminum oxide microcrystals. Some units do not use crystals; instead they use a firm diamond wand to microabrade the skin. Other units use positive instead of negative pressure systems.

During the procedure, the microcrystals strike the skin surface at an angle, and these are drawn across the surface of the skin by negative pressure airflow. Each crystal produces microtrauma to the skin, resulting in microabrasion. The used crystals and the skin debris are simultaneously aspirated by negative pressure from the skin surface into a container, and these are then discarded. The process is repeated as the handpiece is rapidly moved across the skin.

Between each pass, a soft brush is used to wipe away excess crystals. The repetitive movement of the microcrystals across the skin causes intraepidermal injury to the skin, and this in turn causes a dermal response. Patients have to undergo several treatments to achieve the desired results. The time interval between treatments varies from 1 to 4 weeks, depending on the skin type and patient's tolerance. Each session lasts from 20 to 30 minutes.

There are several factors that affect the depth and hence the efficacy of microdermabrasion (Table 16-1). The pressure used, the flow rate of the crystals, the crystal size, and the angle at which the crystals hit the skin will determine the amount of microtrauma to the skin. The larger the crystal size, the greater will be the skin trauma, and the more acute the angle at which the crystals hit the skin, the greater will be the skin abrasion. Increasing the flow rate of crystals and the vacuum suction increases the depth of microdermabrasion. Other factors affecting the depth of microabrasion are the movement of the handpiece across the skin (the longer the dwell time, the greater the injury) and the number of passes.

There are three levels of microdermabrasion that can be achieved (Table 16-2). Level 1 corresponds to a superficial epidermal abrasion. The handpiece is passed across the skin in one to two passes to achieve a cosmetic cleaning of the skin. This is usually done on the whole cosmetic unit. Level 2 is achieved when a higher vacuum pressure and more passes are used to get to the level of the papillary dermis. Here one can see minute pinpoint bleeding. This is usually

---

Table 16-1

Factors affecting depth of microdermabrasion

- Skin type: thin/thick
- Size of crystals
- Impact of the crystals (angle)
- Amount of crystal flow (particle/sec)
- Amount of vacuum created (suction)
- Amount of passes of handpiece
- Dwell time

Table 16-2

Depth of microdermabrasion

Level 1: Down to level of epidermis

Level 2: Down to level of epidermis and in some areas to papillary dermis

Level 3: Down to level of papillary dermis and in some areas of reticular dermis

---

used for improving fine wrinkles, superficial scars, and striae. Level 3 will remove the whole epidermis, as well as a part of the dermis. This is used to improve striae, as well as wrinkles around the lips. Both levels two and three are associated with a higher incidence of side effects and should be performed by the physician. Level 2 and 3 microdermabrasion should be used with extreme care and caution in darker skin types to avoid complications, including hyperpigmentation, hypopigmentation, and scarring (Table 16-3).

INDICATIONS

Microdermabrasion is used to treat a variety of skin problems, including photodamage,[1,2] facial rejuvenation,[3] cutaneous hyperpigmentation,[4] acne,[5] striae,[6] and acne scars.[7]

Photodamage

Microdermabrasion can improve photodamaged skin, especially those with Glogau photoaging class I and II. Tan et al.[1] analyzed the effect of microdermabrasion on skin surface roughness, topography, elasticity, stiffness, compliance, temperature, sebum content, and histology. Ten patients, Fitzpatrick skin types I through III, with photodamage (Glogau

Table 16-3

Side effects of microdermabrasion

Transient erythema

Transient increased sensitivity

Transient skin dryness

Petechiae or purpura

Worsening of telangiectasia or erythema

Posttreatment hyperpigmentation

Corneal trauma

Reactivation of herpes simplex infection

Urticarial reaction

---

scale II and III) were treated at weekly intervals for five to six treatments using the Parisian Peel (Aesthetic Technologies Inc., Colorado Springs, CO). Nine patients had at least five treatments. The face received four passes at a vacuum pressure of 30 mm Hg while the periorbital skin received two passes at a pressure of 15 mm Hg. Improvement was seen in seven patients, six had mild improvement, and one had moderate improvement. The remaining three with no improvement had Glogau photoaging class III. Immediately after the procedure, there was a temporary increase in skin roughness, corresponding to the superficial abrasion, and in skin temperature, consistent with increased blood flow. Surface sebum decreased immediately after the procedure, but this effect did not persist between treatments. Skin stiffness decreased and skin compliance improved where microdermabrasion was done on the cheeks. Histologic studies did not show any change in collagen or elastic content. The epidermis showed some orthokeratosis and reduced rete ridge pattern. The upper reticular dermis showed a perivascular mononuclear cell infiltrate and vascular ectasia.

Microdermabrasion as shown by Shim et al.[2] significantly improved skin roughness/textural irregularities, mottled pigmentation, and overall skin complexion in photodamaged skin. It did not significantly improve fine skin wrinkles.

Facial rejuvenation

Microdermabrasion can improve facial aging and is often used as part of a program for facial rejuvenation. Hernandez-Perez and Ibiett[3] treated seven women, six with Glogau's photoaging class II and one with Glogau's photoaging class III. All had five microdermabrasion sessions, each having three passes per session, repeated at weekly intervals. At the start of treatment, all patients had oily skin, dilated pores, fine wrinkles, and thick skin in varying severity. There were improvements in all clinical variables after each weekly session, and the improvements were considered good to excellent. Patients also reported improvement in their self-esteem. Biopsies taken from these women before and after the fifth microdermabrasion sessions showed histopathological improvements. There was mild to moderate improvement in dermal elastosis and mild improvement in dermal inflammation, edema, and telangiectasias.

Hyperpigmentation

Microdermabrasion can improve the mottled pigmentation associated with photodamaged skin.[2] Cotellessa et al.[4] treated 20 female patients with multiple hyperpigmented macules of the face. Eight patients had complete clearance of the pigmentation after four to eight treatments, whereas ten patients had partial clearance after eight treatments. Two patients did not respond after eight treatments. When 15% trichloroacetic acid peels were combined with microdermabrasion treatments, fewer treatments (four to six) were needed to clear or partially clear the pigmentation (Fig. 16-1 and Fig. 16-2). Microdermabrasion is often

been established.[20,21] To overcome the risk from use of aluminum crystals, some machines use other crystals. Unfortunately, crystals like sodium chloride, being hygroscopic, tend to get stuck in the tubings. In Asia, crystal microdermabrasion units are slowly being replaced with noncrystal units that use a diamond-caped handpiece to abrade the skin. This has the advantage in reducing any perceived risks from inhaled crystals or eye injury. It is also more economical, as the handpiece is easily sterilized and reused without having to replace the used crystals.

CONTRAINDICATION TO MICRODERMABRASION

There are very few contraindications to the use of microdermabrasion. Patients with active skin infections, such as impetigo or viral warts, are relative contraindications. The presence of acute skin inflammation, such as pustular acne or acne rosacea, should be discouraged from the treatment until the skin condition has stabilized.

SUMMARY

Microdermabrasion is a safe and effective superficial resurfacing procedure that can improve a variety of skin problems in darker racial ethnic groups. The improvements are seen within the epidermis and dermis. Microdermabrasion is often used in conjunction with other resurfacing procedures to achieve better results. In addition, after superficially abrading the skin, it improves the penetration of adjuvant topical cosmeceuticals.

REFERENCES

1. Tan MH, Spencer J, Pires L, et al. The evaluation of aluminum oxide crystal microdermabrasion for photodamage. *Dermatol Surg* 2001;27:943–949.
2. Shim E, Barnette D, Hughes K, et al. Microdermabrasion: a clinical and histopathic study. *Dermatol Surg* 2001;27:524–530.
3. Hernandez-Perez M, Ibiett V. Gross and microscopic findings in patients undergoing microdermabrasion for facial rejuvenation. *Dermatol Surg* 2001;27:637–640.
4. Cotellessa C, Peri K, Fargnoli MC, et al. Microdermabrasion versus microdermabrasion followed by 15% trichloroacetic acid for the treatment of cutaneous hyperpigmentations in adult females. *Dermatol Surg* 2003;352–356.
5. Lloyd J. The use of microdermabrasion for acne: a pilot study. *Dermatol Surg* 2001;27:329–331.
6. Tsai RY, Wang CN, Chang HL. Aluminum oxide crystal microdermabrasion: a new technique for treating facial scarring. *Dermatol Surg* 1995;21:539–542.
7. Freedman B, Rueda-Pedraza E, Waddell S. The epidermal and dermal changes associated with microdermabrasion. *Dermatol Surg* 2001;27:1031–1034.
8. Rubin MG, Greenbaum SS. Histological effects of aluminum oxide microdermabrasion on facial skin. *J Aesthetic Dermatol* 2000;1:237–239.
9. Rajan P, Grimes P. Skin barrier changes induced by aluminum oxide and sodium chloride microdermabrasion. *Dermatol Surg* 2002;28:390–393.
10. Karimipour DJ, Kang S, Johnson TM, et al. Microdermabrasion: a molecular analysis following a single treatment. *J Am Acad Dermatol* 2005;52:215–223.
11. Alam M, Omura N, Dover J, et al. Glycolic acid peels compared to microdermabrasion: a right-left controlled trial of efficacy and patient satisfaction. *Dermatol Surg* 2002;28:475–479.
12. Song JY, Kang HA, Kim MY, et al. Damage and recovery of skin barrier function after glycolic acid chemical peeling and crystal microdermabrasion. *Dermatol Surg* 2004;30:390–394.
13. Shelton RM. Prevention of cross-contamination when using microdermabrasion equipment. *Cutis* 2003;72:266–268.
14. Warmuth IP, Bader R, Scarborough DA, et al. Herpes simplex infection after microdermabrasion. *Cosmet Dermatol* 1999; 12(7):13.
15. Farris P, Rietschel R. An unusual acute urticarial response following microdermabrasion. *Dermatol Surg* 2002;28: 606–608.
16. Jederlinci PJ, Abraham JL, Chung A, et al. Pulmonary fibrosis in aluminum oxide workers. Investigation of nine workers with pathologic examination and microanalysis in three of them. *Am Rev Respir Dis* 1990;142:1179–1184.
17. Masalkhi A, Walton SP. Pulmonary fibrosis and occupational exposure to aluminum. *J Ky Med Assoc* 1994;92:59–61.
18. Townsend MC, Enterline PE, Sussman NB, et al. Pulmonary function in relation to total dust exposure at a bauxite refinery and alumina-based chemical products plant. *Am Rev Respir Dis* 1990;142:1172–1178.
19. World Health Organization. Physical and chemical properties of air-borne particles. In: World Health Organization. *Evaluation of Exposure to Airborne Particles in the Work Environment.* Publication #80. Geneva: WHO;1984:360–370.
20. McLachlan DR. Aluminum and Alzheimer's disease. *Neurobiol Aging* 1986;7:525–532.
21. Makjanic J, McDonald B, Li-Hsian Chen CP, et al. Absence of aluminum in neurofibrillary tangles in Alzheimer's disease. *Neurosci Lett* 1998;240:123–126.

17

Superficial Chemical Peels

Pearl E. Grimes, Marta I. Rendon, and Juan Pellerano

The ancient Egyptians were among the first civilizations in recorded history to use chemicals as exfoliating agents for aesthetic purposes. They used alabaster, animal oils, and salt.[1,2] The Greeks and Romans used pumice, myrrh, frankincense, mustard, and sulfur for lightening the skin and improvement of wrinkles. Early reports of chemical peeling in Europe were described by Fox, Hebra, and Unna.[3,4] In 1882, Unna described his experiences using a variety of peeling agents, including resorcinol, phenol, trichloroacetic acid (TCA), and salicylic acid. The experiences of the aforementioned dermatologists pioneered the use of chemical peels in dermatology.

Chemical peeling or chemical exfoliation is a form of skin resurfacing whereby exfoliating chemical agents are applied to the skin surface to induce epidermal and/or dermal injury/destruction. Peeling agents induce controlled wounding of the skin followed by organized repair. The desired outcome of peeling procedures is generation of a new epidermis and dermal collagen remodeling. Dyschromias, photodamage, and rhytides are often improved.

In 1982, Stegman reported the histologic effects of three peeling agents, including TCA, full-strength phenol, Baker's phenol, and dermabrasion on normal and sun-damaged skin of the neck.[5] This study demonstrated that 40% to 60% TCA caused epidermal necrosis, papillary dermal edema, and homogenization to the midreticular dermis 3 days after peeling. Findings were similar in sun-damaged compared with non–sun-damaged skin. Ninety days after peeling, Stegman observed an expanded papillary dermis, which he defined as the *Grenz zone*. The thickness of the Grenz zone increased as the depth of peeling increased. The investigative work of Stegman and others facilitated our understanding of the capacity of medium-depth and deep peeling agents to restore epidermal and dermal order.

Others have assessed the histologic and ultrastructural changes of chemical peeling. Nelson et al.[6] assessed the effects of a combination Jessner's solution and 35% TCA peel. Biopsies were performed at baseline, 2 weeks, and 3 months. Type I collagen increased after peeling. Ultrastructural features of the skin after peeling included markedly decreased epidermal intracytoplasmic vacuoles, decreased elastic fibers, and increased activated fibroblasts. These data further substantiated the effects of chemical peeling agents for improvement of photodamage and rhytides.

Chemical peeling agents are classified as superficial, medium-depth, or deep peels.[7] Superficial peels target the stratum corneum to the papillary dermis (Fig. 17-1). They include glycolic acid, salicylic acid, Jessner's solution, tretinoin, and TCA in concentrations of 10% to 30%. Medium-depth peels penetrate to the upper reticular dermis and include TCA (35%–50%), combination glycolic acid 70%/TCA 35%, Jessner's/TCA 35%, and phenol 88%. Deep chemical peels utilize the Baker-Gordon formula and penetrate to the midreticular dermis. The depth of the chemical peel determines the efficacy, outcome, and safety of the procedure.

INDICATIONS FOR CHEMICAL PEELING IN DARKER SKIN TYPES

Dark skin demonstrates significantly greater intrinsic photoprotection because of the increased content of epidermal melanin (see Chapter 2). Clinical photodamage, actinic keratoses, rhytides, and skin malignancies are less common problems in deeply pigmented skin. However, darker skin types are frequently plagued with dyschromias because of the labile responses of cutaneous melanocytes in deeply pigmented individuals (see Chapter 2). Despite major concerns regarding peel complications such as postinflammatory hyperpigmentation, hypopigmentation, and scarring in darker racial ethnic groups, recent studies suggest that peeling procedures, particularly superficial peeling, can be safely performed in darker skin.

Hence, peel indications differ between light and dark skin (Table 17-1). Key indications in Fitzpatrick's skin types I, II, and III include photodamage, rhytides, acne, scarring, and the dyschromias characterized by hyperpigmentation. In contrast, key indications in darker skin types include disorders of hyperpigmentation, such as melasma and postinflammatory hyperpigmentation, acne, pseudofolliculitis barbae, textural changes, oily skin and wrinkles, and photodamage.

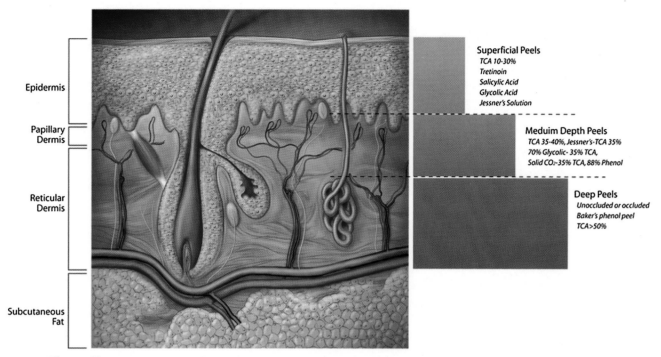

Figure 17-1 Cross section of skin illustrating the depth of wounding caused by chemical peeling agents.

Grimes[8] compared the histologic alterations induced by a variety of chemical peels in 17 patients with skin types IV, V, and VI, including glycolic acid 70%, salicylic acid 30%, Jessner's solution, and 25% and 30% TCA. Peels were applied to 4 × 4–cm areas of the back and 2 × 2–cm postauricular sites. Biopsies were performed at 24 hours (Fig. 17-2A–D). Glycolic acid induced the most significant stratum corneum necrosis. Compared with the other tested peels, salicylic acid and Jessner's peels caused mild lympho-histiocytic dermal infiltrates. The most severe damage was induced by 25% and 30% TCA, which caused deep epidermal necrosis and dense papillary dermal lymphohistiocytic infiltrates. TCA test sites developed postinflammatory hyperpigmentation. These findings corroborate our clinical experience using these agents. In general, glycolic, salicylic acid, and Jessner's peels induce a lower frequency of post-peeling complications compared with 25% and 30% superficial TCA peels.

GENERAL CONSIDERATIONS FOR PATIENT PREPARATION

Peel preparation varies with the condition being treated. Regimens differ for photodamage, hyperpigmentation (melasma and postinflammatory hyperpigmentation), acne vulgaris, and other conditions. In addition, there are special issues to be considered when treating darker racial ethnic groups. A detailed history and cutaneous examination should be performed in all patients before chemical peeling. Standardized photographs are taken of the areas to be peeled, including full-face frontal and lateral views.

Use of topical retinoids (tretinoin, tazarotene, retinol formulations) for 2 to 6 weeks before peeling thin the stratum corneum and enhance epidermal turnover. Such agents also reduce the content of epidermal melanin and

Table 17-1	
Chemical peel indications in skin types I–III versus skin types IV–VI	
Skin types I–III	Skin types IV–VI
Fine wrinkles, rhytids	Postinflammatory hyperpigmentation
Solar keratoses	Melasma
Photodamage	Acne vulgaris
Melasma	Oily skin
Postinflammatory hyperpigmentation	Textural changes
Acne vulgaris	Acne scarring
Rosacea	Fine wrinkles
Superficial scarring	

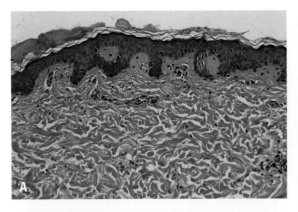

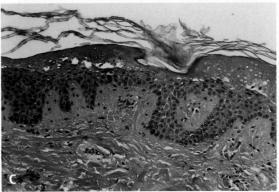

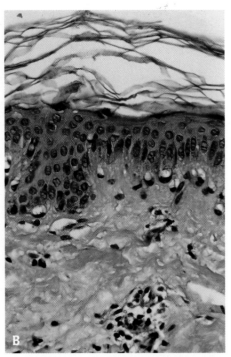

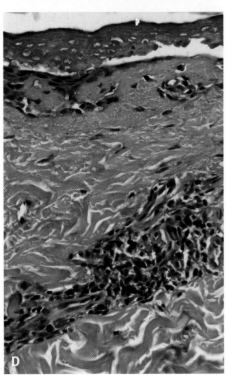

Figure 17-2 Hematoxylin/eosin stains of biopsies of black skin taken 24 hours postchemical peeling. **A:** Glycolic acid 70%. Note stratum corneum necrosis. **B:** Salicylic acid 30%. Note mild lymphohistiocytic infiltrate. **C:** A 25% TCA-peel induced midepidermal wounding/separation. **D:** A 30% TCA peel caused deep epidermal separation. Note lymphohistiocytic infiltrate.

expedite epidermal healing. Retinoids also enhance the penetration and depth of chemical peeling. Optimal effects are demonstrated with these agents when treating photodamage in Fitzpatrick skin types I to III. They can be used until 1 or 2 days before peeling. Retinoids can be resumed postoperatively after all evidence of peeling and desquamation subsides.

In contrast to photodamage, when treating conditions such as melasma and postinflammatory hyperpigmentation, retinoids should either be discontinued 1 or 2 weeks before peeling or completely eliminated from the peeling prep to avoid postpeel complications, such as excessive erythema, desquamation, and postinflammatory hyperpigmentation. These conditions are more common in darker racial ethnic groups, populations at greater risk for post-peel complications. Similar precautions should be taken in acne patients with darker skin types (V and VI).

Topical alpha hydroxy acid or polyhydroxy acid formulations can also be used to prep the skin. In general, they are less aggressive agents in affecting peel outcomes. The skin is usually prepped for 2 to 4 weeks with a formulation of hydroquinone 4% or higher compounded formulations (5%–10%) to reduce epidermal melanin. This is extremely important when treating the aforementioned dyschromias. Although less effective, other topical bleaching agents include azelaic acid, kojic acid, arbutin, and licorice. Patients can also resume use of topical bleaching agents postoperatively after peeling, and irritation subsides. Broad-spectrum sunscreens (UVA and UVB) should be worn daily.

A flare of herpes following a superficial chemical peel is rare. Hence, pretreatment with antiviral therapy is usually not indicated. However, one can prophylactically treat with antiviral therapies including valacyclovir 500 mg twice a day, famciclovir 500 mg twice a day, or acyclovir 400 mg twice a day for 7 to 10 days beginning 1 or 2 days before the procedure.

GLYCOLIC ACID PEELS

Alpha hydroxy acid (AHA) peels have been shown to improve the skin surface by thinning the stratum corneum, promoting epidermolysis, dispersing basal layer melanin, and increasing collagen synthesis within the dermis[9] (Fig. 17-3). The most common AHAs used as peeling agents are glycolic acid, lactic acid, mandelic acid, and, recently, pyruvic acid. Glycolic acid peels decrease hyperpigmentation through a wounding and re-epithelization process. Glycolic acid is the best-known superficial peeling agent, having been used in clinical practice since the 1800s. It is part of the family of alpha hydroxy acids, which occur naturally in foods. Glycolic acid is used in strengths ranging from 20% to 70% to treat a variety of defects of the epidermis and papillary dermis on almost any area of the body.

Moy et al.[10] assessed the efficacy of several commonly used peeling agents, including glycolic acid in a mini pig model. The chemical peels were applied in different concentrations to 2 cm × 2 cm patches and left on the skin for 15 minutes. The following concentrations were used: phenol-Bakers, 25%, 50%, 75%, and 88%; TCA, 25%, 50%, 75%; glycolic acid, 50%, 70%; and pyruvic acid, 50%, 100%. Biopsies were taken from each site at 1, 7, and 21 days postpeel and evaluated for epidermal changes, inflammation, and collagen

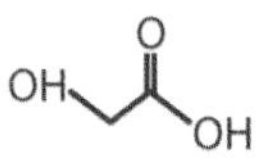

Glycolic acid

Figure 17-3 Chemical structure of glycolic acid.

deposition. The Baker phenol peel caused the most inflammation and nonspecific reaction but also a large amount of new collagen deposition. At 1 day postpeel, larger concentrations of phenol and TCA caused the most epidermal sloughing and inflammation. The extent of the reaction was directly proportional to collagen deposition at 21 days.[10] Although the authors concluded that glycolic acid and pyruvic acid caused the least nonspecific reaction, they found the resulting collagen deposition to be disproportionately large. These findings suggest a direct stimulatory effect by the two acids on collagen production.

Another study assessed the damage and recovery of skin barrier function after glycolic acid chemical peeling and crystal microdermabrasion.[9] Noninvasive bioengineering methods were used in the study. Superficial chemical peeling was conducted with 30%, 50%, and 70% glycolic acid and aluminum oxide crystal microdermabrasion on the forearms of 13 women. Skin response was measured by visual observation and use of an evaporimeter, corneometer, and colorimeter at set intervals before and after peeling. Results of this study suggest that the skin barrier function is damaged by glycolic acid peeling and aluminum oxide crystal microdermabrasion but recovers within 1 to 4 days. Therefore, repeating the superficial peeling procedure at 2-week intervals will allow sufficient time for the damaged skin to recover its barrier function.

Glycolic acid formulations

Glycolic acid peeling agents include buffered, partially neutralized, and esterified formulations. Generally, peeling strengths range from 20% to 70%. The efficacy of glycolic peels can depend on the pH, strength, and time of application. Unbuffered formulations with low pH have the potential to induce greater epidermal and dermal damage.

Indications

Glycolic peels can be used on all body areas and Fitzpatrick skin types. The main symptoms of skin types IV to VI are dyschromias, including melasma and post-inflammatory hyperpigmentation from acne or burns. Other indications are photodamage, rosacea, and pseudofolliculitis barbae.[11,12]

Several studies were conducted to evaluate whether a series of glycolic acid peels would provide improvement in dark-skinned patients when combined with topical regimens, such as hydroquinone, tretinoin, or topical steroids.

Sarkar et al.[13] assessed the efficacy of a series of glycolic acid peels when combined with a topical bleaching agent compared with use of the bleaching formula alone in a series of dark-skinned patients with melasma. The authors compared the efficacy of serial glycolic acid peeling with a series three 30% glycolic peels and three 40% peels in combination with the modified Kligman bleaching formulation (hydroquinone 5%, hydrocortisone acetate 1%, and tretinoin 0.05%) and with the bleaching formula alone. Forty women were included in each group.

Both groups showed a statistically significant improvement in the Melasma Area Severity Index (MASI) score at 21 weeks. However, maximal improvement occurred in the group treated with the series of glycolic acid peels in combination with the topical bleaching regimen.

An 8-week, split-face study of 21 Hispanic women with bilateral epidermal and mixed melasma found no significant difference between combination therapy using glycolic acid peels plus a topical regimen of hydroquinone compared with hydroquinone alone.[14] Patients underwent a glycolic acid peel every 2 weeks plus topical hydroquinone 4% twice daily. Only hydroquinone 4% was applied daily to the opposite side of the face. Both groups showed significant reduction in skin pigmentation compared with baseline. Unfortunately, these two studies used different measurement devices, product concentrations, and frequency of peels. This might explain the differences in results. In our experience, we have noted that the addition of glycolic acid peels to any hyperpigmentation regimen usually accelerates the rate of improvement as well as improves the tone, texture, and color of the skin (Fig. 17-4A,B and Fig. 17-5A,B).

A series of 10 Asian women with melasma and fine wrinkles were treated with 2% hydroquinone and 10% glycolic acid applied to both sides of the face.[15] A series of 20% to 70% glycolic peels were performed on one side for comparison. Greater improvement with minimal side effects were noted on the side treated with glycolic acid

peels. In another study, 40 Asian patients with moderate to moderately severe acne were treated with a series of 35% to 70% glycolic acid peels.[16] The investigators noted significant improvement in skin texture and acne. Side effects were reported in 5.6% of patients.

Nineteen black patients with postinflammatory hyperpigmentation were treated with glycolic acid peeling.[17] The control group was treated with 2% hydroquinone/10% glycolic acid twice a day and tretinoin 0.05% at bedtime, whereas the active peel group received the same topical regimen plus a series of six serial glycolic acid peels. Although not statistically significant, greater improvement was noted in the chemical peel group.

The safety and efficacy of a series of glycolic acid facial peels were investigated in 25 Indian women with melasma.[18] Patients were treated with 50% glycolic acid peels monthly for 3 months. Improvement was noted in 91% of patients with maximal clearing occurring in patients classified with epidermal melasma. Side effects were observed in one patient who developed brow hyperpigmentation.

In patients with photodamage, AHA peels and topical products may be combined with retinoids and other antioxidants for maximum benefit. The synergistic effects of fluorouracil and glycolic acid have been observed in the treatment of actinic keratoses. For patients with melasma, AHA peels and combination products containing bleaching agents such as hydroquinone, kojic acid, and glycolic

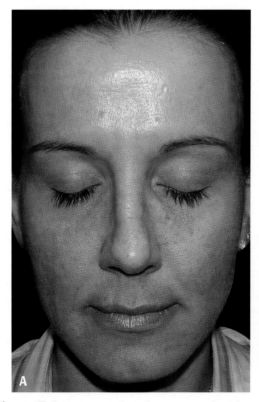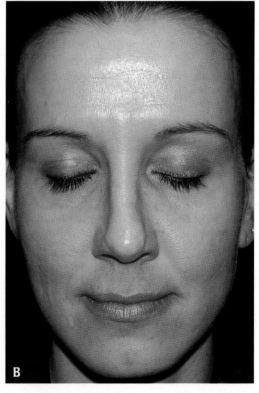

Figure 17-4 Patient with melasma treated with triple combination bleaching agent (Tri-Luma) and a series of glycolic acid peels. **A:** Before. **B:** After.

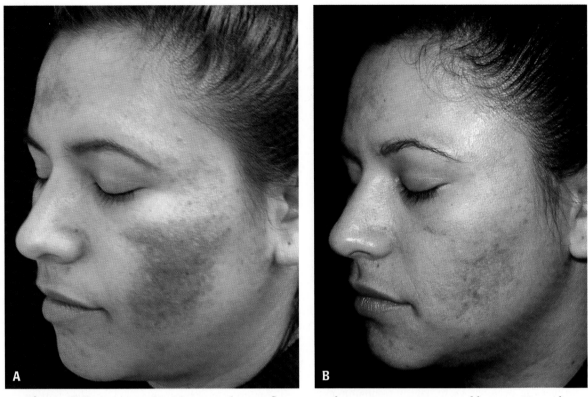

Figure 17-5 Patient with melasma and postinflammatory hyperpigmentation caused by acne. Treated with glycolic acid peeling and triple combination bleaching agent (Tri-Luma). **A:** Before. **B:** After.

acid have increased efficacy. Dark-skinned patients with acne, mild acne scarring, rosacea, and rhytids can obtain results with antibacterial agents and topical retinoids supplemented with AHA peels and lotions.[19]

Contraindications

Absolute contraindications to peels include history of allergy to the peeling solution, neutralizing agent, diluting agent, or any of their components. Relative contraindications can include photosensitization potentially caused from medications or supplements, prior cosmetic surgery, extensive exposure to sun, smoking, poor general physical or mental health, unrealistic expectations, and history of herpetic lesions. There are hypotheses both supporting and contraindicating their use in pregnant women, but evidence is lacking.

Peeling technique

There are general rules that should be followed when applying glycolic acid peels. The area can be cleansed with 70% isopropyl alcohol or acetone using cotton balls, 2 inch × 2 inch gauze, or sponges. The orbicular angles, nasolabial folds, and lips should be protected with white petrolatum. The eyes should be covered with moistened gauze. If working on the eyelids, tetracycline ointment should be applied at the lid margin to protect the eyes. The peeling agent can be applied with cotton balls, sable brush, or 3 inch × 3 inch gauze. The response of the skin should be monitored visually while remaining alert to

mild discomfort, burning, and temporary mild darkening of the skin, which are common during the procedure. Skin contact with glycolic acid should take place for 2 to 6 minutes. Glycolic acid peels are neutralized with 10% sodium bicarbonate solution.

Complications

In general, glycolic acid peels are tolerated well in darker racial ethnic groups. However, hyperpigmentation, hypopigmentation, and scarring can indeed occur with aggressive use of glycolic peeling formulations.[11,19] Side effects can be minimized when concentrations are gradually titrated from the lower concentrations of 20% to 35% to full strength 70% glycolic acid (Fig. 17-6).

SALICYLIC ACID

Salicylic acid (ortho-hydroxybenzoic acid) is a beta hydroxy acid agent (Fig. 17-7). It is a lipophilic compound that removes intercellular lipids that are covalently linked to the cornified envelope surrounding cornified epithelioid cells.[20] Because of its antihyperplastic effects on the epidermis, multiple investigators have used salicylic acid as a peeling agent.[21–23] Recently, histologic assessments using salicylic acid peels in hairless mice reported loss of cornified cells followed by activation of epidermal basal cells and underlying fibroblasts. These findings suggest that salicylic

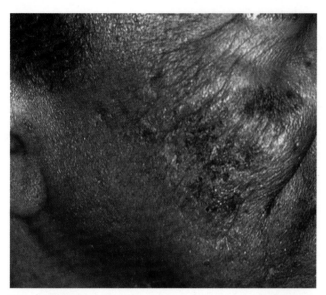

Figure 17-6 Transient hyperpigmentation following a glycolic acid 30% chemical peel in an individual with skin type V.

acid peeling can alter the underlying dermal tissue without directly wounding the tissue or causing inflammation.[24] Salicylic acid has also been shown to have anti-inflammatory and antimicrobial properties.

Formulations

A variety of formulations of salicylic acid have been used as peeling agents. These include 50% ointment formulations[21,22] as well as 10%, 20%, and 30% ethanol formulations.[23,25] More recently, commercial formulations of salicylic acid have become available (BioGlan Pharmaceuticals company, Malvern, PA; Bionet Esthetics, Little Rock, AR).

Indications

The efficacy of salicylic acid peeling has been assessed in several studies. Fifty percent salicylic acid ointment peeling was first used by Aronsohn to treat 81 patients who had freckles, pigmentation, and aging changes of the hands.[22] He reported excellent results. Subsequently, Swinehart[21] successfully used a methyl-salicylate buffered, croton oil-containing, 50% salicylic acid ointment paste for treatment of lentigines, pigmented keratoses, and actinically damaged skin of the dorsal hands and forearms. After pretreatment

Salicylic acid

COOH

OH

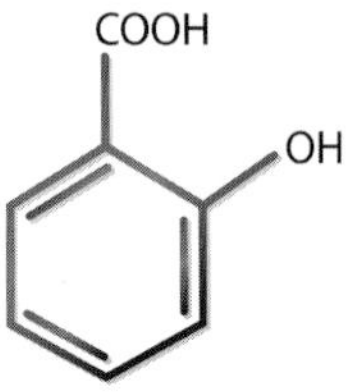

Figure 17-7 Chemical structure of salicylic acid.

with topical tretinoin and localized TCA 20%, the 50% salicylic acid paste was applied to the affected area and occluded for 48 hours. Following dressing removal, peeling and desquamation occurred and was relatively complete by the tenth day. Overall results were described as excellent. Despite these results, salicylic acid peeling did not move into the arena of popular peeling techniques until the mid-1990s when Kligman and Kligman[23] ushered salicylic acid into the current arena of superficial peeling agents. They treated 50 women with mild to moderate photodamage, reporting improvement in pigmented lesions, surface roughness, and reduction in fine lines. Grimes[26] reported substantial efficacy and minimal side effects in 25 patients treated with 20% and 30% salicylic acid peels in darker racial ethnic groups. Conditions treated included acne vulgaris, melasma, and post-inflammatory hyperpigmentation. Thirty-five Korean patients with facial acne were treated biweekly for 12 weeks with 30% salicylic acid peels.[27] Both inflammatory and noninflammatory lesions were significantly improved. In general, the peel was well tolerated with few side effects.

Given these findings, some of the indications for salicylic acid peels include acne vulgaris (inflammatory and noninflammatory lesions), acne rosacea, melasma, postinflammatory hyperpigmentation, freckles, lentigines, mild to moderate photodamage, and texturally rough skin.

Contraindications

In general, there are few contraindications to salicylic acid chemical peeling. Salicylic acid peels are well tolerated in all skin types (Fitzpatrick's I through VI) and all racial ethnic groups. General contraindications include salicylate hypersensitivity/allergy; unrealistic patient expectations; active inflammation/dermatitis or infection at the salicylic acid peeling site; acute viral infection; pregnancy; and isotretinoin therapy within 3 to 6 months of the peeling procedure. One of the authors (Grimes) has performed more than 1,000 salicylic acid peels without observing any evidence of salicylate allergy/hypersensitivity afterward.

Peeling technique

Despite some general predictable outcomes, even superficial chemical peeling procedures can cause hyperpigmentation and undesired results. Popular standard salicylic acid peeling techniques involve the use of 20% and 30% salicylic acid in an ethanol formulation. Salicylic acid peels are performed at 2- to 4-week intervals. Maximal results are achieved with a series of three to six peels.

The initial peel is always performed with a 20% concentration to assess the patient's sensitivity and reactivity. A standard peel tray setup includes a fan, alcohol or acetone for prepping, a spray bottle for water, gauze sponges, cotton-tipped swabs, a soapless cleanser, a bland moisturizer, and a timer. Before treatment, the face is thoroughly cleansed with alcohol and/or acetone to remove oils. The peel is then applied with wedge sponges, 2 inch × 2 inch gauge sponges, or cotton-tipped applicators. Cotton-tipped swabs can also be used to apply the peeling agent to periorbital areas. A total of two to three coats of salicylic acid is usually applied. The acid is first applied to the medial cheeks working laterally, followed by application to the perioral area, chin, and forehead. The peel is left on for 3 to 5 minutes. Most patients experience some mild burning and stinging during the procedure. After 1 to 3 minutes, some patients experience mild peel-related anesthesia of the face. Portable handheld fans substantially mitigate the sensation of burning and stinging.

A white precipitate, representing crystallization of the salicylic acid, begins to form at 30 seconds to 1 minute following peel application (Fig. 17-8A–E). This should not be confused with frosting or whitening of the skin, which represents protein agglutination. Frosting usually indicates that the patient will observe some crusting and peeling following the procedure. This may be appropriate when treating photodamage. However, it is best to have minimal to no frosting when treating other conditions. After 3 to 5 minutes, the face is thoroughly rinsed with tap water, and a bland cleanser, such as Cetaphil, is used to remove any residual salicylic acid precipitate. A bland moisturizer is applied after rinsing. Efficacious bland moisturizers include Cetaphil, Purpose, Theraplex, and SBR Lipocream (Fig. 17-9A,B, Fig. 17-10A,B, and Fig. 17-11A,B).

Bland cleansers and moisturizers are continued for 48 hours or until all postpeel irritation subsides. Patients are then able to resume the use of their topical skin care regimen, including topical bleaching agents, acne medications, and/or retinoids. Postpeel adverse reactions, such as excessive desquamation and irritation, are treated with low- to high-potency topical steroids. Topical steroids are extremely effective in resolving postpeel inflammation and mitigating the complication of postinflammatory hyperpigmentation. Any residual postinflammatory hyperpigmentation usually resolves with use of topical hydroquinone formulations following salicylic acid peeling.

Side effects

Side effects of salicylic acid peeling are mild and transient (Fig. 17-12). In a series of 35 Korean patients, 8.8% had prolonged erythema that lasted more than 2 days.[27] Dryness occurred in 32.3%, responding to frequent applications of moisturizers. Intense exfoliation occurred in 17.6%, clearing in 7 to 10 days. Crusting was noted in 11.7%. There were no cases of persistent postinflammatory hyperpigmentation or scarring. In a series of 25 patients comprising 20 African Americans and 5 Hispanics, 16% experienced mild side effects.[26] One patient experienced temporary crusting and hypopigmentation that cleared in 7 days. Three patients had transient dryness and hyperpigmentation that resolved in 7 to 14 days.

Salicylism, or salicylic acid toxicity, is characterized by rapid breathing, tinnitus, hearing loss, dizziness, abdominal cramps, and central nervous system reactions. It has been reported with 20% salicylic acid applied to 50% of the body surface, and it has also been reported with use of 40% and 50% salicylic acid paste preparations.[28] One of the authors (Grimes) has peeled more than 1,000 patients with the current 20% and 30% marketed ethanol formulations and has observed no cases of salicylism.

Advantages and disadvantages

Salicylic acid is one of the best peeling agents for patients who have skin types IV to VI in that it is efficacious with minimal complications. It is an excellent peeling agent in patients with acne vulgaris. Given the appearance of the white precipitate, uniformity of application is easily achieved. After several minutes, the peel can induce an anesthetic effect, increasing patient tolerance. However, the agent has a limited depth of peeling and minimal efficacy in patients with significant photodamage.

JESSNER'S PEEL

Jessner's solution has been used for more than 100 years as a therapeutic agent to treat hyperkeratotic epidermal lesions.[29] This superficial peeling agent constitutes a mixture of salicylic acid, resorcinol, and lactic acid in 95% ethanol (Fig. 17-13). Jessner's solution causes loss of corneocyte cohesion and induces intercellular and intracellular edema. Jessner's typically induces wounding to the level of the papillary dermis. Historically, resorcinol (a key component of Jessner's peels) was used in concentrations of 10% to 50% in the early 20th century. High concentrations of resorcinol were associated with side effects such as allergic contact dermatitis, irritant contact dermatitis, and skin discoloration. Subsequently, Jessner's solution was formulated by Dr. Max Jessner to lower the concentrations of any one agent contained in the mixture and to enhance its overall effects as a keratolytic agent.

Each component of Jessner's solution has specific effects. Salicylic acid (orthohydroxy benzoic acid) is a beta-hydroxy acid agent.[30] It is a lipophilic compound that removes intercellular lipids that are covalently linked to the cornified envelope surrounding epithelial cells.[20] It also enhances penetration of other agents. Resorcinol (m-dihydroxy benzene) is structurally and chemically similar to phenol. It disrupts the weak hydrogen bonds of keratin.[31] Lactic acid is an alpha hydroxy acid that causes corneocyte detachment and subsequent desquamation of the stratum corneum.[32] It has been used to treat acne, melasma, postinflammatory hyperpigmentation, lentigines, freckles, and photodamage.

Formulations

The standard formulation of Jessner's solution contains resorcinol (14 g), salicylic acid (14g), and lactic acid (85%, 14 g) mixed in a sufficient quantity of ethanol to make 100 mL. Solutions are also available that do not contain resorcinol (Delasco, Council Bluffs, IA). Modified Jessner's

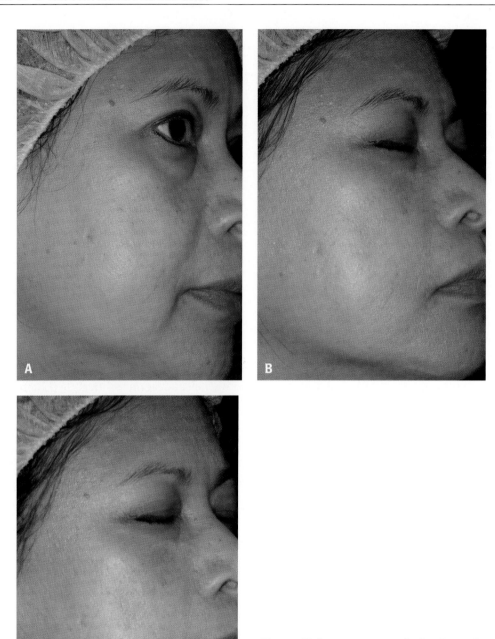

Figure 17-8 Progression of salicylic acid peel. **A:** Baseline before application of peel. **B:** One minute after peel application. **C:** Two minutes after peel application (note more intense precipitate representing complete crystallization of salicylic acid).

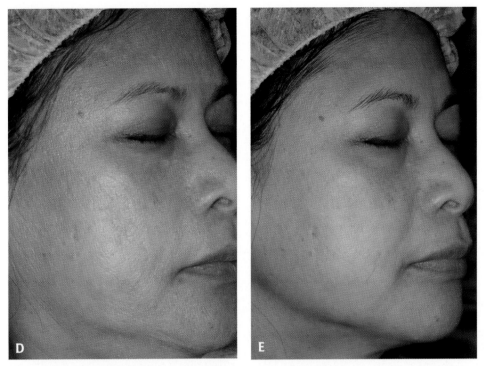

Figure 17-8 (*Continued*) **D:** Complete crystallization of salicylic acid precipitate achieved 4 minutes after peel application. **E:** Postpeel after salicylic acid precipitate removed.

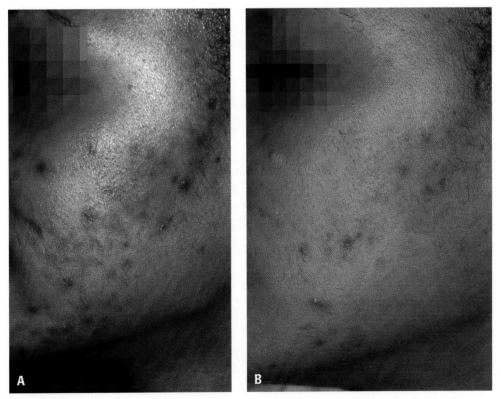

Figure 17-9 Before and after series of five salicylic acid peels for postinflammatory hyperpigmentation. **A:** Baseline. **B:** After.

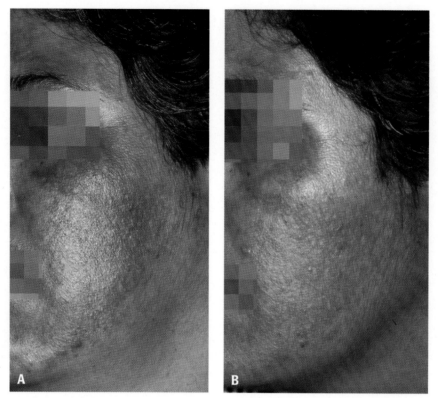

Figure 17-10 Before and after series of five salicylic acid peels for treatment of melasma. **A:** Baseline. **B:** After.

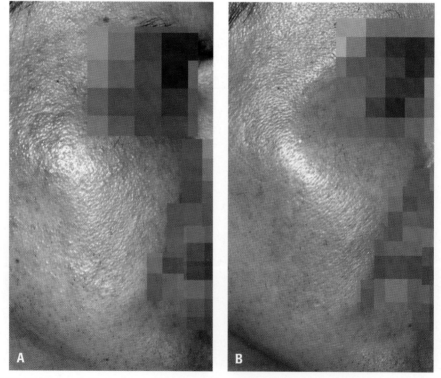

Figure 17-11 Before and after series of five salicylic acid peels for textural changes in oily skin. **A:** Baseline. **B:** After.

The deep phenol chemical peel does offer some advantages. It acts as an excellent tool in providing a striking improvement of advanced photoaging skin, wrinkles, and especially in the perioral area and acne scars (Table 18-2), despite the advent of resurfacing lasers in cosmetic surgery. A single deep chemical peel is required to achieve the desired results, and the effect is long lasting. The disadvantages are that the recovery time for a deep chemical peel is the longest and rather uncomfortable as the patient experiences discomfort, swelling, erythema, oozing, crusting, and peeling for more than a week at least. For about 2 to 3 months following a deep chemical peel, the skin will appear sunburned in appearance. The side effects are more pronounced in persons with darker and oily skin and those with freckles. Side effects include permanent pallor of the skin with inability to tan, scarring, and uneven skin pigmentation with lines of demarcation between peeled and nonpeeled skin. Cardiac arrhythmias, renal toxicity, and laryngeal edema are other limiting systemic side effects.[21–23] As the risks of deep chemical peels far outweigh the advantages, this procedure is usually not carried out in darker-skinned patients.[9]

Each ingredient of the Baker-Gordon phenol peel serves a specific function. Because of the sulfide bond disruption, phenol causes keratolysis and protein coagulation. Septisol is a surfactant, which offers a more uniform penetration through the skin by decreasing the skin surface tension. Croton oil also further enhances phenol absorption by causing epidermolysis.[12] All these ingredients are mixed in a clean glass cup just before the peel procedure. The other ways to increase the absorption of phenol peels, besides croton oil and Septisol, are by diluting the phenol concentration from 88% to 55% and by occlusion or taping. Recently, Hetter changed the concentration of croton oil in his version, the phenol croton oil peel, to make a less destructive and safer version of the Baker-Gordon phenol peel.[24,25] This provided a more natural-appearing skin color and texture. The method of performing a deep peel follows.

Prepeel evaluation and preparation

The prepeel evaluation and priming of the skin is essentially the same as for a medium peel. Perioperative antibiotics and antiviral agents may be started a night before the procedure and may be continued for 10 days thereafter. A full-face deep chemical peel takes 1 to 2 hours to perform, and a more limited procedure (treatment of wrinkling above the lip) may take less than half an hour. The presence of cardiac and hepatorenal disease should be ruled out. It is advisable to perform an electrocardiogram (ECG), a complete blood cell count, hepatorenal profile, serum electrolytes, and chest x-ray examination before the procedure.

Sedation and anaesthesia

The deep chemical peel is carried out by a trained cosmetic surgery professional in a doctor's office, hospital, or surgery center. Heavy sedation or general anaesthesia must administered for the procedure.

The deep chemical peel procedure

It is advisable to carry out the deep peel procedure in a medically supervised environment, where emergency cardiopulmonary resuscitation equipment is available and the patient can be monitored for blood pressure, pulse, and cardiac activity to avoid the arrhythmic complications of phenol toxicity.[21–23] Before the procedure, an ECG is performed. To decrease phenol absorption and lower serum phenol levels, two procedures are carried out. First, the face is divided into five to eight cosmetic units, and each segment is peeled sequentially at 15-minute intervals, allowing the procedure to be spread out over 60 to 120 minutes. Second, the patient is hydrated with a liter of lactated Ringer's solution before the procedure and another liter of the fluid during and after the peel. The peel solution is applied to the area to be treated (avoiding the eyes, brows, and lips). There can be a slight burning sensation, but it is usually minimal as the solution also acts as an anesthetic. After leaving the peel solution on for the desired effect, it is neutralized with copious amounts of water. Thymol can also be used to stop the phenol peel. In case a deeper peel is desired, occlusion in the form of either taping or a nonpermeable membrane or thick petroleum jelly is used. About 1 hour after the procedure, a thick coating of petroleum jelly is layered over the patient's face, covering the protective crust that develops rapidly over the area. Alternatively, the patient's face can be covered by a "mask" composed of strips of adhesive tape with opening for the eyes and mouth. The patient is released from the hospital after the procedure and allowed to recover at home.

Postpeel period

The patient can experience discomfort, swelling, erythema, oozing, crusting, flaking, and peeling. A few days after the peel, new skin with bright pink color will emerge and then fade within a few days. After about 2 weeks, this coloration can be covered with makeup. Postoperative swelling and difficulty in opening the eyes also subsides in a few days, but the skin remains sensitive. Analgesics can be given in the postpeel period to decrease the discomfort and swelling. Sun protection and use of broad-spectrum sunscreens are extremely important after a deep chemical peel and should be continued for 6 months after the peel along with a good bleaching maintenance regime. The patient can resume normal work schedule and other activities after 2 weeks. For about 2 to 3 months following a deep chemical peel, the skin has a sunburned appearance as re-epithelialization takes place. At the end of this period, the skin appears extremely pale. After re-epithelialization occurs, maintenance therapy with bleaching agents can be started. Follow-up visits should be done every 2 to 3 days after re-epithelialization is complete, then every week for the next 2 to 3 months. Steroids must be avoided in the postpeel period as they interfere with the thickening process of the new skin. Deep chemical peels should not be performed before 1 year after the prior peel.

Combination procedures

For facial rejuvenation procedures, to obtain a natural appearance of the skin, the cosmetic units of the face are blended together. Deep chemical peels or laser resurfacing are usually applied to the perioral and periorbital areas. The forehead, cheeks, and chin are treated with a medium-depth peel and the neck is treated with a superficial chemical peel. The blending of these cosmetic units avoids demarcation lines and shortens the postoperative healing period.

Combined chemical peels with dermabrasion, laser, and dermasanding

Chemabrasion—or applying 50% TCA to the entire face followed by dermabrasion with topical cryoanesthesia, which was used for acne pitting and scarring—has been discarded because of postoperative scarring and pigmentary alterations that resulted from 50% TCA.[12] Pulsed CO_2 laser resurfacing system, as opposed to medium-depth and deep chemical peels, can eradicate the deeper wrinkles in the perioral and periorbital regions more effectively. A combined procedure is used for photoaging skin to obtain improved results: CO_2 laser for perioral and periorbital units, Jessner's plus 35% TCA for the remaining facial skin, and only Jessner's solution for the neck. The peel is performed first, followed by the laser. If one drop of diluted peel solution accidentally falls into a laser area, it may produce a scar.

Harris and Noodleman have demonstrated that combining dermasanding (silicone carbide sandpaper) with medium-depth chemical peeling is an effective method for treating fine to moderate rhytides.[26] TCA is applied first, and this is followed by abrading the skin in a circular motion with two 2 × 2–inch gauze pads rolled up into a cylinder over which autoclaved silicone carbide sandpaper is folded and moistened with normal saline. Once fine bleeding points are visualized, the dermasanding is stopped. Hemostasis is obtained by using 1:10,000 epinephrine droplets to coat the affected area. Acetic acid soaks and a moisturizer are used in the postoperative period. Scarring and hypopigmentation are the complications of this procedure.

COMPLICATIONS OF MEDIUM-DEPTH AND DEEP CHEMICAL PEELING

Proper patient selection, performance of the procedure by an experienced dermatologist or cosmetic surgeon, proper knowledge of the peeling agent, good prepeel preparation, and postpeel care are important factors in preventing

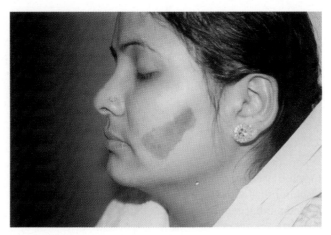

Figure 18-8 Postinflammatory hyperpigmentation after spot medium-depth peel.

complications with peeling agents.[8] However, the dermatologist must be aware of the complications that can occur and how they can be tackled in darker-skinned patients. The common complications of medium-depth and deep chemical peeling are pigmentary alterations: postinflammatory hyperpigmentation and hypopigmentation, persistent erythema, scarring, infections, pruritus, atrophy, textural changes, accentuation of telangiectasias, enlargement of pilosebaceous pores, and increased sensitivity to wind, sunlight, and changes in temperature.[8,10–13,27] In addition, phenol peels also have systemic complications, such as arrhythmias, renal toxicity, and laryngeal edema.

Postinflammatory hyperpigmentation is seen commonly in darker-skinned patients and is one of the limiting factors in conducting chemical peels in darker races.[10,12] It is seen commonly with medium-depth chemical peels and may take months to years to return to normal (Fig. 18-8). In a study of medium-depth peels to treat acne scars in Iraqi patients, although 73.4% of the patients developed postinflammatory hyperpigmentation, none of them had permanent sequelae.[10] The pigmentation faded away in all after a maximum of 3 months. In patients with a family background of dark skin, hyperpigmentation can occur despite reasonable avoidance of sun exposure. This is due to melanocytic sensitivity caused by the irritating effect of the chemical peel.[10] Therefore, in susceptible individuals, treatment of this possible hyperpigmentation must be considered before its appearance.[28] A pretreatment as well as a maintenance regime of 2% to 4% hydroquinone, retinoic acid 0.025%, and 2% hydrocortisone cream (a modification of Kligman's regime) can be used to prevent and treat postinflammatory hyperpigmentation in dark-skinned patients.[29] This combination appears to be well tolerated by darker-skinned patients. Moreover, factors that exacerbate hyperpigmentation—including oral contraception, sunlight, pregnancy, and photosensitizing drugs—should be avoided for 6 months. Postpeel hypopigmentation is an

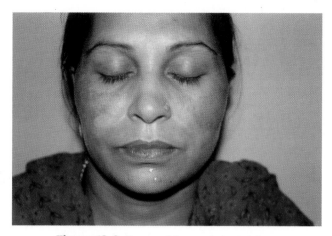

Figure 18-9 Postpeel hypopigmentation.

undesirable side effect with phenol peel.[13,26] and seen less commonly with medium-depth peels (Fig. 18-9). This is dependent on the amount of peel applied, occlusion, and depth of injury. Other pigmentary alterations with deep chemical peels are visible lines of demarcation between the treated and untreated areas, inability of the skin to tan, and uneven skin pigmentation. Careful application of camouflage makeup and foundation as well as sun protection may be required for aesthetic reasons.

Persistent erythema, a complication of medium-depth chemical peels, is almost always a transient phenomenon and may require no treatment in its mild form (Fig. 18-10). It usually lasts for 2 to 3 weeks after medium-depth peeling and 3 months after deep chemical peeling. Risk factors for this complication are genetic background, excess alcohol consumption, and a recent use of isotretinoin or topical tretinoin. In the author's practice, only 0.025% tretinoin is used in the prepeel and maintenance regime in darker-skinned patients. Higher concentrations of tretinoin are associated more frequently with this compli-

cation. Prolonged erythema may also be an early sign of potential scarring and pigmentation. It should be treated early with mild topical steroids, oral antihistamines, systemic corticosteroids, or camouflage makeup.[10,12] In a study of medium-depth TCA peels for treatment of acne scars in dark-skinned patients, persistent erythema occurred only in two patients but resolved spontaneously.[10]

Scarring is a common complication of medium-depth or deep chemical peels. Chemical peels using 50% TCA can cause increased scarring.[14] This can be avoided by using combination medium-depth chemical peels or using 50% TCA only at the edges of depressed acne scars. Hypertrophic scars usually occur on the skin of the neck, dorsal aspects of the hands and arms, and other areas not rich in cutaneous adnexa. On the face, it may occur on the upper lip and near the mandible.[8] Prior dermabrasion or chemical peeling, peeling over undermined skin, and isotretinoin use within the previous 6 months predispose a patient to scarring. A test spot may be helpful to prevent this complication. Scarring could be treated with gentle massage, topical or intralesional steroids, silicone gels, or pulsed dye laser.[12]

Streptococcal and staphylococcal folliculitis can occur as a result of use of occlusion in deep chemical peels and should be prevented with 0.25% acetic acid soaks in the postpeel period. If bacterial infection occurs, appropriate antibiotics should be given. For pseudomonas infection, oral ciprofloxacin should be given. Because latent herpes simplex infection can be reactivated by chemical peels, patients with a history of herpes simplex should be given prophylaxis with valacyclovir 500 mg three times daily, 1 day before and for 7 to 10 days after peeling. In case herpes infection occurs during the postpeel period, a higher dose will have to be used. Atrophy and textural changes are other postpeel complications with medium-depth or deep chemical peeling. These complications can be prevented by avoiding the application of deep peels in the periorbital area and repeeling with superficial peeling agents.

CONCLUSIONS

Medium-depth chemical peels and deep chemical peels have changed the face of cosmetic surgery and dramatically improved the aesthetic quality and appearance of the skin, especially in cases of acne scars, photoaging skin, wrinkles, and recalcitrant pigmentary dyschromias. However, their complications, like pigmentary alterations and scarring, are more pronounced in darker-skinned patients, making them unsuitable candidates for such peels. Thus peels should be mainly reserved for fair-skinned patients. Medium-depth peels may still be performed by experienced dermatologists and cosmetic surgeons who have a good knowledge of the peeling agents as well as expertise in their technique in select, highly motivated, darker-skinned patients, using a good prepeel and postpeel topical

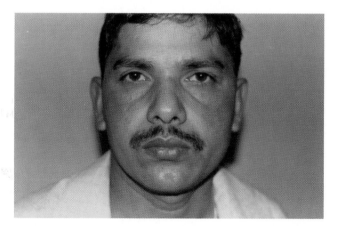

Figure 18-10 Postpeel persistent erythema after medium-depth peels.

maintenance regimen to minimize the postpeel complications; but deep peels are hardly ever performed in this group of patients because of the undesirable side effects. Overall, the risks far outweigh the advantages in the case of medium-depth or deep chemical peels in darker-skinned patients, and the patient must be counseled realistically about the outcome of these procedures.

REFERENCES

1. Brody HJ, Monheit GD, Resnick SS, et al. A history of chemical peeling. *Dermatol Surg* 2000;26:405–409.
2. Mackee GM, Karp FL. The treatment of post acne scars with phenol. *Br J Dermatol* 1952;64:456–459.
3. Stegman SJ. A comparative histologic study of the effects of three peeling agents and dermabrasion on normal and sun damaged skin. *Aesthetic Plast Surg* 1982;6:123–135.
4. Brody HJ, Hailey EW. Medium depth chemical peeling of the skin: a variation of superficial chemosurgery. *J Dermatol Surg Oncol* 1986;12:1268–1275.
5. Monheit G. The Jessner's + TCA peel: a medium-depth chemical peel. *J Dermatol Surg Oncol* 1989;15:945–950.
6. Brody H. Variations and comparisons in medium depth chemical peeling. *J Dermatol Surg Oncol* 1989;15:953.
7. Rubin MG. What are skin peels? In: Winters SR, James M, Caputo GR, eds. *Manual of Chemical Peels: Superficial and Medium Depth.* 1st ed. Philadelphia: JB Lippincott Co.;1995: 17–25.
8. Roenigk RK. Facial chemical peel. In: Baran R, Maibach HI, eds. *Textbook of Cosmetic Dermatology.* 2nd ed. London: Martin Dunitz Ltd.;1994:585–594.
9. Savant SS. Superficial and medium depth chemical peeling. In: Savant SS, ed. *Textbook of Dermatosurgery and Cosmetology.* 2nd ed. Mumbai: ASCAD;2005:177–195.
10. Al-Waiz M, Al-Sharqi AI. Medium depth chemical peels in the treatment of acne scars in dark skinned individuals. *Dermatol Surg* 2002;28:383–387.
11. Coleman W, Brody H. Advances in chemical peeling. *Dermatol Clin* 1997;15:20–26.
12. Monheit GD, Kayal JD. Chemical peeling. In: Nouri K, Leal Khouri S, eds. *Techniques in Dermatologic Surgery.* 1st ed. St. Louis: Mosby;2004:233–244.
13. Monheit GD. Medium depth chemical peels. *Dermatol Clin* 2001;19:413–425.
14. Collins PS. Trichloroacetic acid peels revisited. *J Dermatol Surg Oncol* 1989;15:933–940.
15. Brody HJ. *Chemical Peeling and Resurfacing.* St. Louis: Mosby;1997:109–110.
16. Rubin MG. Basic concepts in skin peeling. In: Winters SR, James M, Caputo GR, eds. *Manual of Chemical Peels: Superficial and Medium Depth.* 1st ed. Philadelphia: JB Lippincott Co.;1995:44–59.
17. Nanda S, Grover C, Reddy BSN. Efficacy of hydroquinone (2%) versus tretinoin (0.025%) as adjunct topical agents for chemical peeling in patients of melasma. *Dermatol Surg* 2004;30:385–389.
18. Saraf V. *Chemical Rejuvenation of the Face and Nonfacial Areas in Asian Skin.* 1st ed. Mumbai: Saraf Vinay;2003.
19. Coleman WP, Futrell JM. The glycolic and trichloroacetic acid peel. *J Dermatol Surg Oncol* 1994;20:76–80.
20. Baker TJ. The ablation of rhytides by chemical means: preliminary report. *J Fla Med Assoc* 1961;48:451–454.
21. Stagnone GJ, Orgel MG, Stagnone JJ. Cardiovascular effects of topical 50% trichloroacetic acid and Baker's phenol solution. *J Dermatol Surg Oncol* 1987;13:999–1002.
22. Beeson WH. The importance of cardiac monitoring in superficial and deep chemical peeling. *J Dermatol Surg Oncol* 1987;13:949–950.
23. Alt TH. Occluded Baker-Gordon chemical peel: review and update. *J Dermatol Surg Oncol* 1989;15:980–993.
24. Hetter GP. An examination of the phenol croton oil peel: Part 1. Dissecting the formula. *Plast Reconstr Surg* 2000;105 (1):227–239; discussion 249–251.
25. Hetter GP. An examination of the phenol croton oil peel: Part III. The plastic surgeons' role. *Plast Reconstr Surg* 2000;105 (2):752–762.
26. Harris DR, Noodleman RR. Combining manual dermasanding with low strength trichloroacetic acid to improve actinically injured skin. *J Dermatol Surg Oncol* 1994;20: 436–442.
27. Cassano N, Alessandrini G, Mastrolonardo M, et al. Peeling agents: toxicological and allergological aspects. *J Eur Acad Dermatol Venereol* 1999;13:14–23.
28. West T, Alster T. Effect of pretreatment on the incidence of hyperpigmentation following cutaneous CO_2 laser resurfacing. *Dermatol Surg* 1999;25:15–17.
29. Sarkar R, Kaur C, Bhalla M, et al. The combination of glycolic acid peels with topical regimen in the treatment of melasma in dark-skinned patients. *Dermatol Surg* 2002;28 (9):828–832.

20

Surgical Tightening Procedures

Matthew R. Kaufman, Reza Jarrahy and Michael Jones

AGING

Facial aging is a gradual process that typically begins in the fourth decade of life. The process, however, can be accelerated by excessive sun exposure, cigarette smoking, radiation therapy, or certain genetic disorders (e.g., progeria, pseudoxanthoma elasticum). Histologically, aging is characterized by multiple changes that occur primarily in the dermis and at the dermal/epidermal junction. There is loss of the dermoepidermal papillae and a gradual reduction in the melanocyte population. The thickness of the reticular dermis is substantially reduced as overall dermal organization is degraded. A decrease in total collagen content results in thinning of the skin with age; the normal ratio of type I to type III collagen is also altered. Total dermal thickness decreases with age by an average 6% per decade of life in both men and women.[1]

There are alterations in both the facial skeleton and soft tissues that contribute to age-related changes in the face. With age, there is a remodeling of the facial skeleton that involves a rotation of the facial structures downward and inward with respect to the cranial base. Wrinkles, gravitational descent, and atrophy constitute the significant soft-tissue changes that occur over time. There are three causes of wrinkles in the human face: repetitive mimetic muscle action, disruption of the elastic structural network, and sun damage. Although sun damage is preventable to a certain degree and is often more limited in individuals with darker skin color, the other two noted factors contribute to the aging process in virtually all human populations. The increased melanin present in darker-skinned individuals limits actinic damage and slows the development of age-related stigmata. Darker-skinned ethnicities often do not exhibit the same degree of facial wrinkling and furrowing as their lighter-complected counterparts. If they do, it is usually at a much later age.

HISTORY

Early facelift procedures involved a limited elevation of the skin and subcutaneous tissues, placing the burden of tension on the skin. Innovative surgeons were eager to reduce the skin slough and scarring that was believed to be at least partly due to tension on the skin flaps and incisions. There was also a desire to improve the longevity and aesthetic results of the procedures. To improve outcomes, other methods were developed, especially following the description of the superficial musculoaponeurotic system (SMAS) in 1976 by Mitz and Peyronie.[2] Skoog and others developed techniques that involved dissection and suspension of the SMAS, thereby transferring tension from the skin closure to deeper tissues.[3–7] The literature was soon replete with various descriptions of SMAS procedures (plication, imbrication, strip SMASectomy) aimed at achieving the most aesthetically pleasing results.[8–10] The deep-plane facelift and composite rhytidectomy pioneered by Hamra were both extensions of the SMAS procedures, involving extensive sub-SMAS dissections and suspension.[11,12] The next landmark in the evolution of rhytidectomy surgery was the description of the subperiosteal facelift, in which the soft tissues of the face are elevated off the facial skeleton.[13,14] Over time, techniques were popularized that involved progressively deeper planes of dissection. The increased complexity of these procedures was believed to be warranted by improved and longer-lasting results.

Interestingly, in the new millennium, there has been a change of focus to minimally invasive procedures. The application of the endoscope to facial surgery has inspired facelifting procedures that limit incisions and minimize recovery times. Through exposure by the mass media and a wider acceptance of plastic surgery by the public in general, these procedures have become some of the most sought after, especially in the younger age groups. It is imperative for practitioners to describe to their patients the benefits as well as the limitations of these less invasive techniques; they certainly cannot achieve the results of a more traditional facelift and may only have applications for a specific subset of patients with more limited degrees of facial aging.

The wider acceptance of plastic surgery in the United States has led to an increased demand for facelift procedures in almost every ethnic group. Whereas surgeons previously focused almost exclusively on issues related to Caucasian skin types, they now have to be intimately familiar with issues related to wound healing, scarring, and skin care in darker-skinned individuals. Surgeons must understand these issues for surgical planning to achieve optimal results in these patient populations.

PATIENT SELECTION AND EVALUATION

Ethnic patients presenting for facial rejuvenation require a thorough evaluation before a surgical plan can be established. In addition to taking a full history that includes documentation of comorbidities, prior surgery, medications, family history of aging, sun exposure, and tobacco history, there must be an inquiry as to how the patient heals wounds (i.e., a history of keloids or hypertrophic scars) and whether the patient has problems related to nonuniform skin pigmentation or other medical skin conditions. Furthermore, it is necessary to ask the patient targeted questions regarding hairstyle and care, such as how they style their hair, whether they wear wigs, and if they frequently receive hair-conditioning treatments. Contraindications to surgery that could be elicited in the history include cardiovascular disease, autoimmune diseases (e.g., lupus, sarcoid, sickle cell anemia), and prior radiation therapy to the face or neck.

As with any plastic surgery patient, there must be a clear and realistic expectation of goals. It is important to allow the patient to express in their own words exactly what result he or she hopes to obtain with facial rejuvenation surgery. An invaluable part of the initial exam is providing the patient with a mirror and asking him or her to point out areas for which he or she is seeking specific improvement. This should be followed by a complete physical examination, including skin color and thickness, assessment of actinic damage, amount/location of skin laxity, assessment of facial bony skeleton, cranial nerve exam, assessment of hairline, and inspection of previous surgical or traumatic scars.

Medical photodocumentation is an integral part of the initial consultation that allows the surgeon to reanalyze the patient before surgery. It also provides a basis for postoperative comparison. The standard preoperative photographic views for facelift surgery include the full-face frontal view, full-face left and right oblique views, and left and right profiles.

The physician must process all of this information to recommend a procedure that can be performed safely and provide the results that will most closely match the expectations of the patient. For example, patients who are obese and/or have extremely thick skin must be informed that the results of rhytidectomy may be less than satisfactory. Ultimately, the best outcomes can be expected in those patients who have moderately thick skin, minimal sun damage, and some preservation of skin elasticity. In addition, patients with strong facial bony structures and a well-defined, acute cervicomental angle will exhibit more dramatic postoperative enhancements than those without such pre-existing features.

OPERATIVE TECHNIQUES

Subcutaneous facelift

The original surgical tightening procedure involves a preauricular incision extending posteriorly around the lobule of the ear into the postauricular sulcus. The incision is often carried into the postauricular hair-bearing region of the scalp or, alternatively, it may follow the hairline inferoposteriorly toward the neck. The skin is elevated, preserving some subcutaneous fat on the flap so as not to compromise its vascularity. Although the pioneers of this procedure would perform limited undermining before skin excision and closure, it was soon realized that unless the flap was elevated for some distance medially and inferiorly, the excessive skin tension would result in skin slough and widened scars.

Although there are now few indications for a purely subcutaneous lift given the development of other safe and effective techniques, there are certain patients in whom this indeed may be the appropriate procedure. In patients who have previously had facelifting procedures and are presenting years later for revision surgery, the subcutaneous lift may provide a safe, effective way of refining the recurring effects of aging. It is believed that in these patients, the skin flaps have improved vascularity from previous elevation that minimizes ischemic complications and that a SMAS or sub-SMAS dissection would be difficult and perhaps treacherous if planes of dissection are scarred and obscured because of previous surgery. Furthermore, the thicker skin often present in darker-complected individuals would provide an additional margin of comfort when elevating and retracting facial skin flaps. However, the procedure is generally not an ideal option in patients with a history of cigarette smoking because of the compromised vascularity in the skin.

Subcutaneous facelift with superficial musculoaponeurotic system manipulation

Facelifting procedures based on SMAS manipulation begin with the dissection of a skin flap as described for the subcutaneous lift. (The original Skoog procedure was described as elevation of the skin and SMAS as a single unit). Once the SMAS is identified, it should be followed into the neck, where it becomes continuous with the platysma. Elevation of the SMAS-platysma in unison permits a rejuvenation of the midface, jowls, and neck that produces an effective surgical enhancement. Once dissected, methods of lifting and tightening the SMAS include plication (suture infolding), imbrication (incision, advancement, and overlapping), or strip SMASectomy (excising a strip of SMAS). Regardless of the specific method, adequate suspension of the SMAS using multiple points of suture fixation must be performed to produce the desired tightening.

Once the fascial lift has been completed, the skin flaps can be redraped and modified as necessary. As the excess skin is trimmed, the surgeon should place great importance on stable skin fixation in both the preauricular temporal region and along the postauricular incision. An effort should be made to minimize skin tension to avoid alterations to the final position of the hairline, the tragus, and the lobule of the ear.

The various methods of subcutaneous dissection with SMAS manipulation undoubtedly account for the most commonly performed facelifting procedures. Critics argue that separation of the SMAS from the skin limits perfusion of the skin flap by the underlying fascia system and that ultimately the dermis still bears the burden of tension during skin closure. Furthermore, a lengthy subcutaneous flap dissection may still result in unacceptably high rates of wound-healing complications when performed in smokers. However, in trained hands and with appropriate patient selection, there is abundant evidence that these techniques yield exceptional, long-lasting results.

Deep-plane/composite facelift

The deep-plane and composite techniques for facelifting consist of a limited subcutaneous dissection from the initial incision (2–3 cm), followed by an extensive sub-SMAS elevation extending anteromedially above the zygomaticus major muscle to include the lower orbicularis oculi muscle. The platysma undergoes a more thorough dissection to permit its suspension to the preauricular fascia near the lobule of the ear. Essentially, the skin, subcutaneous tissue, SMAS, and platysma are elevated as one thick flap extending from the site of SMAS incision laterally to a point medial to the nasolabial folds. Imbrication is then performed at the level of the SMAS to achieve suspension, allowing the skin to be redraped, trimmed, and inset as in other facelifting procedures.

The aesthetic results that can be achieved with these procedures are attributed, at least in part, to the widespread SMAS undermining, as well as extension of the dissection across the nasolabial folds. Whereas in other procedures the nasolabial folds are often not sufficiently tightened, the deep-plane/composite procedures emphasize elevation and suspension in this area of the face. Extensive undermining in the sub-SMAS plane permits suspension of a thick musculofasciocutaneous flap and is believed to produce longer-lasting results and be safer in smokers. On the contrary, the procedure may have a higher rate of nerve injury that is due to the deeper plane of dissection, with longer operative times and a somewhat prolonged recovery compared with procedures that are characterized by more limited dissection.

Subperiosteal facelift

Extensive dissection in the subperiosteal plane of the temporal and malar regions is the basis for the subperiosteal facelift. The soft tissues are mobilized with suture suspension, and the results can be enhanced with deep periosteal tacking sutures. In the temporal region, the dissection is carried deep to both layers of temporalis fascia, thereby reducing the risk of injury to the frontal branch of the facial nerve. The procedure is beneficial for redraping of the forehead and malar areas but may be insufficient for rejuvenation of the perioral areas and neck unless direct skin suspension is included. In fact, patients with significant redundancy in the lower third of the face are probably not candidates for a subperiosteal facelift. The critics of this procedure argue that an extensive subperiosteal dissection may disinsert mimetic muscles and thereby actually accentuate cheek ptosis.

Although the subperiosteal facelift has not been accepted as widely as the aforementioned procedures, it has been the foundation for some of the newer, minimally invasive procedures designed to rejuvenate the midface.

MINIMALLY INVASIVE TECHNIQUES

In the last 15 years, there have been numerous descriptions of procedures designed to surgically tighten the face. These are characterized by smaller incisions and quicker recovery times compared with traditional facelifts. Many of these are based on the techniques of the subperiosteal facelift but incorporate the use of the endoscope to minimize incision length. One of the popular techniques for endoscopic midface rejuvenation was popularized by Hester, who described the transblepharoplasty subperiosteal cheek lift.[15,16] The procedure consists of a lower blepharoplasty incision to access the subperiosteal plane over the maxilla, followed by an endoscopically assisted dissection of the midface and suture suspension of the malar soft tissues in a superior vector of elevation. Other authors have described a similar procedure using a temporal incision to achieve a more superolateral vector of soft tissue suspension.[17–19] The most appropriate candidate for endoscopic-assisted composite rhytidectomy would be a patient with minimal skin redundancy, as the limited incisions would prohibit aggressive skin resection and redraping.[20]

Recently, there has been great interest in surgical tightening procedures that use transcutaneous needles and barbed sutures to elevate the midface and neck, thereby obviating the need for skin incisions altogether. These products have been marketed under several different brand names, and there has been widespread interest from patients looking for a minimally invasive method of facial rejuvenation. These procedures generally do not involve any soft-tissue undermining; the suspension sutures must therefore counteract the soft-tissue attachments of the face. Short durations and quick recovery

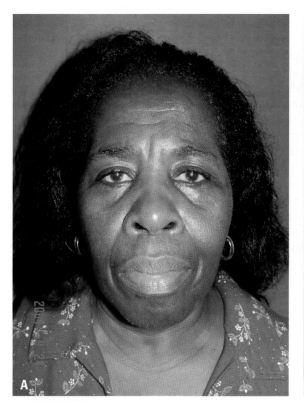 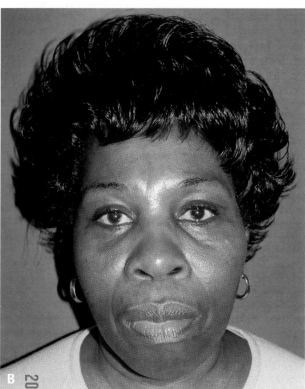

Figure 20-1 Pre- **(A)** and **(B)** postoperative photos of a patient undergoing endoscopic browlift and midfacelift.

times render these procedures quite attractive to patients, but there is still no consensus as to the longevity of the results. Furthermore, the patients who may indeed be candidates for these techniques are not necessarily the same patients who would benefit from more traditional facelifts.

Although it is desirable for surgeons to incorporate minimally invasive techniques into their practices to provide patients with a greater number of options, they must do so carefully during this time of ongoing evolution of these types of procedures.

ISSUES SPECIFIC TO ETHNIC FACELIFTING

Between 1999 and 2001, the number of African Americans who had cosmetic surgery quadrupled, along with other darker-complected ethnic groups.[21] The increased demand for surgical tightening procedures in these populations has encouraged physicians to analyze how best to achieve surgical success and patient satisfaction. Whereas a successful facelift in a Caucasian patient may involve one set of criteria, it does not necessarily apply to other ethnic groups. For example, African American patients seeking facial rejuvenation may not want to eliminate the natural characteristics of their ethnicity, seeking instead a natural-appearing restoration of more youthful African American

features (Figs. 20-1, 20-2, and 20-3). Therefore, any surgeon caring for ethnic patients must understand what are considered to be attractive features in each group.

The skin characteristics of darker-complexioned ethnicities must be considered in the preoperative evaluation of a cosmetic surgery patient. Obviously, there is a concern for scarring that often may be more of a risk than in Caucasian patients. A thorough history and examination of previous surgical or traumatic scars will sometimes elicit whether the patient is likely to develop postoperative hypertrophic scars and/or keloids. There are, however, some patients who will develop keloids and hypertrophic scars despite a negative history (Fig. 20-4). This is especially relevant in the traditional rhytidectomy incision. People of color must be counseled about the prominence of the incision in the pre- and postauricular region, and those patients who wear their hair short or back may not be the ideal candidates for a traditional facelift incision. Surgical planning may have to be modified based on the severity of the risk, and patients must receive a detailed explanation of the risk of scarring and possible remedies if it occurs.

African American patients and other dark-skinned ethnicities often present for facial rejuvenation procedures at a later age than their Caucasian counterparts. The effects of aging may present later in life, and there may be fewer signs of facial aging present at younger ages. The

21

Nonsurgical Tightening Procedures

Sorin Eremia

IMPORTANT DIFFERENCES BETWEEN LIGHTER AND DARKER SKIN TYPES

The detailed histologic and physiologic characteristics of darker skin types are beyond the scope of this chapter.[1-4] Chapter 2 provides an overview of the structural and physiologic features of darker skin types. It is, however, important to understand three key differences between lighter and darker skin types that are relevant to the aging process and to methods of skin tightening discussed in this chapter.

Presence of increasing amounts of melanin

The amount of melanin is the very basis of the skin type I to VI classification. More melanin translates, on one hand, into better photoprotection and delays the appearance of the photoaging changes seen earlier in lighter-skinned individuals. On the other hand, melanocyte response to epidermal and superficial dermal tissue injuries is more severe, with potential permanent or at least long-lasting and difficult-to-treat pigmentary changes. Therefore, when aging changes begin to appear in darker-skinned individuals and these patients seek treatment, much greater care must be taken when using the concept of tissue injury to trigger rejuvenating changes, such as new collagen and elastic tissue formation and collagen tightening and remodeling in general.

Treatment methods that involve significant epidermal tissue injury, methods that are defined as ablative skin resurfacing—be they the more modern laser or broadband light-based methods or the older chemical and mechanical abrasive methods—are not well suited for darker skin types. Such treatment techniques are in fact considered largely contraindicated for anyone with skin darker than what is defined as a relatively light type IV. The increased presence of skin pigment also generally limits the wavelengths that can be used for photorejuvenation treatments to longer wavelengths outside the melanin absorption spectrum. Epidermal cooling to protect superficial skin injury that may trigger melanocytes to respond also becomes of greater importance the darker the skin type that is being targeted for treatment.

Increased thickness of skin associated with dark skin types

The increased thickness of skin associated with darker skin types appears to be primarily due to increased dermal thickness and amounts of collagen present. Combined with better melanin photoprotection, it delays the appearance of fine wrinkles associated with actinic damage, typically seen in lighter skin type individuals. It contributes to differences in skin appearance at a given age, according to skin type characteristics, and makes larger wrinkles a greater concern for non-Caucasian patients, especially those with types V and VI skin. In the author's experience, thicker, non-Caucasian type skin tends to experience better tightening following the use of nonablative rejuvenating devices that heat the dermis.

Risk of hypertrophic and keloid scar formation and generally greater visibility of incisional scars

These risks make incisional-based, especially traditional long incision, tissue-resection–based skin tightening less desirable for non-Caucasian skin patients. It raises some concerns even for minimal incision lifts, although in the author's experience, relatively small incisions placed inside the hairline and closed without tension do not present a significant problem. Increased tendency to scar formation also increases the risk of serious complications secondary to heat-generating energy–based nonablative rejuvenating devices, from what would have been only a minor superficial burn in lighter skin type patients. Therefore, greater caution must be exercised with such devices for darker, non-Caucasian patients. Many of the published and conference presented reports of good skin tightening results achieved with such devices also include, in the complications section, a certain number of minor burns that healed without or with minimal scarring. Unless otherwise specifically mentioned in the reports, most likely those injured were lighter skin type patients, and far more serious consequences could have developed in comparably burned darker skin type patients.

As of August 2006, there are two categories of relatively nonsurgical, minimally invasive treatment methods and devices that are available for skin tightening in darker-skinned, non-Caucasian patients: (a) the use of energy-delivering devices to achieve tissue tightening, and (b) the use of minimal incision suspension sutures, including the newer small barbed or larger multianchor type suture. These sutures elevate the tissues into position and rely either on natural postinsertion skin contraction or on inducement of subcutaneous fibrous tracts or fibrosis in a plane above or below the elevated tissues to hold up the lift long term. To improve long-term results, increased tissue fibrosis and contraction is induced through various methods, including the combined use of energy-delivering devices with suspending sutures.

ENERGY-DELIVERING DEVICES USED FOR NONABLATIVE OR MINIMALLY ABLATIVE SKIN TIGHTENING

The concept behind these devices is to deliver sufficient energy to the superficial and middermal tissue without creating any—or at least very little—injury to the epidermis, hence the terms *nonablative* and *minimally ablative*. The energy is transformed into heat as it is absorbed by the target tissue. The desired thermal injury occurs in the area of maximum energy absorption. The injury triggers formation of new collagen and elastic tissue; it is hoped, in sufficient amounts, to achieve a clinically significant improvement. Sufficient heating of the collagen fibers can also trigger some dermal "remodeling" through instant shrinkage of these protein fibers. The trick is to limit the thermal injury to the targeted dermal tissues and to avoid significant injury to the epidermis, either from direct epidermal absorption of the energy beam as it traverses the epidermis to reach the dermis or from diffusion of the heat superficially. Selection of suitable energy parameters and delivery methods, such as wavelengths and pulse widths, can minimize or virtually eliminate the absorption of energy by the epidermal tissue and determine the depth of maximal dermal absorption. The use of epidermal cooling technologies can protect the epidermis from injury resulting from a certain degree of unavoidable energy absorption by epidermal tissue and from heat diffusing up from the dermis.[5]

From a wavelength point of view, properly delivered far infrared and radiofrequency energy can pass through the epidermis with very little absorption by epidermal tissue, including melanocytes. Wavelength selection also takes into consideration its scatter characteristics as it passes through tissue. Some wavelengths in the infrared spectrum, such as 1,319 nm and 1,450 nm, also have more scattering characteristics as they penetrate through the dermis than 1,064 nm, so most if not all the energy is delivered to the desired dermal target area. On the other hand, when the target area is deeper—such as with hair follicles, which are deeper in the subcutaneous fat—a wavelength with low scatter characteristics is better suited. The delivery of energy in pulses can also vary the target tissue. Various components of the skin have different thermal relaxation times. Larger targets, related to the surface-to-volume ratio of the target, dissipate absorbed heat more slowly than smaller targets. Therefore, when energy is delivered more slowly over time (longer pulse width), smaller targets with short thermal relaxation times have the time to dissipate the heat before the next pulse of energy hits the target, and the heat does not accumulate. Larger targets, with longer thermal relaxation times, accumulate heat, eventually reaching the critical temperature that triggers thermal injury. Skin-cooling strategies also need to take into account the source of heat reaching the epidermis. When some of the energy is absorbed by the epidermis as it passes through, precooling as well as contemporaneous cooling of the epidermis is very important to prevent epidermal injury. When the heat is not the result of direct absorption by the epidermis but instead rises up from the dermis, postcooling or continuous cooling may be more effective at preventing epidermal injury. Continuous cooling is obviously effective at protecting the epidermis, but on one hand can carry the risk of excessive cooling and freeze injury to the epidermis and on the other hand can diffuse into the dermis and negate the desired thermal injury there.

Although device manufacturers obviously take all such factors into consideration when building their machines, patent restrictions and technical and cost considerations sometimes limit their ability to provide the most effective energy delivery and cooling system. In the author's opinion, it is important for physicians using such devices to have a thorough understanding of the science behind them to be better able to judge and choose the most appropriate device for the physician's patient population needs.

First-generation nonablative devices

The first-generation devices specifically designed for nonablative skin tightening were lasers delivering light energy in the far infrared spectrum. CoolTouch (NewStar Lasers, Rosemont, CA) using a 1,320-nm Nd:YAG–generated wavelength and a fixed 50-millisecond pulse width was introduced in 1997. The availability of cryogen spray pre- and postcooling, the addition of a temperature sensor, and a relatively large 10-mm treatment spot set CoolTouch apart from the SmoothBeam (Candela Lasers, Boston, MA), a smaller, less sophisticated, but less expensive, 1,450-nm diode–generated wavelength laser and the European-developed Aramis Erbium:Glass 1,540-nm laser, which never quite caught on in the United States. As is too often the case with new devices, the laser manufacturers and some physicians promoting these lasers made unrealistic claims that as few as four treatments could produce significant skin tightening and improvement in acne scars and even improve acne. In time, it was determined that many treatments (for example, in the author's experience, 10 to 14 monthly treatments with the CoolTouch laser) were needed to achieve modest long-term skin tightening or acne-scarring improvement. Overaggressive treatments also resulted in rare but annoying scarring thermal injuries. Both the CoolTouch and SmoothBeam lasers are still available and have proven to be generally reliable, low-operating-cost lasers. Very similar to the CoolTouch, but technologically more advanced, is a Sciton 1,319-nm Nd:YAG laser that presents several advantages. It has a variable pulse width, which allows great flexibility as to how the energy is delivered; a fast, large treatment area with a scanned 6-mm spot; and excellent adjustable contact window cooling. One of the chief complaints about the CoolTouch, and the SmoothBeam lasers is significant patient discomfort. Use of longer pulse widths decreases treatment pain, and, when compared with the 10-mm CoolTouch spot size, so does the randomly scanned smaller 6-mm Sciton spot. The unit can operate on a platform that can support multiple lasers (such as 1,064-nm Nd:YAG and an Er:YAG, and pulsed broadband light units). The wavelength used by all these lasers has virtually no melanin absorption.

Other lasers and early broadband light devices

The concept of nonablative thermal skin injury to induce formation of new collagen and elastic tissue led to attempts to use other existing lasers, such as the 595-nm pulse dye laser, the 1,064-nm Nd:YAG with long pulse width, alone or in combination with the 532 Nd:YAG to induce skin tightening. In general, these results have been very modest. The use of the 532-nm and the 595-nm wavelengths in darker skin is contraindicated. The use of selectively filtered pulsed broadband light was also attempted for purposes of skin tightening. The earliest version was the "photofacial" treatment with the Lumenis intense pulsed light units. Skin tightening results were very disappointing. Newer units are discussed below.

Radiofrequency devices

In 1999, the ThermaCool device (Thermage Inc., Hayward, CA) was introduced. Volumetric dermal heating is accomplished using a skin-cooling tip with capacitive coupling monopolar radiofrequency (RF) technology. The device converts electrical energy to RF spectrum wavelength energy. These waves of energy are delivered in monopolar fashion to the skin through a square tip that is also equipped with surface chilling to help cool and protect the epidermis. A coupling gel is used to decrease epidermal impedence and allow the energy to get through to the dermis with minimal absorption. Dermal tissue resistance/impedance converts the RF spectrum energy waves to heat, which has been shown to produce various degrees of tissue-tightening results. FDA approval for periorbital skin tightening use was obtained in 2002 amid much fanfare and claims of impressive documented skin tightening and lateral brow elevation. This was followed with claims on national television shows of impressive tissue tightening and appearance improvement in the jowls area of the face. Unfortunately, these results seemed largely exaggerated, or at best unpredictable, and limited to a small percentage of treated patients. Claims were also made of significant acne scarring improvement as well as long-term improvements in acne as well. Misguided attempts to produce such results through use of high-power settings led to some highly publicized burns with permanent scars.[6] The treatment tips initially developed by Thermage were small (1 cm) and delivered the energy slowly and quite painfully. Newer generations of tips and improved treatment protocols that involve multiple passes at lower energy settings[7] have decreased risks, improved treatment speed, and, with the most recent 3-mm tips, significantly decreased patient discomfort and operator fatigue. These large tips have also rendered more practical the use of the Thermage unit for nonfacial areas, such as the abdomen and arms, with studies ongoing.

The newest Thermage tip is specially designed for treatment of the eyelids, which was previously contraindicated with the older tips. This tip is much smaller, delivers much less energy, and is designed specifically for the thin upper-lid skin. The use of a plastic (not metal) eye shield is essential. The eyelid tip was introduced in April 2006, and preliminary results appear to be better and more predictable than results on the face. Because RF waves are not absorbed by melanin, non-Caucasian skin is well suited to it (Fig. 21-1A,B). Also, the thicker dermis of certain ethnicities appears to respond better to this device than thinner skin. The cost of the ThermaCool unit is much lower than most other tissue-tightening devices. It is relatively small and portable as well as reliable and less expensive to maintain than laser and light units. However, the cost of the tips, which are single-use disposable devices, is quite high—$500 to $600 or more per treatment (about $175 for the eyelids tip)—and has been one of the obstacles for greater use. Thermage was once promoted its product as an independent, one-time, effective treatment. More likely, several treatments at 1- to 3-month intervals are needed for best results. Although not as much a concern with types V to VI skin, the RF-induced skin-tightening effects do little if anything for fine facial wrinkles nor does it improve any pre-existing dyschromia. The author is using Thermage both as an independent procedure and in combination with the knotted multianchor suspension suture lift (AnchorLift) discussed later in this chapter.

In 2005, Aluma (Luminis, Santa Clara, CA) introduced a bipolar RF unit using vacuum to press the tissues to the treatment head. This keeps the skin in contact with the parallel electrodes, decreasing the risk of arcing and accidental skin burns. It is claimed this vacuum-negative pressure, which pulls the tissues tight onto the RF current–generating electrodes, reduces the fluences needed to heat the desired

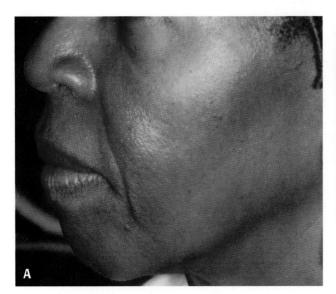
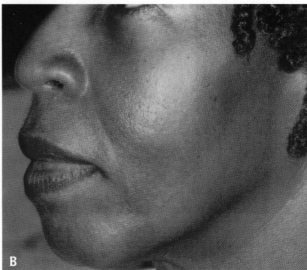

Figure 21-1 A: Pretreatment of lower face rhytides, type VI skin, African American patient. **B:** Six months posttreatment of the lower face with a Monopolar RF device. (Courtesy of Dr. Mark Nestor and Thermage Inc.)

volume of dermis, reducing patient discomfort. As with other RF units, a coupling gel is also used.

The tip is disposable and works for only 300 pulses, rendering treatment costs relatively high. The initial manufacturer-supported studies claim impressive results, but, as with most of these units, early results have yet to be independently confirmed as truly clinically significant.

Accent (Alma Lasers, Caesarea, Israel), still awaiting FDA approval, has two separate handpieces—one for monopolar and one for bipolar RF technology—to provide variable penetration depths and heating. The monopolar handpiece heats the dermis up to 2 mm in depth and appears to be designed for tissue tightening. The bipolar handpieces heats deeper, between 2 and 4 mm, and may be able to cause adipocyte lipolysis. The released fatty components are absorbed and eliminated. The bipolar component is more designed for treatment of cellulite. Treatment pain has been reported to be a significant factor, and results are variable. The unit is thus a dual-purpose one, designed to induce facial skin tightening and for treatment of cellulite on the rest of the body. Care must be taken not to use the bipolar component on the face where it could lead to subcutaneous fat loss. Alma also makes a fractional delivery device (Pixel) using an Er:YAG laser (not to be confused with the Er:Glass lasers used by Fraxel and Palomar) and a pure pulsed broadband light device.

Combined radiofrequency and broadband light devices

Shortly after Thermage introduced pure volumetric monopolar RF dermal heating as a skin-tightening modality,

Polaris (Syneron Medical Ltd., Yokeam, Israel) was introduced as a nonablative tissue-tightening device that combines the use of 780- to 980-nm light energy with RF energy, delivered with a contact cooling tip. Claims have been made of a synergistic effect,[8] but whether such synergy has been demonstrated remains subject to debate. Lower levels of RF energy are delivered by this unit, resulting in smaller volumes of dermal heating per pulse. At the very least, the 780- to 980-nm light treatment portion has some effect on the epidermis and very superficial dermis, primarily because of melanin absorption, and can generate minor, probably temporary improvements in fine wrinkles and dyschromia. There are published reports claiming skin-tightening results, and many users are happy with the patient response. Given the use of melanin-absorbed optical energy with this device, its use for darker skin types is probably contraindicated. A newer device is ReFirme, combining the use of bipolar RF with broadband (700–2,000 nm) light energy. It is more powerful than Polaris, delivering up to 120 J/cm^3 of RF energy and 20 J/cm^2 of light energy. It is too early to judge how much more effective this newer unit will be. Early reports from manufacturer-supported studies are, as with most new devices, optimistic. Presence of melanin-absorbed wavelengths suggests caution for darker skin types.

Pure broadband light devices

Titan (Cutera, Brisbane, CA) is the flagship of this technology. It emits infrared light energy in the 1,100- to 1,800-nm range. It uses a 1.5 × 1 cm tip with a cooled sapphire skin contact window to help protect the epidermis.

Noninvasive Wrinkle Correction

22

Botulinum Toxin

Doris M. Hexsel, Camile L. Hexsel, and Leticia T. Brunetto

The value of facial and corporal aesthetic image plays an important role in society and has grown with the development of numerous minimally invasive procedures. Patients are looking for safe, new, and less invasive techniques for facial rejuvenation as they search for quick results with low incidence of side effects. Certain minimally invasive procedures are also practical, as patients can immediately return to their activities.

Repeated facial movements, caused by contraction of the muscles of facial expression, are one of the most important etiologic factors of facial expression lines and rhytides. Such repeated movements also play a role in the development of redundant skin around these lines and rhytides. Botulinum toxin (BT) injections represent one of the latest and most revolutionary treatments in facial rejuvenation, targeting hyperkinetic muscles of facial expression. They are currently considered the best alternative for the treatment of dynamic wrinkles.[1] BT can be used alone or in combination with other minimally invasive or invasive techniques.[2–4]

In the last decade, the results of the therapeutic and cosmetic use of BT types A and B have been published in many articles and chapters. The cosmetic use of BT has permitted better understanding of the physiopathology of the aging process, specifically of the role of muscular contraction in aging.

HISTORY OF CLINICAL USE

In 1817, Justinus Kerner described botulism, a new disease characterized by muscle paralysis caused by the intake of poisoned food, probably spoiled sausage (from the Latin *botulus,* sausage).[5,6]

In 1897, Emile Pierre Van Ermengen isolated an anaerobic bacteria from contaminated food and injected the toxin of this bacteria, promoting disease in laboratory animals.[6,7] He identified this anaerobic Gram-positive bacillus as the etiological agent of botulism and called it *Bacillus botulinus*.[5,7] As bacillus identified aerobic organisms, in 1922, *Bacillus botulinus* received a new denomination of *Clostridium botulinum,* indicating its anaerobic nature.[5,8] *Clostridium botulinum* produces botulinum toxin, the most potent neurotoxin known in nature.[9] There are seven different serotypes of botulinum neurotoxins. Botulism in humans is most commonly caused by BT types A, B, and E.[5]

In 1949, it was demonstrated that BT inhibits the release of acetylcholine (Ach) from nerve endings.[10]

In 1973, Scott reported the use of BT in monkeys, demonstrating reversible ocular muscle paralysis during 3 months. In 1980, the toxin was introduced as a therapeutic agent when the same author published a study demonstrating BT injections as a successful adjunctive or alternative treatment to the surgical treatment of strabismus.[8,11] After that, the clinical use of BT advanced to the treatment of other muscular disorders, characterized by excessive or inappropriate contraction, such as focal dystonia, blepharospasm, achalasia, anal spasm, vaginismus, and nystagmus.[12,13]

The cosmetic use of BT type A began in the late 1980s, when Carruthers and Carruthers noted an improvement in the glabellar lines after injections of BT for the treatment of patients with blepharospasm.[14,15] At the beginning, only the upper third of the face was treated.[16,17] Later, the cosmetic use advanced to applications in the mid- and lower face and neck.[4,16,18–21] Other important uses in dermatology, such as hyperhidrosis[22,23] and gingival smile,[16] among others, have been developed in recent years.

The therapeutic use of BT for migraine and tension-type headache has also been described,[16] and they include the treatment of some muscles of facial expression.

AVAILABLE BOTULINUM TOXINS

Seven neurotoxin serotypes were purified and identified. They are denominated as A to G. The serotype A has been shown to be the most potent. Currently not only the serotype A but also the serotype B are commercially available and authorized for therapeutic use.[24] Only the serotype A is currently used for cosmetic purposes. Other serotypes are under investigation, as well as other toxins,[17,25–28] and perhaps new toxins will be available in the near future. The serotype B has shown to be an option for the treatment of patients resistant to serotype A.[24,29]

Botulinum toxin type A is available in three commercial preparations that are authorized for cosmetic use in some

Table 22-1

Characteristics of Botox and Reloxin

	Reloxin	Botox cosmetic
Composition	*Clostridium botulinum* toxin type A hemagglutinin complex 125 μg (0.125 mg) human serum albumin 2.5 mg lactose	*Clostridium botulinum* toxin type A hemagglutinin complex 500 μg (0.5 mg) human serum albumin 0.9 mg sodium chloride
Molecular Weight (neurotoxin)	150 kDa	150 kDa
Bulk Active Substance (total protein content)	~5 ng	~5 ng
Vial Size	500 Units	100 Units
Recommended Storage (postreconstitution)	2°–8°C (2°–8°C/use within 8 hours)	–5°C (2°–8°C/use within 4 hours)

countries, including Brazil: Botox (Allergan Inc., Irvine, California, USA), Dysport (Ipsen Limited, Paris, France), and Prosigne (Lanzhou Institute of Biological Products, China). Dysport is currently under investigation in the United States by the Food and Drug Administration (FDA), and its approval is expected for the next year. The commercialization of Dysport in the United States may go by the name of Reloxin. All these products produce similar and comparable effects in muscles and sweat glands, although they have distinct characteristics.[2,16] Other BT type As are currently under investigation, such as Xeomin (Merz Pharmaceuticals, Frankfurt, Germany)[30,31] and Neuronox (Meditox/Comedix, Seoul, South Korea).

Botulinum toxin type B is commercially available as Myobloc/NeuroBloc (Élan Pharmaceuticals Inc., South San Francisco, California, USA). Its use was approved by the FDA for the treatment of cervical dystonia in 2000[24,32] and was investigated in patients who have developed antibodies to type A.[29,33] Studies have shown the safety and efficacy of BT type B for the treatment of axillary hyperhidrosis,[34,35] although it is not currently approved for cosmetic use.[32] The data in the literature evaluating the safety and efficacy of BT type B for the treatment of facial wrinkles is sparse.[32]

MECHANISM OF ACTION

Botulinum A exotoxin prevents the release of Ach from the presynaptic neuron of the neuromuscular junction of striated muscles, producing chemical denervation and consequently reversible paralysis of the muscles.[16,25,26,36,37]

There are three steps involved in the inhibition of the release of neurotransmitter Ach from the presynaptic nerve terminal at the neuromuscular junction:[37,38]

1. *Binding:* The toxin binds to a receptor at the surface of the cell membrane of the presynaptic neuron.
2. *Internalization:* The toxin is internalized within the neuron.
3. *Blockage:* The release of Ach-containing vesicles is blocked by the interaction of the toxin with intracellular proteins that are responsible for vesicle release.

Weakness of affected muscles begins 6 to 36 hours after injections of BT, depending on the dose,[26] and is clinically evident 3 to 7 days after treatment, rarely later. This action lasts for 3 to 6 months, when the formation of new neuromuscular junctions (neurogenesis) occurs, permitting muscular function.[5,16,25,37,39–41]

The chemical denervation is also effective for excessive sweating, as it can affect the eccrine sweat glands leading to transient anhidrosis.[22,23,42]

PHARMACOLOGY, CONSERVATION, DILUTION, AND STORAGE

Botox, Reloxin, and Prosigne are marketed in a vacuum-dried lyophilized form, but only Botox and Prosigne are vacuum sealed.[43,44] Any vial of Botox or Prosigne[45] without vacuum seal should be discarded.[43] The expiration date indicated on the package of all these toxins should be respected.[43–46]

Myobloc is provided as a clear and colorless to light yellow sterile injectable solution in 3.5 mL glass vials.[46]

The particular characteristics of Botox and Reloxin are shown in Table 22-1.

Prosigne is made with *Clostridium botulinum* toxin type A hemagglutinin complex, 5 mg gelatin, 25 mg dextran, and 25 mg sacarose.[45]

Myobloc is made with *Clostridium botulinum* toxin type B in 0.05% human serum albumin, 0.01 M sodium succinate, and 0.1 M sodium chloride at an approximately pH 5.6. The neurotoxin complex is recovered from the fermentation process and purified through a series of precipitation and chromatography steps.[46] Myobloc vials contain 5,000 units (U) of BT type B per milliliter.[46] It is available in three vial presentations of 2,500, 5,000, and 10,000 U.[47]

The vials of Botox and Prosigne contain 100 units of BT type A.[43,45] The vials of Reloxin contains 500 units of BT type A.[44]

The storage temperature recommended by the manufacturers are 2°C to 8°C (35°–45°F) for Reloxin,[44] Prosigne,[45] and Myobloc[46] and –5°C (25°F) for Botox.[43]

Myobloc has shown stability for months when stored appropriately at this temperature.[48] Its manufacturer recommends to avoid freezing or shaking the vial of Myobloc.[46]

The recommended therapeutic doses of Botox and Reloxin are different,[49] and there are divergences about their equivalence.[50] Some publications consider that 1 U of Botox is equivalent to 3 U to 5 U of Reloxin.[21,50–53] The equivalence ratio use is 1:2.5 U between Botox and Reloxin, and similar results can be achieved. A recent pilot study performed by two of the present authors (Hexsel and Hexsel) demonstrated similar action halos between Botox and Reloxin at a conversion ratio of 1:2.5 U when injections are performed using the same volume and at the same depth on frontal muscles.[54] It is important to emphasize that side effects are more frequent when higher conversion rates, such as 1:3 or 1:4 or more, between Botox and Reloxin are used.[53,55]

Botox and Prosigne have 100 units of BT type A per vial and seem to be equivalent, although there is currently no evidence of this equivalence in the literature.

Manufacturers of all BT type A recommend the reconstitution of their products, with 0.9% preservative-free saline solution.[43–45,56,57]

Myobloc does not require reconstitution.[47] However, it also can be diluted with normal saline if necessary. Once diluted, the product must be used within 4 hours, as the formulation does not contain a preservative.[46]

Some studies tested the effects of the use of preservatives in BT type A dilutions.[26,58–60] In 2002, a double-blind, randomized controlled trial demonstrated no difference in the efficacy of the treatment when comparing results of BT type A reconstituted using isotonic sodium chloride with and without preservative. This indicated that reconstitution with preserved saline solution does not impair the stability of the toxin.[60] The use of BT type A reconstituted with preserved saline would also have additional advantages, such as longer periods of storage after reconstitution, reduced risk of bacterial contamination,[26] and less

painful when compared with preservative-free saline reconstitution.[26,59,60]

To date, only one fatal case of anaphylaxis was described in a patient who received Botox with lidocaine.[61] Mixtures of BT with local anesthetics should be avoided because it may change the tertiary structure of the toxin and interfere with its pharmacokinetics.[62]

The dilution of Botox, Prosigne, or Reloxin may be performed with 1 mL, 2 mL, 5 mL, or 10 mL of preservative-free saline, aiming a concentration of 10 U/0.1 mL; 5 U/0.1mL; 2 U/0.1 mL; or 1 U/0.1 mL, respectively, for Botox and Prosigne or 50 U/0.1 mL, 25 U/0.1 mL, 10 U/0.1 mL, or 5 U/0.1 mL for Reloxin. Dilution of the commercially available toxins depends on the physician's preference. For cosmetic purposes, dilution of the products with a smaller amount of volume is recommended because it results in higher concentration and allows the injection of smaller volumes. Additionally, it is safer and more precise, reducing the risk of complications and increasing the duration of the effects.[5,16,17,27,41,63,64] To achieve a 1:2.5 U equivalence dose between Botox (or Prosigne) and Reloxin, an easy and practical way to go is to dilute Reloxin in double the amount of volume of saline used for Botox, which allows physicians to inject same exact volumes of both product for the same indications by same technique, reducing the possibility of conversion mistakes. This equivalence ratio allows the achievement of similar results regarding potency and duration of effects.[54] However, proper to the high sensitivity of the muscles for BT, in some cases, especially at the lower face, the equivalence of Botox for Reloxin must be modified for 1:2 or lower.

The recommended doses of BT type A and B are different. The equivalence doses between BT type B (Myobloc) and BT type A (Botox) have been described as a conversion ratio of 50 U of Myobloc/1 U of Botox.[65]

BT type A may be inactivated by heat, freezing, shaking, excessive dilution, and surface tension generated from bubbles when the toxin is reconstituted.[37]

The reconstituted vial should be used within 4 hours according to the manufacturers' instruction for Botox[43] and Prosigne[45] and 8 hours for Reloxin.[44] They can be stored in the refrigerator at 2°C to 8°C. In 1996, a study demonstrated that reconstituted Botox refrigerated for up to 1 month had no substantial loss of potency.[58] More recently, Hexsel et al. demonstrated in a multicenter, double-blind study that reconstituted Botox stored in the recommended conditions may be applied up to 6 weeks without losing its effectiveness.[66] A similar study with Reloxin is being done, and the results will be available soon.

Any reconstituted BT type A should be clear, colorless, and free of particles.[43,45,67]

A comparative study using BT type A (Botox 5 U) and BT type B (Myobloc 500 U) for the treatment of forehead wrinkles described that BT type B produced a greater area of diffusion and a more rapid onset of action than type A.[68]

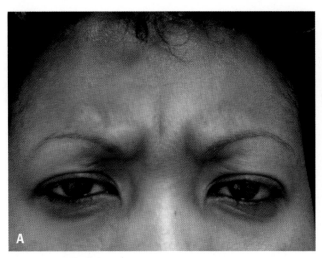 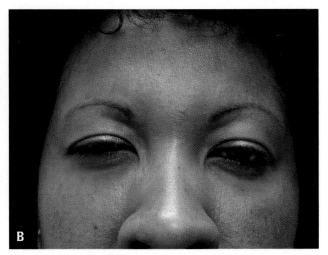

Figure 22-1 Before **(A)** and after **(B)** pictures of the glabellar area, showing the efficacy of the treatment with botulinum toxin.

INDICATIONS OF BOTULINUM TOXIN INJECTIONS IN DARK-SKINNED PATIENTS

The cosmetic use of BT is recognized as an effective and efficient treatment for dynamic wrinkles, independently of sex, age, or race.[18,69] Some characteristics that are unique

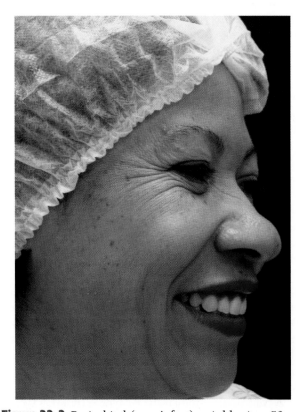

Figure 22-2 Periorbital (crow's feet) wrinkles in a 50-year-old patient. She also recruits her nasal muscles when smiling.

to darker ethnic skin patients are relevant for BT injections in these individuals. They include the rounded facial phenotype, fuller upper and lower lips, and broader and flattened nostrils. Dark skin patients (DSPs) have fewer facial wrinkles than fair-skinned patients when comparing patients of similar age. Dynamic wrinkles in these individuals are also predominantly found in the upper face, especially in glabellar area (Fig. 22-1A).

In the glabellar area, BT injections can erase or diminish lines[70] and promote better position[17,71,72] and shape of the brow (Fig. 22-1B).[16,56,73–75] Repeated injections of BT can also prevent the physiologic brow ptosis.

Periorbital wrinkles are one of the earliest signs of the normal aging process. They are mainly caused by a combination of photodamage and muscular hyperactivity. Periorbital wrinkles appear after the age of 40 in DSPs and can be treated by injections of BT type A (Fig. 22-2).[58,76,77] Nasal wrinkles can appear in these patients when smiling, but they are usually associated with excessive activity of glabellar muscles (Fig. 22-2).

Most DSPs present late physiologic blepharoptosis. However, eye bulging seems to be as frequent as in fair-skinned patients, because this condition is basically caused by anatomical configuration of the eyelid and subcutaneous fat.

Perioral injections of BT are rarely needed or performed in DSPs. BT can correct perioral wrinkles (Fig. 22-3), increase the fullness of the lips, and cause slight eversion of the upper lip.[78] These effects are usually undesirable. Perioral wrinkles appear late in life and are rare in DSPs.

As the mentalis muscles can be very expressive in some DSPs, this is often an indication for BT injections for these individuals. The mentalis muscles have synergistic movements with the depressor angulis oris (DAO) muscles, so mentalis muscles relaxation determines less action of the DAO muscle.

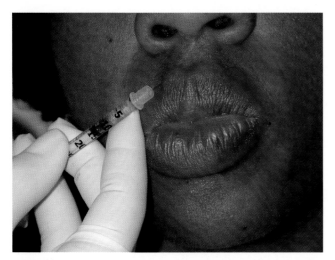

Figure 22-3 Small doses of BT injections can be used in the treatment of perioral wrinkles, such as 0.5 to 1 U of Botox or 1.25 to 2.5 U of Dysport/Reloxin.

Aging neck is characterized by signs of photodamage, including wrinkles, laxity, loose skin, and poikiloderma of Civatte. These findings are more frequent in Caucasians and can be treated adjunctively by other techniques, such as surgical lift of the neck and tightening. Other signs of aging neck are wrinkles caused by the action of the platysmal bands. Selected cases in whom the platysmal bands are expressive can be successfully treated by BT type A applications.[19,20,77,79] DSPs present fewer signs of photoaging, but the action of the platysmal bands seems to be similar to fair-skinned patients.

Independent of skin color, all patients develop the same response to BT injections. In the phase III BT type A clinical trials, 21 of the 405 enrolled were African American. An analysis was conducted looking at the overall efficacy and safety in the 21 African Americans compared with Caucasian subjects. There were no statistically significant differences in the efficacy or safety responses[80] (Fig. 22-4A–C).

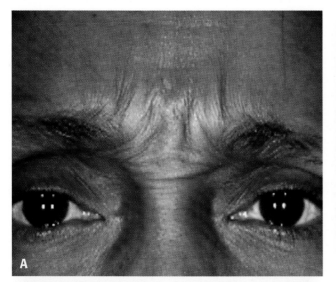

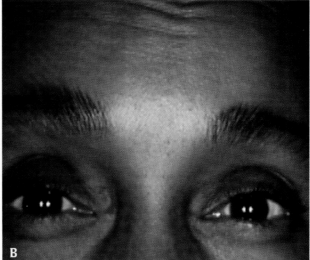

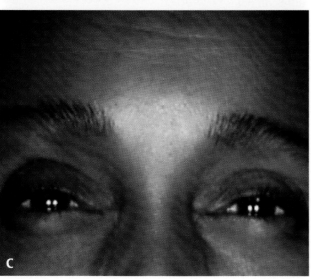

Figure 22-4 Glabellar lines at baseline **(A)**. Patient treated with 20 units of botulinum toxin A. Note responses at day 30 **(B)** and day 60 **(C)**.

Doses and treatment should be individualized for each patient, according to the muscles to be treated, their location and size, as well as their potency of contraction. Cultural and other particular aspects, such as patients' desires and needs, should also be taken into account.

CONTRAINDICATIONS

The complete medical history of the patient is required to identify any contraindications to BT injections. BT is not recommended in patients who are psychologically unstable, overly anxious, or have unrealistic expectations.[5,27,62] It should not be used in the presence of infection at the proposed injection sites.[17,43,45] Previous history of neuromuscular disease is a relative contraindication.[21,26,37,43] It is not known if BT type A affects the reproduction capacity or causes harm to the fetus when administered to a pregnant woman; therefore, it is classified as a category C drug in pregnancy.[27,28,41,45,81] It is also unknown if it is excreted in human milk.[43] Therefore, its use in pregnancy or breastfeeding women is not recommended.[21,26–28,37,41,56]

The administration of BT type A must be avoided in patients known to be allergic to any ingredient of the formulation, such as botulinum toxin, lactose, gelatin, saline, or human albumin.[5,26,45,56]

Simultaneous administration of BT type A and aminoglycosides or other agents interfering with neuromuscular transmission, such as quinine and calcium channel blockers, should only be performed with caution, as they can potentate the effects of the toxin.[21,26–28,41,45,82]

One case of death caused by anaphylaxis to Botox-lidocaine mixture has been described.[61] An important precaution of not reconstituting the toxin in any fluid different than 0.9% saline should be taken and the history of previous reaction to drugs, especially lidocaine, should be investigated before the injections.

PRE- AND POSTOPERATIVE CARE

Preoperative instructions should be given to all patients. Certain drugs that may cause prolonged bruising, such as anticoagulants, analgesics, steroidal and nonsteroidal anti-inflammatory agents, vitamin E or beta-blockers, if possible, should be stopped 7 to 10 days before the injections.[27,41,56,83,84]

Photographs should be taken before and after the procedure, preferably at rest and at maximum contraction of the facial muscles.

Special caution should follow the application of BT type A for any cosmetic purpose to minimize the risk of side effects and complications. The recommended advice includes to avoid pressing, massaging, or manipulating the treated area in the following 3 to 4 hours after injections,[5,64,85] to avoid physical extenuating activities during

the rest of the day,[74,85] and to maintain vertical posture in the 4 hours following injections.[5,41,64,85] Some authors believe that the toxin works better in actively contracted muscles after injections, so they recommend patients contract the treated muscles repeatedly a few hours after the injections.[5,21,37,64,85,86]

TECHNIQUES OF INJECTIONS

Patients are positioned sitting upright on a chair with the upper part of the body elevated.[5]

After cleaning the skin, the points to be injected are marked using a marking pen while the facial musculature is examined. Antisepsis of the area to be treated must be performed carefully, usually with 70% alcohol or iodinated alcohol.[17]

Local anesthesia is usually not necessary. Pain upon injection is slight but may be further minimized by previously using topical anesthetics[28] or by cooling the area before and after the injections, if necessary.[5,21,41,67]

The use of an 1-mL or smaller syringe with a 30-gauge needle is preferable and minimizes patient's discomfort.[39,50] The BD Ultra-Fine II short-needle 0.3-cc syringe is considered the ideal syringe to deliver precise units of botulinum toxin to the underlying musculature for cosmetic treatment of the aging face.[87] BT type A should be injected slowly, followed by gentle massage at the injection site.

All toxins once active provoke the formation of an action halo around the injected points. Percutaneous injections of BT type A deposit the toxins into or adjacent to the overactive muscles, relaxing the target muscles and eliminating overlying rhytides of the skin. It is important to emphasize that Botox and Reloxin have similar action halos when the equivalent dose of 1:2.5 U between Botox and Reloxin in the same volume, depth, and technique are used. These action halos are sometimes misinterpreted as diffusion halos.[54]

ANATOMIC CONSIDERATIONS FOR BOTULINUM TOXIN INJECTIONS AND INDICATIONS

The knowledge of the facial muscular anatomy is extremely important for correct and successful treatments with BT. Facial lines and wrinkles are usually perpendicular to the direction of the fibers of the muscles.[5]

Upper face
Horizontal forehead wrinkles

The function of frontalis muscles is to raise the skin of the forehead, elevating the eyebrows.[5,74,88] The fibers of these muscles are oriented vertically, and their contraction leads

Captique	Nonanimal streptococci	For injection into the mid- to deep dermis for correction of moderate to severe facial wrinkles and folds (e.g., nasolabial folds)	No	Cross-linked using DVS Similar to Restylane but softer	Immediate effect May last up to 1 year	FDA approved for filling moderate to severe facial wrinkles and folds (e.g., nasolabial folds)
Hylaform Fineline/ Hylaform/ Hylaform Plus	Nonanimal Rooster combs	Hylaform Fineline for superficial papillary placement to treat fine lines (e.g., periorbital and perioral lines) Hylaform for midreticular placement to treat glabellar lines, oral commissures, moderate nasolabial folds, and acne scars Hylaform Plus for deep reticular placement above the subcutis to treat deeper folds (e.g., deep nasolabial folds), lip enhancement, facial contouring, and deeper scars	No	5.5 mg/mL HA Cross-linked using DVS Mean HA particle size larger in Hylaform Plus than Hylaform	Immediate effect Lasts several months	Hylaform and Hylaform Plus are FDA approved for moderate to severe facial wrinkles and folds (e.g., nasolabial folds) Hylaform Fineline is in use outside the U.S.
*Juvéderm 18/ 24/30/24HV/30HV Ultra (U.S.) Ultra Plus (U.S.)	Nonanimal streptococci		No	Cross-linked using BDDE Monophasic	Immediate effect Lasts several months	PMA for 24HV (Ultra, 30HV (Ultra Plus) and 30 formulations FDA approval in December 2006 Also, use outside U.S.

(continued)

227

Table 23-1

Hyaluronic acid fillers (Continued)

Injectable	Source	Skin test needed?	Main uses	Characteristics	Duration of effect	FDA approval status
Teosyal	Nonanimal streptococci	No	Meso formulation for preventing wrinkles and reducing deficits in elasticity and hydration in the face and neck 27G formulation for nasolabial folds, lip augmentation, and facial contouring 30G formulation for linear wrinkles and peribuccal contours	Meso is 15 mg/g HA 27G and 30G are 25 mg/g HA Cross-linked using BDDE Monophasic	Immediate effect Lasts several months	In use outside U.S.
Esthelis	Nonanimal streptococci	No	"Soft" formulation is for fine lines "Basic" formulation is for at least medium lines	HA is double cross-linked using BDDE "Soft" formulation contains 20 mg/g HA "Basic" formulation contains 25 mg/g HA	Immediate effect Lasts several months	Not FDA approved but in use outside U.S.
Puragen/Puragen Plus	Nonanimal bacterial	No	For adding volume, smoothing wrinkles, and restoring fullness in the glabellar lines, nasolabial folds, and lips Also suitable for wrinkles, lines, depressions, scars, and facial contouring in most areas of the face	Puragen Plus contains lidocaine	Immediate effect Lasts several months	Puragen Plus under review at FDA Puragen in use outside U.S.

| Dermalive/ Dermadeep | 60% HA of nonanimal origin and 40% acrylic hydrogel | No | For nasolabial folds, marionette lines, lip contours, cheeks, chin, and facial scars Dermalive is for dermal injection Dermadeep is for subcutaneous injection | Permanent injectable implants | Immediate effect Lasts years | Not FDA approved but in use outside U.S. |

BDDE, butanediol-diglycidyl-ether; DVS, divinyl sulfone; FDA, Food and Drug Administration; HA, hyaluronic acid.

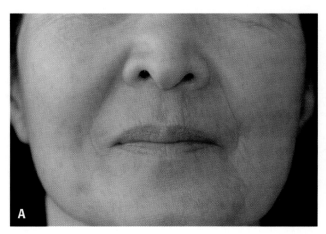 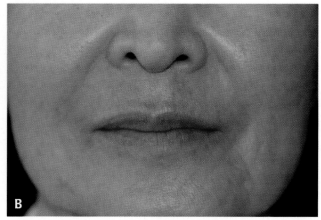

Figure 23-1 A: Baseline nasolabial folds of and lips of an Asian patient. **B:** Three weeks post hyaluronic acid injection (Restylane) to lips and nasolabial folds.

needs to be met. These subtypes commonly differ in rate of cross-linking, size, and formulation of HA strands or particles, and HA concentration. Typically one formulation is intended for the treatment of fine lines, a middle formulation is intended for treating medium-depth lines, and one formulation is intended for resolving deeper defects or replacing volume. Statistics from the American Society for Aesthetic Plastic Surgery indicate that the use of HA fillers in the United States grew almost 700% between 2003 and 2004.[1]

COLLAGEN FILLERS

Bovine collagen

Bovine-derived collagen fillers were first approved for soft-tissue augmentation in the 1980s in the United States. These fillers set the standard in filler materials for smoothing facial lines, wrinkles, and scars and in providing lip border definition until HA products became available recently. More than a million treatments have been performed with bovine collagen, and the most widely used products include Zyderm I, Zyderm II, and Zyplast (Table 23-2). The content of collagen concentration varies in these products. For example, Zyderm I contains 95% to 98% type I collagen with some type III collagen. It has 3.5% bovine collagen by weight. Zyderm II is similar to Zyderm I except that it contains 6.5% collagen by weight. Neither Zyderm I nor II are cross-linked. Zyplast has 3.5% bovine collagen cross-linked by glutaraldehyde to form a latticework and is considered less immunogenic and more resistant to degradation than Zyderm I and Zyderm II. All three products contain 0.3% lidocaine and therefore are contraindicated in persons who have lidocaine allergy. Furthermore, these products are contraindicated in patients with hypersensitivity to bovine collagen. Approx-

imately 5% of patients may experience hypersensitivity to injectable bovine collagen and so skin testing is required before treatment. At least two skin tests should be performed at least 2 weeks apart, with the last test at least 2 weeks before treatment for new patients or anyone who has not received the same product within 2 years. A positive test result is defined as erythema, induration, tenderness, or swelling that persists for more than 6 hours after implantation. If any hypersensitivity occurs, it is usually within 1 to 2 weeks of treatment and manifests as erythema and induration, with or without pruritus in the area treated. Treatment of hypersensitivity may include topical immunomodulatory calcineurin inhibitors, topical steroids, intralesional steroids, systemic steroids, and systemic cyclosporine. Observation alone may be enough in mild cases. Contraindications to injectable bovine collagen include a history of an anaphylactic event of any cause, previous sensitivity to bovine collagen, lidocaine sensitivity, pregnancy, and active infection at the treatment site. Although no formal testing has been completed, patients undergoing hormonal fluctuation (e.g., during pregnancy or the menopause) may have an increased risk for hypersensitivity.

Bovine collagen treatments reportedly last between 3 and 18 months, with an average duration of 2 to 6 months, depending on location. In the authors opinion, bovine collagen lasts approximately 2 to 3 months in the nasolabial folds and significantly less in the lips. Zyderm I is injected into papillary dermis to correct superficial facial rhytides. Zyderm II is injected slightly deeper to treat moderate rhytides and scars. Zyplast, injected into the deeper dermis for treatment of moderate to severe rhytides and scars, can be expected to last longer than Zyderm I or II. However, Zyplast is contraindicated in the glabellar area due to reports of skin necrosis after injection into this area.

Table 23-2

Collagen fillers

Injectable	Source	Skin test needed?	Main uses	Characteristics	Duration of effect	FDA approval status
Zyderm I/ Zyderm II/ Zyplast	Bovine	Yes	Zyderm is for fine lines, wrinkles, shallow scars, and thin-skinned areas Zyplast is for pronounced lines and wrinkles, scars, and thicker-skinned areas	Contains lidocaine Zyderm I is 3.5% collagen by weight Zyderm II is 6.5% collagen by weight Zyplast is 3.5% collagen cross-linked by glutaraldehyde	Immediate effect Lasts for a few months	Approved for the correction of contour deformities of the dermis in non–weight-bearing areas
Evolence	Porcine	No	For wrinkles; nasolabial folds; scars; atrophy from disease or trauma; defects secondary to rhinoplasty, skin graft, or other surgically induced irregularities; and other soft-tissue defects or deficiencies	Cross-linking of collagen achieved without use of potentially toxin chemicals Theoretically more immunocompatible with human collagen because of removal of telopeptides (the most antigenic part of collagen) during production	Immediate effect Lasts for at least 1 year	Not FDA approved but in use outside U.S.
Cymetra (micronized AlloDerm)	Human cadaver collagen matrix	No	For lips, nasolabial folds, and deep wrinkles and lines	Multiple treatments needed to build tissue and achieve stable level of defect correction; lasts 2 months	Immediate effect Lasts for a few months	Not required

(continued)

Table 23-2

Collagen fillers (Continued)

Injectable	Source	Skin test needed?	Main uses	Characteristics	Duration of effect	FDA approval status
Cosmoderm/ Cosmoplast	Human foreskin	No	For the correction of soft-tissue contour deficiencies, such as wrinkles and acne scars. Cosmoderm is injected into the superficial papillary dermis. Cosmoplast is injected into the mid- to deep dermis	35 mg/mL collagen. Contains lidocaine. Cosmoderm is not cross-linked and is used for superficial lines. Cosmoplast is cross-linked and is primarily used for more pronounced wrinkles	Immediate effect. Lasts for a few months	Approved
Fascian	Human cadaver fascia	Usually unnecessary	Stimulates collagen formation, adds bulk	A very thick suspension of solid pieces of fibrous material	Lasts for a few months	Not required
Autologen	Autologous dermal matrix	No	For wrinkles and other skin irregularities. An alternative to traditional collagen injections	Small pieces of patient's own skin are harvested (2 square inches required per mL product) and processed. Typically, two or three treatments needed over a 6- to 8-week period to correct most depressions of the skin	More than 1 year	Approval not required but product is no longer available

| Isolagen | Autologous fibroblasts | No | For facial rhytides and dermal defects | 3-mm punch biopsy is sent to a laboratory. After 6–8 weeks, cultured fibroblasts are returned to the physician (need to be injected within 48 hrs of leaving laboratory). Usually three sets of injections, 2 weeks apart. Fibroblasts may continue to multiply and create collagen in vivo, thus inducing a gradual and continual improvement | Effects visible within 1–3 months. Results may theoretically persist indefinitely as autologous cells are unlikely to be degraded by the body. However, long-term clinical data are awaited | Anticipated Biologics License Application filing in 2006 |

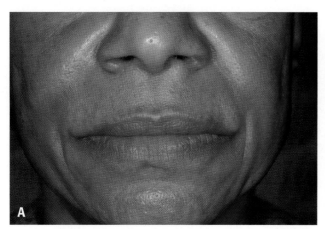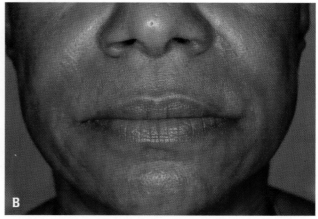

Figure 23-2 A: Baseline lower face nasolabial folds. **B:** One month postinjection with human collagen (Cosmoplast). (Courtesy of Pearl E. Grimes, MD.)

Porcine collagen

Evolence is a porcine-derived collagen filler available in some countries outside the United States. It is claimed that a novel cross-linking procedure (Glymatrix technology) used in the production of the material slows the rate of collagen biodegradation and results in a more prolonged clinical improvement. Therefore, maintenance of the effect may be achievable with only one treatment session each year (manufacturer's information). The most antigenic part of the collagen molecule is removed during the production process, so theoretically, the product should be highly immunologically compatible with human collagen. At this time, no public data is available on the duration of the product, which is likely to be critical in determining the demand by physicians and patients.

Autologous collagen

Bovine-derived collagen fillers have been the most widely used type of collagen, but attempts made at reducing the potential for hypersensitivity reactions have resulted in formulations derived from autologous tissue. By using only material derived from the patient's own body, autologous fillers aim to avoid any potential issues of biocompatibility and to use autologous cultured fibroblasts to stimulate long-term collagenesis in vivo. In addition, cryogenic preservation of the source material may offer patients the ability to receive treatment in later years from material harvested when they were younger. Whether this might offer any clinical benefit is unknown.

The manufacturer of Autologen provided autologous collagen, but the product is no longer available. Preliminary phase III data for Isolagen were announced in 2005, and the manufacturer plans to conduct one additional trial before submitting a complete regulatory package to the Food and Drug Administration (FDA) in 2006. Isolagen needs to be injected into the patient within 48 hours of leaving the laboratory. This can create scheduling challenges. Although initially, the idea of autologous collagen was viewed favorably, this technique has not been used to any great degree in the United States despite the technology having been available for years. There have been several drawbacks—mostly, this is a time-consuming and expensive technology to use, the effects may take several weeks to become evident, and long-term data are not available for an adequate assessment of their longevity potential.

Other human collagen

Cosmoderm and Cosmoplast are derived from human collagen and are the human-derived counterparts of bovine-derived Zyderm and Zyplast. Cosmoderm contains 35 mg/mL collagen, is a non–cross-linked formulation, and is used in the treatment of superficial rhytides. Cosmoplast also contains 35 mg/mL collagen, is cross-linked with glutaraldehyde, and is primarily used for the treatment of moderate to deep rhytides (Fig. 23-2A,B). They have little cross-reactivity, and therefore skin testing is not needed. On the other hand, they contain 0.3% lidocaine and therefore are contraindicated in patients who have hypersensitivity to lidocaine. Overcorrection of approximately 20% to 30% is required for optimal improvements, and few studies have evaluated long-term results.

AlloDerm (FDA approved for cosmetic corrective use) is an acellular dermal matrix derived from donated human cadaver skin tissue supplied by U.S. American Association of Tissue Banks–compliant tissue banks. It has been used for a variety of surgical reconstructive procedures. Because it is human derived, no skin test is recommended by the manufacturer. Cymetra is a micronized particulate form of AlloDerm. This material is rehydrated with lidocaine in the physician's office before injection, so the procedure is far less painful. Similar to AlloDerm, Cymetra contains collagen, elastin, other proteins, and proteoglycans. Because of the small particle size, Cymetra can be delivered by injection as a minimally invasive tissue graft. It is not recommended for use in the glabellar or periorbital region.

NONCOLLAGEN AUTOLOGOUS FILLERS

Autologous fat can be used for lip augmentation and to fill moderate to deep wrinkles and scars. Fat cells from the patient's own thighs, abdomen, or buttocks are processed and then reinjected. The duration of improvement can vary tremendously between patients, from months to years. Neither FDA approval nor skin testing is required. The drawbacks are that an additional surgical procedure to harvest fat cells from patients is required, increasing the risks of surgical complications, such as bleeding and infection. Furthermore, it is more difficult to inject fat with a controlled flow, and this may increase lumpiness at the injection site (e.g., the lips). Although fat cells are derived from the patient's own body, it is unclear from studies whether the injections last any longer than other fillers, such as HA injections.[5,6] Additionally, the harvesting procedure itself can result in temporary or permanent problems, such as hyperpigmentation or scars.

Plasmagel is an emulsion of the patient's own plasma and vitamin C. It has been used to add volume, and its effects are reported to last for up to 3 months. Significant scientific data are not currently available about this product.

PERMANENT FILLERS

Long-lasting and permanent fillers are also available. The lack of biodegradability of these fillers assures that their effects are long term. The corollary to this is that any adverse effects are also likely to be long term, perhaps permanent. Additionally, even when permanent fillers are placed correctly, the face continues to age and change, and what may be in the right place today may be in the wrong location in the future. Therefore, permanent fillers or very long-lasting fillers should only be used with extreme caution in persons with great skill in the use of the specific filler if used at all. It may be worth forsaking the apparent convenience of long-term treatment to avoid the risk of permanent problems or patient dissatisfaction.

Hydroxylapatite (Radiesse, formerly Radiance)

Radiesse is composed of smooth microspheres of synthetic calcium hydroxylapatite suspended in a polysac-charide gel. The gel is resorbed, leaving the particles. It is hypothesized that collagenesis occurs around the particles,[7] but data to substantiate this are not available. The product results in immediate clinical improvements and longer-lasting results, although as is the case with most of the so-called semipermanent fillers, published data on duration are scant. The hydroxylapatite is reported by the company to form a scaffold through which the body's own collagen forms, but fibrosis and foreign body reactions may be the mechanism by which a longer-term filling effect occurs. This longevity may also be a disadvantage in that the product is not easily cleared by the body, and therefore, in the event of excessive injection, tissue reaction, or a poor cosmetic result, the effect cannot be easily corrected. For adverse effects, such as nodules, corticosteroid injections have been used, but the adverse effect may still persist. Radiesse is FDA approved for correction of moderate to severe facial wrinkles and folds, and facial lipoatrophy. Radiesse is used for facial contouring in areas including nasolabial folds, marionettes lines, cheeks, and chin. Because of possible unpredictable tissue reactions, many authors caution against its use in the lips.

Poly-L-lactic acid (Sculptra)

Sculptra contains absorbable non–animal-derived poly-L-lactic acid, and it is FDA approved for restoration and for correction of HIV-induced facial lipoatrophy. It is also used to treat wrinkles and acne scars, as well as to improve facial and lip contouring. Although it has been used for wrinkles and other cosmetic enhancements in several countries for some years, it has not been approved for such use by the FDA. Results are not immediate and usually require multiple treatments spaced 2 to 4 weeks apart. Sculptra induces an immediate local inflammatory response, which leads to a progressive increase in volume. Indeed, the product is promoted as a "volume enhancer" as opposed to "wrinkle filler." Nodules have been reported frequently, and this may be related to technique (dilution, level, and amount of injection). After several injections, the effects can last for up to 1 to 2 years, but touch-ups are usually required.

Silicone

Multiple studies have documented the efficacy of silicone for the correction of wrinkles and volume restoration. However, silicone no doubt is one of the most controversial of all filling agents. Its use has been associated with the migration of silicone particles, causing undesired side effects years after the injection. Other complications of silicone include persistent nodules, ulceration, and cellulitis. In 1994 and 1997, Adatosil 5000 and Silikon 1000 were approved by the FDA for intraocular tamponade to treat retinal detachment. Hence, off-label use of silicone has been permitted since 1997. However, many physicians remain fearful of its complications and potential litigation.

Silicone has recently been used for treatment of human immunodeficiency virus associated facial lipodystrophy,[8] but further studies are warranted to determine long-term safety and efficacy.

INJECTION TECHNIQUE

There is wide variation in the way one injects fillers. The technique will vary depending on the location of the injection site, the types of fillers used, and on the individual patient. There are several general guidelines that are useful. Having the patient in an upright position allows the injector to accurately evaluate the rhytides or defects. Almost everyone has asymmetry in the face, and this should be pointed out to patients before injection and documented with pre- and postprocedure photographs. Applying a topical anesthesia for at least 30 to 60 minutes before injection will reduce the pain of injection. Local nerve blocks, particularly the infraorbial and mental nerve blocks for the mid- and lower face injections, are useful, but care should be taken not to distort the tissues in which the filler will be placed. Waiting at least 20 minutes will allow the block to be more effective. Cosmoderm/Cosmoplast and Zyderm/Zyplast have lidocaine in the formulations and are much less painful to inject than currently avialable HA fillers.

In general for injection of collagen or HA, there are at least two different techniques that are used commonly. A threading technique in which the filler is injected along the entire length of the defect can be used. This allows for a smooth contiguous layering of the filler substance. One advantage of this technique is that there are fewer needle punctures, however, it can lead to a cordlike feel if the injection is not deep enough or too much filler material is placed. The serial puncture technique uses multiple punctures to inject a small amount of filler at a time. This allows for more precise injection into a given area but requires more needle punctures and can lead to a more lumpy result if careful technique is not used. In general, for HAs and collagens, a 27- or 30-gauge needle is used, though each product comes with a specifically recommended needle based on the product's physiological characteristics. For poly-L-lactic acid injection into cheeks, using a 25-gauge needle for the injection will help avoid clotting within the needle. The fanning technique works well for injecting poly-L-lactic acid into the cheeks for lipoatrophy. This technique involves placing the needle through a single entry point in the skin and injecting the material in a linear fashion. From this single entry point, the needle is redirected in a fanlike pattern. In general, the poly-L-lactic acid is injected in a retrograde fashion.

The depth of injection depends on the fillers being used. For example, Zyderm and Cosmoderm are injected into the superficial dermis. The needle should be placed very superficially and with minimal force on the plunger.

On the other hand, Zyplast, Cosmoplast, and HA are injected into the mid- to deep dermis by directing the needle in a 45-degree angle. Often, the threading technique is used to inject into the deeper dermis along the nasolabial folds or into the lips for volume. This is followed by a superficial injection using a serial puncture technique to place a small amount of the Zyderm or Cosmoderm to fill the lines and to create definition of the lips. In treating the nasolabial crease, fillers should be placed medial to the crease to avoid further accentuating the cheeks. In the glabella, Zyplast and Cosmoplast should be avoided because of the risk of vascular injury leading to skin necrosis. This complication has also been reported with HAs. Hydroxylapatite and poly-L-lactic acid are usually placed in the deep dermis at the dermal-subcutaneous junction or subdermal plane. Following treatment with fillers, massage and ice applied to the treated area can reduce erythema, ecchymoses, and swelling. In general, there are no specific precautions in injecting patients with darker skin types, but some recommend using fewer needle punctures to decrease the possibility of injection site erythema and postinflammatory hyperpigmentation. However, there are no studies to support use of the threading technique versus the serial puncture technique in darker skin.

USING FILLERS IN DARKER RACIAL ETHNIC GROUPS

There is wide variation in the color and texture of the skin between darker skin types and that of Caucasian skin. In general, darker skin color is due to an increase in melanin and melanosome distribution. The melanin in skin types IV through VI has been reported to provide an inherent sun protection factor of 13, which may result in less skin aging being evident at an early age compared with paler skin.[9] The fine-to-deep rhytides that are characteristic of Caucasian skin are less prevalent in darker skin. Photoaging is minimal in darker racial ethnic groups. As a result, younger patients with darker skin tend to have a lower need for fillers than Caucasian patients, and care should be taken not to overcorrect. On the other hand, the midface aging of darker skin type, in particular African Americans, warrants the use of filler substances to correct nasolabial lines and elemental lines. The thicker and more fibrous dermis of ethnic skin also may have a tendency toward a more vigorous fibroblastic response during wound healing. This may promote hypertrophic scars and keloid formation. Darker skin types are also more prone to dyschromic conditions, including ephiledes, melasma, and postinflammatory hyperpigmentation. Because darker skin types are more prone than Caucasian skin to dyspigmentation, keloid formation, and abnormal scarring, patient selection is important. Thorough exams and detailed patient histories can help to exclude patients who are most prone to scar formation and hyperpigmentation. All injections

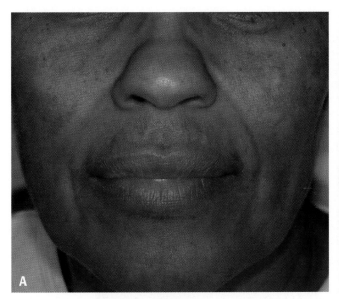
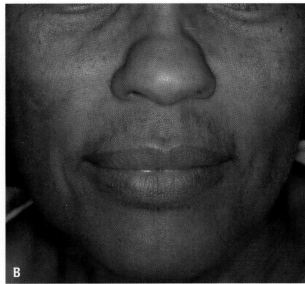

Figure 23-3 A: Baseline nasolabial folds in an African American patient. **B:** One month post–hyaluronic acid (Restylane) injection to nasolabial folds and cheeks. (Courtesy of Pearl E. Grimes, MD.)

should proceed gingerly to avoid traumatizing the skin. An initial small test dose followed by a waiting period of a few weeks is not unreasonable in patients for whom the risk of reactions is thought to be possibly high. However, this is not generally needed for skin types IV through VI patients unless recommended for the specific product by the manufacturer. There are no fillers known to be specifically unsuitable for darker skin types. Nevertheless, if fillers are injected too superficially or in thin skin, such as is found in the periorbital areas, they can give the skin a bluish appearance.

Currently, there is no evidence that darker racial groups experience a higher incidence of problems with fillers than Caucasians (Fig. 23-3A,B and Fig. 23-4A,B). Of note, the FDA has been requiring that companies trying to obtain approval for fillers do postmarketing studies in patients of color if they do not include enough of these patients in their registration trials. Current evidence and clinical experience of using fillers in darker skin types suggest that these products are associated with very few adverse events in both Caucasians and non-Caucasians. It appears that any individual demonstrating an inflammatory response is at risk of pigmentation problems regardless of the color of their skin. Thus, Caucasians who show prolonged erythema also have the potential to develop dyspigmentation. For patients with darker skin, injection site dyschromia may persist, and the possibility of this problem should be discussed with patients before treatment. Also, injection technique using fewer injections with a threading technique rather than multiple injections to treat an area should be considered (Fig. 23-5A,B). No reports of keloid formation or

hypertrophic scars post–filler injection in darker skin types were found. Any hyperpigmentation that does arise can be treated with the standard therapeutics using bleaching agents, retinoids, and exfoliating agents.

Clinical trials involving more than 400 subjects treated with either Juvederm (30, 24HV, or 30HV) or Zyplast have been completed and reveal some useful information on skin of color treated with fillers. Among patients treated with Juvederm in a split-face study with Zyplast in the treatment of nasolabial folds, no differences in efficacy or adverse events were seen between Caucasians and non-Caucasians. Also, among patients treated with Zyplast, no differences in efficacy or adverse events were seen between Caucasians and non-Caucasians. Hypersensitivity was seen in only one non-Caucasian patient treated with Zyplast and no patients treated with Juvederm. No postinflammatory hyperpigmentation or abnormal scarring was seen in any patient in the trial. These data suggest that both Juvederm and Zyplast are very safe and effective in both Caucasians and non-Caucasians and would not imply that any special precautions are needed in darker skin types (data on file, Allergan, Inc.).

In the U.S. census for 2000, 25% of the population was reported to be nonwhite.[10,11] The percentage of people in the United States with darker skin types has been increasing in recent years, and some shifts have been particularly rapid. For example, between 1980 and 2000, the Hispanic population more than doubled, and the Asian and Pacific Islander population tripled. Furthermore, the proportion of all individuals undergoing cosmetic procedures who are not white has also been increasing (from

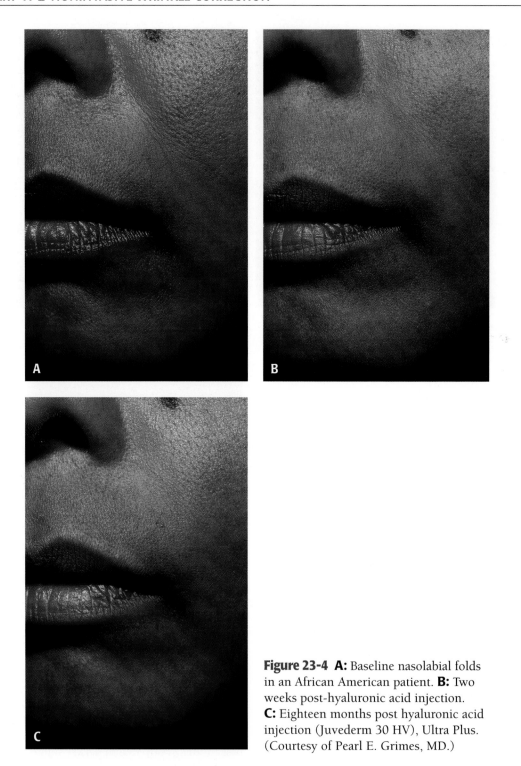

Figure 23-4 A: Baseline nasolabial folds in an African American patient. **B:** Two weeks post-hyaluronic acid injection. **C:** Eighteen months post hyaluronic acid injection (Juvederm 30 HV), Ultra Plus. (Courtesy of Pearl E. Grimes, MD.)

15% in 2000 to 17% in 2001, 19% in 2002, and 20% in 2003 and 2004). Despite the trend for more people with darker skin types to undergo cosmetic procedures, there are few data evaluating the use of fillers specifically in patients with skin of color. This is largely because the vast majority of patients in clinical trials have been Caucasians. For example, of 137 patients in a trial that resulted in the approval of Restylane by the FDA in 2003, only 8% were

Hispanic, 1.5% were Asian, and 1.5% were black. As a result, and to increase the knowledge base concerning the use of such fillers in darker skin types, the FDA approved Restylane only on condition that its manufacturer conduct a postmarketing study of an additional 100 patients with Fitzpatrick skin type V or VI.[12] The aim of the study was to assess the likelihood of keloid formation, pigmentation changes, and hypersensitivity reactions in such patients

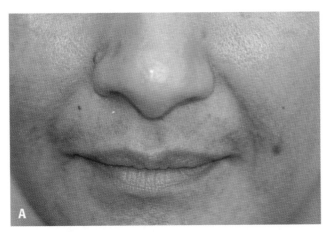
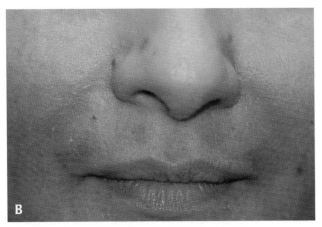

Figure 23-5 A: Baseline nasolabial folds of a Hispanic patient. **B:** Immediately after hyaluronic acid injection (Restylane). A threading technique using fewer injections was used to treat the nasolabial folds to minimize injection site dyschromia.

during nasolabial fold treatment. The study required a 6-month follow-up, but no results had been released in print at the time of this writing. A similar requirement for a postmarketing study was also required by the FDA when it approved Hylaform in 2004 because the trial that resulted in its approval had included relatively few non-white patients (of 261 patients, 13% were Hispanic, 3% were Asian, 2% were African American, and 2% were other non-Caucasians).[13,14] The postmarketing study was designed to evaluate the incidence of dermal keloid and pigmentation disorders, hypertrophic scarring, and hypersensitivity reactions (Fig. 23-6A,B).

CULTURAL CONSIDERATIONS

The potentially different desires and facial features of various patients of different ethnic backgrounds means that it is important to adjust the goal of treatment to each patient's wishes and to understand both what is culturally acceptable to them and what they particularly desire. They may want to maintain the features that they see as part of their ethnicity and thus treatment should not aim to create the same look in all patients. Also, some races are more likely to opt for certain cosmetic procedures than others. Lip augmentation is particularly common in Caucasian patients. In contrast, few African American women request lip augmentation. Individualization is key, as there is natural variation that can affect treatment decisions.

COMBINATION THERAPIES

The best results in dermatology are often achieved through combination therapy, and cosmetic dermatology is no exception. Different types of fillers can be used

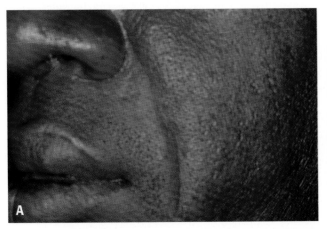
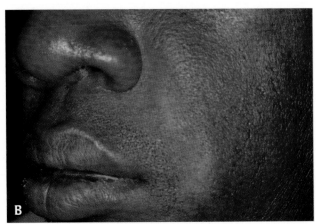

Figure 23-6 A: Baseline nasolabial fold of an African American patient. **B:** Immediately after injection of two syringes of hyaluronic acid (Hylaform). (Courtesy of Pearl E. Grimes, MD.)

together with excellent results, and many physicians are using HA fillers and collagen fillers in combination therapy.[15] The HA provides skin volume, and the collagen provides structural support and definition to the skin. Fillers are also used successfully in conjunction with other treatment options, such as botulinum toxin type A. Fillers and botulinum toxin A complement each other particularly well because of their different mechanisms of action. Botulinum toxin type A is most appropriate for dynamic lines associated with facial expressions, and fillers are most appropriate for static wrinkles caused by aging rather than hyperkinesis. Because of this, combination therapy can offer important and dramatic synergies. In a study of glabellar lines, patients who received botulinum toxin type A 1 week before Restylane treatment achieved dramatically greater and more prolonged efficacy than those who received Restylane alone. The median time for return to pretreatment furrow status was 32 weeks with botulinum toxin type A plus Restylane in comparison with 18 weeks with Restylane alone. Furthermore, patients experienced less pain and fewer adverse events.[16]

CONCLUSIONS

Fillers are gaining popularity in all ethnic and racial categories. The growth of cosmetic procedures among darker racial ethnic groups is increasing more rapidly than in Caucasians. Thus far, fillers appear to be equally safe and effective in ethnic populations and Caucasians, but more data are needed and should be forthcoming. Cultural differences and desires should be taken into account when treating all patients with fillers, and such preferences will help determine the optimal treatment. Although hyperpigmentation and aberrant scarring are concerns when instituting any invasive procedure in darker racial ethnic patients, to date there is no evidence that such risks are higher when treating such skin types.

REFERENCES

1. The American Society for Aesthetic Plastic Surgery. 2004 Cosmetic Surgery National Data Bank Statistics. Available at: http://www.surgery.org/download/2004-stats.pdf. Accessed December 9, 2005.
2. Andre P. Hyaluronic acid and its use as a "rejuvenation" agent in cosmetic dermatology. *Semin Cutan Med Surg* 2004; 23:218–222.
3. Lindqvist C, Tveten S, Bondevik BE, et al. A randomized, evaluator-blind, multicenter comparison of the efficacy and tolerability of Perlane versus Zyplast in the correction of nasolabial folds. *Plast Reconstr Surg* 2005;115:282–289.
4. Narins RS, Brandt F, Leyden J, et al. A randomized, double-blind, multicenter comparison of the efficacy and tolerability of Restylane versus Zyplast for the correction of nasolabial folds. *Dermatol Surg* 2003;29:588–595.
5. Coleman SR. Long-term survival of fat transplants: controlled demonstrations. *Aesthetic Plast Surg* 1995;19:421–425.
6. Ersek RA. Transplantation of purified autologous fat: a 3-year follow-up is disappointing. *Plast Reconstr Surg* 1991;87: 219–227.
7. Marmur ES, Phelps R, Goldberg DJ. Clinical, histologic and electron microscopic findings after injection of a calcium hydroxylapatite filler. *J Cosmet Laser Ther* 2004;6: 223–226.
8. Jones DH, Carruthers A, Orentreich D, et al. Highly purified 1000-cSt silicone oil for treatment of human immunodeficiency virus–associated facial lipoatrophy: an open pilot trial. *Dermatol Surg* 2004;30:1279–1286.
9. Jesitus J. Ethnic skin: handle with care: dark skin is more protected from sun, but vulnerable to hyperpigmentation, scarring. *Cosmetic Surgery Times* 2004;21–25.
10. Grieco EM, Cassidy RC. Overview of race and Hispanic origin. Census 2000 brief. Available at: http://www.census.gov/prod/2001pubs/c2kbr01-1.pdf (page 3). Accessed December 9, 2005.
11. Hobbs F, Stoops N. Demographic trends in the 20th century. Census 2000 special reports. Available at: http://www.census.gov/prod/2002pubs/censr-4.pdf (page 73). Accessed December 9, 2005.
12. General and Plastic Surgery Devices Panel 64th meeting, November 21, 2003. Available at: http://www.fda.gov/ohrms/dockets/ac/03/transcripts/4004T1_01.DOC. Accessed December 9, 2005.
13. Hylaform labeling. Available at: http://www.fda.gov/cdrh/pdf3/p030032c.pdf. Accessed December 9, 2005.
14. Hylaform letter of approval. Available at: http://www.fda.gov/cdrh/pdf3/p030032a.pdf. Accessed December 9, 2005.
15. Baumann L. Cosmoderm/Cosmoplast (human bioengineered collagen) for the aging face. *Facial Plast Surg* 2004; 20:125–128.
16. Carruthers J, Carruthers A. A prospective, randomized, parallel group study analyzing the effect of BTX-A (Botox) and nonanimal sourced hyaluronic acid (NASHA, Restylane) in combination compared with NASHA (Restylane) alone in severe glabellar rhytides in adult female subjects: treatment of severe glabellar rhytides with a hyaluronic acid derivative compared with the derivative and BTX-A. *Dermatol Surg* 2003;29:802–809.

Correction of Specific Anatomic Imperfections

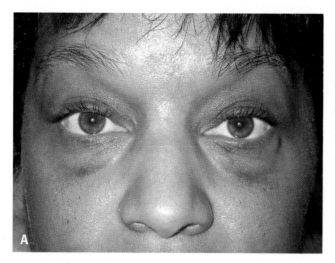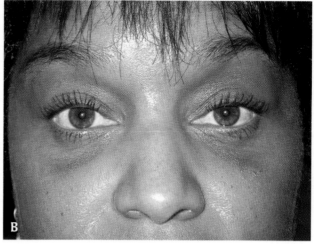

Figure 25-5 A: Preoperative photo of an African American woman with herniated lower orbital fat and skin hyperpigmentation. **B:** Postoperative photo of an African American woman after lower transconjunctival blepharoplasty. The hyperpigmentation remains.

True complications of lower blepharoplasty include orbital hemorrhage, infection, conjunctival chemosis, and wound dehiscence. Suboptimal surgical results of lower blepharoplasty include undercorrection, overcorrection, asymmetry, lid retraction, canthal dystopia, and ectropion. Lid retraction, canthal dystopia, and ectropion occur from a transcutaneous, skin-muscle flap lower blepharoplasty (Fig. 25-8); these complications can be avoided using a transconjunctival approach. Lid retraction, canthal dystopia, and ectropion may also rarely occur after a "pinch" skin lower blepharoplasty if horizontal laxity is not properly assessed preoperatively, and additional procedures, such as a canthopexy or canthoplasty

with lateral tarsal strip, are not performed concurrently. Indeed, many patients who are seen in referral have lower eyelid retraction, scleral show, canthal dystopia, eyelid rounding, and/or frank ectropion after having previous skin-muscle flap lower blepharoplasty.

Some black patients may have prominent eyes and shallow orbits, and the relative exophthalmos may be concealed with the full eyelids. Careful preoperative evaluation for the prominent eye is necessary, and blepharoplasty in the patient with a prominent eye must be extremely conservative because aggressive skin, muscle, and fat excision of the upper and/or lower eyelids will make the eyes appear more prominent and proptotic postoperatively.

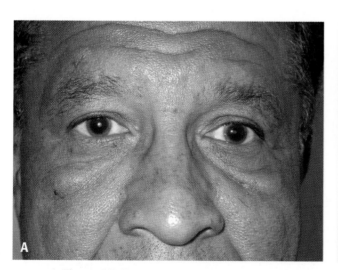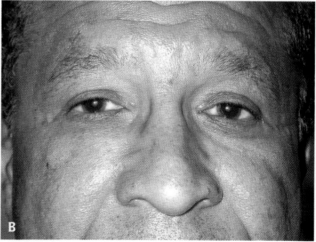

Figure 25-6 A: Preoperative photo of an African American man with herniated lower orbital fat, excess skin, lower eyelid laxity, festoons, and midface ptosis. **B:** Postoperative photo of an African American man after skin-muscle-flap lower blepharoplasty, pinch-skin excision, lateral canthopexy, preperiosteal midface lift, and Restylane injection.

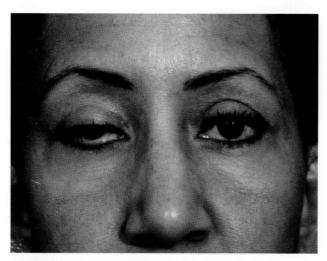

Figure 25-7 African American woman referred for complications. Right upper blepharoptosis occurred after upper blepharoplasty. There is also overcorrection of left upper lid with a high eyelid crease and scaphoid appearance.

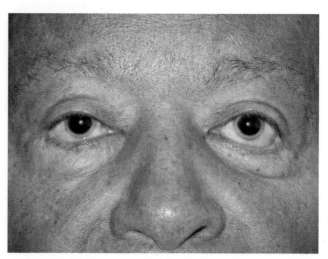

Figure 25-8 African American man referred for complications after four-eyelid blepharoplasty. Lower lid retraction and ectropion are present after transcutaneous, infraciliary, skin-muscle-flap lower blepharoplasty. Note the feminization of the male upper eyelids after upper blepharoplasty.

CONCLUSION

Blepharoplasty in patients with darker skin tones is performed similarly to other patients with a few specific variations and considerations. Upper blepharoplasty should be performed with appropriate, moderate skin and fat excision, with preservation of the orbicularis oculi muscle to preserve the blink mechanism, insure adequate eyelid closure, and preserve a natural, nonsurgical appearance. Transconjunctival lower blepharoplasty should be used whenever possible to prevent postoperative lid retraction, canthal dystopia, and ectropion. Keloid formation after blepharoplasty is extremely rare. Each patient's surgery should be personally tailored to his or her own needs, desires, ethnicity, sex, and individual anatomy.

REFERENCES

1. Saadat D, Dresner SC. Safety of blepharoplasty in patients with preoperative dry eyes. *Arch Facial Plast Surg* 2004;6 (2):101–104.
2. Migliori ME, Gladstone GJ. Determination of the normal range of exophthalmometric values for black and white adults. *Am J Ophthalmol* 1984;98(4):438–442.
3. De Juan E Jr, Hurley DP, Sapira JD. Racial differences in normal values of proptosis. *Arch Intern Med* 1980;140(9): 1230–1231.
4. Chrisman BB. Blepharoplasty and browlift with surgical variations in non-white patients. *J Dermatol Surg Oncol* 1986;12 (1):58–66.

26

Ethnic Rhinoplasty

Matthew R. Kaufman, Reza Jarrahy, and Michael Jones

The demand for cosmetic rhinoplasty within ethnic populations has risen dramatically in the last two decades. Evidence of this trend was provided by a 2005 survey conducted by the American Academy of Facial Plastic Surgery, which revealed that African Americans and Hispanics were more likely to seek rhinoplasty than any other facial cosmetic procedure.[1] Concomitant with this increasing interest in rhinoplasty among ethnic populations has been a shift in the surgical approach to the ethnic nose by rhinoplasty surgeons.

The surgeon attempting to successfully treat the ethnic rhinoplasty patient must appreciate that variations exist not only between Caucasian and non-Caucasian noses, but also between each of the non-Caucasian ethnic groups. In fact, the term *ethnic rhinoplasty* is too simplistic; it tends to group together individuals with vastly different features. A detailed understanding of nasal anatomy and the specific differences that exist between all non-Caucasian groups (African American, Asian, Hispanic, Mediterranean, and Middle Eastern) is the only way to effectively treat these patients. Even within the African American population, morphological differences have been subcategorized into three groups: African, Afro-Caucasian, and Afro-Indian.[2]

Among the most challenging aspects of rhinoplasty surgery is the ability to precisely identify any structural abnormalities that exist and reconcile these anatomic realities with the patient's perception of what the problem is. No two rhinoplasty procedures are the same; each intervention must be customized to the anatomy and desired outcome of each individual patient. However, there are some general surgical approaches to different nose types—often categorized by ethnicity—that may be broadly applied. For example, one relatively common goal of the Caucasian rhinoplasty is to decrease the overall nasal size in the pursuit of an aesthetic ideal. This may be accomplished, for example, by reduction of the dorsal hump or trimming of the lower lateral cartilages.

Historically, the Caucasian model of nasal reduction was applied to the African American nose. Results were often unsatisfactory, reflecting a lack of sensitivity to the impact of ethnicity on "ideal" outcomes in rhinoplasty. A misunderstanding existed regarding the disparity between excessive bulky soft tissues and deficient osteocartilaginous support.[3] As surgeons came to understand that it was rarely desirable to create the ideal Caucasian nose in an African American patient, but rather to correct structural abnormalities while preserving favorable ethnicity-specific features, a unique set of rhinoplasty techniques for this patient population evolved. For example, rather than prioritizing reduction of the size of the nose to achieve an aesthetic ideal, rhinoplasty in most ethnic groups today often incorporates some degree of augmentation to achieve desired aesthetic outcomes.

The primary lesson to be learned—and the underlying principle behind all truly successful rhinoplasty surgery—was eloquently elaborated by Pitanguy in 1972, who stated that the nose must be in harmony with the rest of the face *as well as* the race of the individual.[4]

NASAL ANATOMY

Nasal anatomy may be divided into the internal framework and the external soft-tissue envelope. The osseocartilaginous structures that make up the internal framework include the paired nasal bones and bony septum in the upper third of the nose, the upper lateral cartilages in the middle third, and the lower lateral cartilages in the lower third (Fig. 26-1). The midline cartilaginous septum provides structural support to the midvault and lower third of the nose. It is also functionally important in regulating nasal airflow. The soft-tissue envelope consists of the subcutaneous tissues and overlying skin. Skin quality varies among different parts of the nose (e.g., nasal skin is thicker and more sebaceous at the tip than over the dorsum). Variations in both osseocartilaginous and soft-tissue elements seen in ethnic groups, although not uniformly present, are common enough to distinguish the particular ethnicities from typical Caucasian noses.

The literature is replete with detailed descriptions of and comparisons between Caucasian and African American nasal anatomy.[5-7] Fundamental differences are noted in both structural and coverage components. For example,

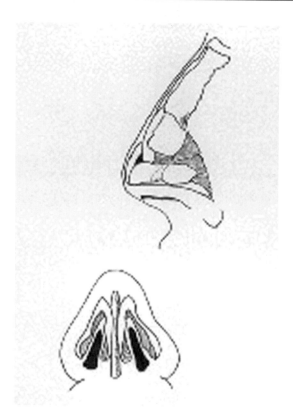

Figure 26-1 Internal nasal anatomy depicting the paired nasal bones, the upper and lower lateral cartilages, and the midline nasal septum.

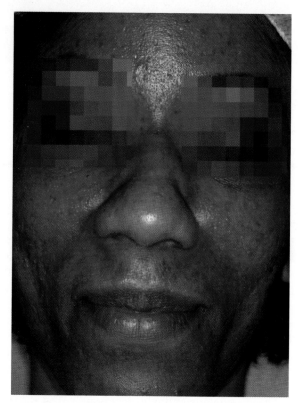

Figure 26-2 This patient has many of the commonly described African American nasal features, including short, widely based nasal bones, an amorphous nasal tip, and flared ala.

the bony pyramid that accounts for the structural support of the upper third of the nose is very different in many African American noses when compared with the typical Caucasian nose: The nasal bones are often smaller, and there is a widened angle between them, creating the appearance of a flattened nasal bridge and dorsum and a deep nasofrontal angle. Additionally, in African Americans, the premaxilla and nasal spine are often relatively underdeveloped. This bony variation results in a foreshortened columella and contributes to a poorly projecting nasal tip. Furthermore, the thick skin and dense subcutaneous tissues present at the tip produces an amorphous appearance. Finally, flared ala and a widened pyriform contribute to poor definition in the lower third of the nose (Fig. 26-2).

There are several similarities between the general characteristics of Asian and Hispanic noses and the African American nose. The nasal skin and subcutaneous tissues of Asians and Hispanics are often moderately to very thick. There is often weak tip support, a widened lobule, and a foreshortened columella. The dorsum is often shallow, and the nasal bridge appears wide. By comparison, Mediterranean patients traditionally demonstrate a straight to convex nasal dorsum and a plunging tip, whereas Middle Easterners often exhibit a high arching dorsum with a long nasal contour on profile.[8]

PREOPERATIVE ASSESSMENT

Patients presenting for ethnic rhinoplasty must express their desires to the surgeon, who must in turn decide whether these are indeed realistic. Although the majority of ethnic patients will indicate the importance of preserving their ethnic features, occasionally patients will have expectations that reveal an underlying wish to eliminate features of ethnicity from their faces. These patients require extensive counseling by the physician regarding why such an approach risks disturbing overall facial harmony. They may also benefit from preoperative psychological analysis. Ultimately, patients whose expectations prove to be unrealistic or irrational should not be considered for surgery.

Following a complete medical history, the physician should perform a thorough examination of the nose, including an internal and external assessment. Using inspection and palpation, a systematic inspection should include quality of skin, amount of tip support, alar width, dorsal height and width, internal valve angle, septal shape, and the relationship between the nose and other facial elements (e.g., nasofrontal and nasolabial angles). The findings on physical examination should be reassessed and corroborated with photodocumentation, which should include frontal, oblique, lateral, and basal views. All of this information should be documented in the medical record, along with a description of the informed consent that is obtained.

SURGICAL TECHNIQUES

There are several different approaches that allow for surgical access to the structural and soft-tissue elements of the nose. The open rhinoplasty approach provides optimal visualization of the internal nasal framework, permitting accurate graft placement and easy fixation. There is, however, increased risk associated with the transcolumellar incision in ethnic patients, as their thick sebaceous skin may be more prone to scarring. Closed rhinoplasty offers an opportunity to access the bony-cartilaginous framework without external incisions. When limited tip work is planned, the nondelivery closed rhinoplasty approach with an intercartilaginous incision is sufficient to access the nasal dorsum. This may be combined with a retrograde dissection of the lower lateral cartilages to modify portions of the lower third of the nose. For improved access to the nasal tip, the delivery approach is a better option. This technique involves performing intercartilaginous and marginal incisions, permitting a full dissection and exposure of the lower lateral cartilages and nasal tip without the need for a skin incision.

As noted above, rhinoplasty for the ethnic patient often incorporates some degree of augmentation. Dorsal augmentation is a key component whenever there is a broad, flat nasal dorsum (Fig. 26-3). Although there remains some debate about the value (and risks) of nasal bone osteotomies, most surgeons do agree that dorsal grafts are necessary. There are many available options for dorsal grafts, including autologous tissue and allograft options. Despite the fact that most surgeons prefer to use autologous tissues, some investigators have proposed algorithms in which the choice of graft substrate is predicated upon the amount of desired augmentation: autologous cartilage for up to 3 mm, allograft for 3 to 8 mm, and autologous bone for more than 8 mm.[9] Septal and auricular grafts are the most common sources of autologous cartilage; preferred sites for harvesting bone grafts are calvarium, iliac crest, and rib. A variety of alloplastic materials have been used as dorsal nasal implants. Currently, the most common are solid silicone (Silastic) and high-density porous polyethylene (Medpor).

Treatment of the poorly defined and poorly supported nasal tip involves multiple sequential steps. Routinely, the thick fibrofatty tissue present in the subcutaneous layer of the nasal tip is thinned (it is important not to devascularize the skin or dermis while performing this maneuver). The lower lateral cartilages are modified with domal suture techniques and cartilaginous tip grafts that enhance projection and improve definition (Fig. 26-4). Columellar strut grafts placed in pockets between the medial crurae anterior to the nasal septum help improve tip support. Alternatively, aggressive use of the cephalic strip technique is not recommended, as it has been attributed to alar collapse and instability of the external nasal valva. A

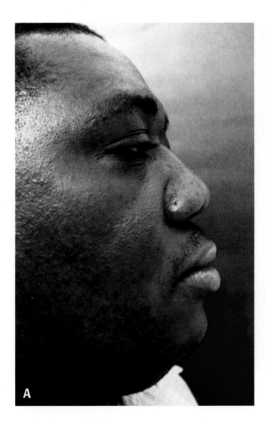
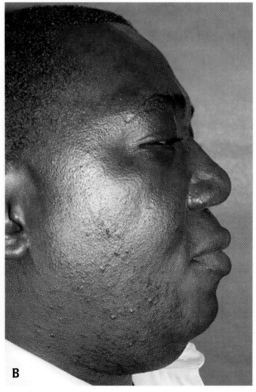

Figure 26-3 Pre- **(A)** and postoperative **(B)** views of rhinoplasty patient with dorsal grafting to improve dorsal height and contour.

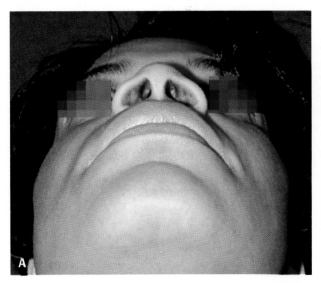 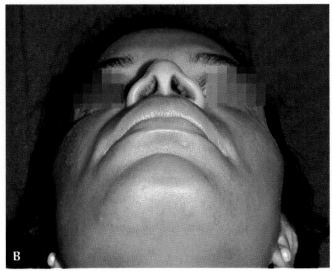

Figure 26-4 Pre- **(A)** and postoperative **(B)** views of a rhinoplasty patient using tip-defining techniques, such as domal sutures and cartilage grafting.

"plumping" graft of fibrofatty tissue or cartilage placed into a premaxillary pocket will reduce the appearance of the contracted columella and improve the contour of the nasolabial angle.

Alar base reductions are often performed to reduce the width of the nose to fall within the boundaries of a vertical line drawn from the medial canthi (Fig. 26-5). It is important to maintain symmetry on both sides by removing the same amount of tissue while still preserving the natural alar groove. Small monofilament sutures should be used and subsequently removed early to minimize the risk of scarring. Another technique used to minimize visible scars is to perform internal alar reductions by placing the incision in the nasal sill.

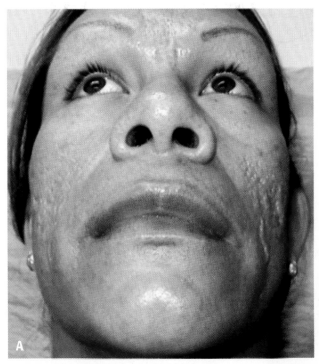 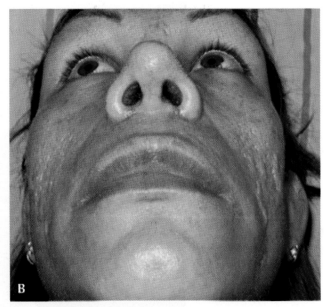

Figure 26-5 Pre- **(A)** and postoperative **(B)** view of patient who had tip-defining rhinoplasty with alar base reduction.

COMPLICATIONS

Ethnic rhinoplasty is associated with certain postoperative complications unique to this procedure. This is in addition to the more generalized problems of bleeding, infection, functional abnormalities, and poor aesthetic outcome, which are occasionally observed in all cosmetic nasal surgery.

Alloplastic dorsal nasal implants, especially those made of silicone, have an established rate of extrusion, usually through the nasal tip. Patients should understand that threatened exposure almost always requires early removal of the implant to prevent further complications. Alteration in skin color, either hyperpigmentation or hypopigmentation, may result from incisions or minor trauma. Treatment of these problems may require adjunctive topical therapies, depending on their temporal relationship to surgery and the specific type of pigment abnormality. Although it is rare to see true keloids forming at the sites of open rhinoplasty incisions or alar base reductions, hypertrophic scars have been reported. Additionally, a thickened scar along the columella incision may result in an inadvertent visible notching.

SUMMARY

Rhinoplasty in ethnic populations has been a challenge to plastic surgeons for many years. There was previously a misconception regarding nasal morphology that led to overresection of nasal structures, yielding poor surgical outcomes. With a greater understanding of nasal anatomy in different ethnic groups, surgical techniques that permit nasal refinement without losing facial harmony have been developed. These techniques are often very different than those used in traditional rhinoplasty for Caucasian populations and must be mastered to achieve optimal results.

REFERENCES

1. American Academy of Facial Plastic and Reconstructive Surgery 2005 Membership Survey: Trends in Facial Plastic Surgery. http://www.aafprs.org/media/stats_polls/. Accessed September 2006.
2. Ofodile FA, Bokhari FJ, Ellis C. The black American nose. *Ann Plast Surg* 1993;31:209–218.
3. Hoefflin SM. *Ethnic Rhinoplasty: Blacks, Asian and Hispanics.* New York: Springer-Verlag;1997:181–195.
4. Pitanguy I. The negroid nose. In: Conley J, Dickinson J, eds. *First International Symposium on Plastic and Reconstructive Surgery of the Face and Neck.* New York: Grune & Stratton Inc.;1972:147–152.
5. Romo T III, Abraham MT. The ethnic nose. *Facial Plast Surg* 2003;19:269–277.
6. Kontis TC, Papel ID. Rhinoplasty on the African-American nose. *Aesthetic Plastic Surgery* 2002;26(1):12.
7. Porter JP, Olson KL. Analysis of the African American female nose. *Plast Reconstr Surg* 2002;111:620–626.
8. Trenite GJN. Considerations in ethnic rhinoplasty. *Facial Plast Surg* 2003;19:239–245.
9. Zingaro EA, Falces E. Aesthetic anatomy of the Non-Caucasian nose. *Clin Plast Surg* 1987;14:749–765.

27

Reduction and Augmentation of the Breasts

Matthew R. Kaufman, Reza Jarrahy, and Michael Jones

REDUCTION MAMMAPLASTY

Although it is not altogether clear why many women in certain racial ethnic populations suffer from breast hypertrophy, the etiology is suspected to be some combination of hormonal, genetic, and developmental factors. Large-breasted women often have significant functional and psychosocial impairments, prompting them to investigate surgical options. In addition, these patients are prone to developing comorbid conditions, such as chronic back and neck pain, and often there are multiple medical professionals involved in the search for effective treatments.

Because reduction mammaplasty offers a cosmetic and functional resolution to the consequences of large breasts, it is associated with high rates of patient satisfaction. During the initial patient assessment, the physician must determine the patient's desired breast size and be able to meet this desire using one of the various descriptions of surgical techniques.[1–3] Some of the more common surgical methods are the inferior and superior pedicle techniques, whereas partial breast amputation with free nipple grafting is reserved for patients with massive breasts or significant risk factors.

Darker-complexioned women presenting for breast reduction surgery must be informed of the risk of unsightly breast scars and the possibility of needing scar revision treatments in the months to years that follow the initial procedure. Despite the increased risk of scarring that is present in these patient populations compared with their lighter skinned counterparts, most women will still undergo the procedure and achieve satisfaction because of the significant functional improvements.

Patient assessment and selection

Candidates for breast reduction surgery encompass a wide range of age groups, including young girls with virginal hypertrophy to elderly women seeking to reverse the effects of aging on large, uncomfortable, sagging breasts. During the initial assessment, a full history must be obtained, including age of breast development, pregnancy and lactation history, previous breast surgery, weight change, smoking, family history of breast cancer, and how

past scars have healed. The patient should specifically state her goals regarding the desired breast size. During the physical assessment, a full breast exam must be performed. The physician should determine the degree of breast symmetry (or asymmetry) and the distances from the sternal notch to the nipple and from the nipple to the inframammary fold. These measurements will be important in determining the vertical lift requirements and the safest method of accomplishing the reduction; a common rule is that when the nipple to inframammary fold distance is greater than 17 cm, the inferior pedicle is less likely to support survival of the nipple. Another important consideration, especially pertinent in the darker-skinned patient, is the diameter of the nipple-areolar complex. In many women with mammary hyperplasia, this diameter will be greater than normal, and patients must be informed that it too will be reduced, along with the breast volume. Objective signs of breast hypertrophy should be elicited, such as bra-strap grooving, skin rashes or irritations, striae, postural abnormalities, and early kyphosis of the cervicolumbar spine. Preoperative assessment should include screening mammograms, especially for women older than 30 and for patients with a personal or family history of breast disease. It is also recommend that patients undergo mammography 6 months after surgery to establish a postoperative baseline. Patients with comorbid back pain conditions should be evaluated by an appropriate specialist and may require magnetic resonance imaging to objectify the chronic effects of breast hypertrophy on the spine.

Appropriate candidates for breast reduction surgery usually present with long-standing symptoms of back and neck pain resulting from large, pendulous breasts. Skin rashes, or intertrigo, and bra-strap grooving make up some of the cutaneous manifestations of breast hypertrophy. Women with severe breast asymmetry will also desire breast reduction to alleviate the unilateral symptoms plaguing their daily lives. Just as important are the psychosocial effects of breast hypertrophy that are especially disturbing to younger women or teenage girls suffering from virginal hypertrophy. The daily embarrassment that is often associated with this condition can be detrimental

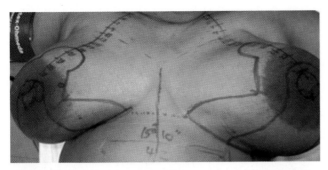

Figure 27-1 This patient had been previously marked for surgery, using an inferior pedicled technique, while in a standing position.

to a teenager or young woman, thus negatively affecting both physical and mental development.

The prevalence of obesity in ethnic populations has increased the number of people seeking breast reduction surgery as a way of treating the effects of weight gain on the breasts. Unfortunately, it is inappropriate to view reduction mammaplasty as a weight reduction procedure, and the best course of action is to recommend the patient lose weight before breast surgery. Ideally, a woman should be within 30 pounds of her ideal weight to be a surgical candidate. Abiding by this philosophy will improve patient satisfaction and reduce the rate of perioperative complications associated with surgery in obese patients.

Surgical techniques

Arguably, the most common method of breast reduction surgery is the inferior pedicle technique, whereby the majority of parenchyma is removed from the medial, lateral, and superior quadrants, and the blood supply to the nipple-areolar complex is maintained from the inferiorly based soft tissues. The key to achieving surgical success is

careful, accurate preoperative markings made with the patient seated or standing, usually in the holding area (Fig. 27-1). A complete technical description of the markings is beyond the scope of this chapter, so the reader is referred to previous publications that thoroughly outline the procedure.[4–5] Notable aspects of the preoperative markings include setting the new nipple-areolar position by transposing the inframammary fold onto the breast mound and use of the keyhole pattern to design the resultant shape of the new nipple-areolar complex and determine the extent of skin resection. The markings will ultimately guide the surgeon toward the resultant breast scars, which include a periareolar incision and an "inverted T" incision at the base of the breast (Fig. 27-2). During the surgery, it is important to proceed in a systematic way, as even the most experienced surgeons can sometimes lose sight of the three-dimensional nature of the reduction procedure. It is also critical that there be attention to detail to achieve absolute breast symmetry and minimize resultant scarring (Fig. 27-3).

There are many other techniques available, some of which have been developed in an attempt to minimize incisions. For example, the vertical mammaplasty, popularized by Lejour, accomplishes reduction of the breast parenchyma and skin excision without a resultant horizontal incision at the base of the breast.[6] Although this technique may have applications for smaller-volume breast reductions, the skin "bunching" and increased tension that is often required along the vertical limb of the incision may not be ideal for darker-skinned patients in whom there may be a higher chance of hypertrophic scarring.

For patients with massive breast hypertrophy, a safe, reliable method of reduction involves partial breast amputation with free nipple grafting. The basic design is similar to the inferior pedicle technique, but the glandular

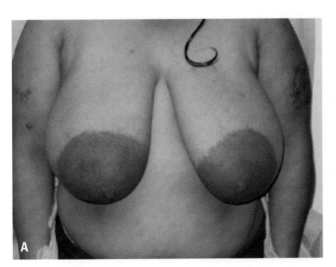
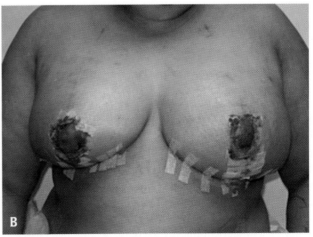

Figure 27-2 A: Preoperative photo. **B:** Two days post breast reduction. Note the Steri-strips along the incision lines, including the periareolar incision and the inverted "T" at the base of the breast.

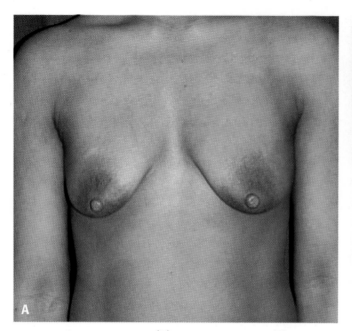
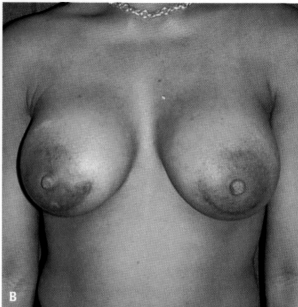

Figure 27-3 Pre- **(A)** and postoperative **(B)** photos of a patient undergoing breast augmentation. In this patient, the implants were placed in a subglandular position. Because she has moderate breast ptosis, subglandular implant placement was suggested by her surgeon to avoid an unnatural ("double-bubble") appearance.

resection includes the inferior pole, and the nipple-areolar complex is excised completely and replaced at the end of the procedure as a full-thickness graft. The main advantage of this technique is avoiding problems with nipple-areolar necrosis that may occur in a large-volume breast reduction when there is an excessively long distance of the inferior pedicle. The obvious consequences of complete nipple excision are the loss of sensation to this area and the inability for subsequent lactation. Other breast reduction techniques often will preserve nursing functions, especially when an effort is made to limit parenchymal excision directly under the nipple.

BREAST AUGMENTATION

Although physicians have been using various materials to augment the breasts for more than a century, the modern age of augmentation mammaplasty began in 1962, when Cronin and Gerow first performed silicone gel–filled prosthesis augmentation.[7] Since that time, breast augmentation has become one of the most common plastic surgery procedures in women. In 2005, the number of breast augmentation procedures in ethnic patients increased dramatically, especially in Hispanic and Asian women. In these groups, breast augmentation surgery was among the three most commonly requested cosmetic procedures.[8] The type of implants most commonly used are saline filled. After a prolonged moratorium due to concerns raised about the safety of implantable silicone, the Food and Drug Admin-

istration recently re-approved silicone filled breast implants. Preoperative discussion is necessary to elicit a realistic expectation on the part of the prospective patient, as well as a clear understanding of the risks and limitations of breast implants.

Patient assessment and selection

Patients seeking breast augmentation must have a clear understanding of the procedure and the possible adverse sequelae, especially those related to the implants themselves. In addition, the desired outcome of the patient should be elicited so the physician can determine if it is a realistic expectation. A thorough patient interview should include pregnancy and lactation history, as well as the prevalence of breast cancer in family members. Physical examination should focus on—amongst other things— breast shape, symmetry, and degree of ptosis. Furthermore, the physician should assess the quality of the skin overlying the breast and the thickness of the pectoralis muscle to determine the optimal implant recipient site (subglandular or submuscular).

Discussion of the surgical plan should commence with the options for surgical access: periareolar, inframammary, transaxillary, or transumbilical (transumbilical breast augmentation, or TUBA). The choice depends on several factors, including body habitus, site of previous scars, patient desire, and surgical expertise. The issue of surgical access is especially important in ethnic patients, in whom scarring is almost always a significant concern. It is the author's opinion that the periareolar incision is preferable to the inframammary incision because the scar is camouflaged in the junction between the outer edge of the areola and the adjacent breast skin. The transaxillary and TUBA approaches also limit visible scars; however, they tend to provide less visibility of the pocket and thus may be less forgiving when attempting to adjust implant position to achieve ideal breast symmetry. The patient should be informed whether she would be a better candidate for a subglandular or submuscular procedure, with a clear rationale justifying one or the other. For example, patients with extremely well-developed pectoralis major muscles may be poor candidates for submuscular implantation, whereas in those patients with extremely thin, pliable skin, it may not be suitable to perform subglandular implantation. Furthermore, in patients with mild-to-moderate breast ptosis, subglandular placement of implants may reduce the chances of a "double-bubble" or "snoopy" deformity—an unsightly condition in which the epicenter of the breast parenchyma is at a different level than that of the implant (Fig. 27-3).

Until just recently saline implants were the only option for women presenting for primary augmentation, whereas silicone-gel implants were restricted to patients with prior breast surgery, breast ptosis, or breast reconstruction patients following cancer ablation. As of this writing, silicone-gel breast implants have been FDA approved for use in primary breast augmentation. The major advantage of silicone-gel breast implants over saline implants is their natural shape and feel, however they require a larger incision for placement because, unlike saline implants, they are manufactured in a prefilled state.

Surgical techniques

Patients should be marked in the preoperative holding area. Marks should delineate the vertical midline between the two breasts as well as the location of the inframammary folds bilaterally. Many surgeons also delineate the borders of the pocket dissection to guide accurate subglandular or subpectoral pocket development. In patients undergoing TUBA, additional marks are made extending superolaterally from the umbilicus to demarcate the path of tunnel creation from the surgical access site to the lateral inframammary fold.

Surgery is performed either with local plus sedation, or general anesthesia, with special care to use strict sterile technique, especially during handling and insertion of the implants. The sequence of steps involves making the appropriate incision, creating the subglandular or submuscular pocket, irrigating the pocket, achieving hemostasis, and placing the deflated saline implant (or sizer). The implant is then inflated to the appropriate size, and the same maneuvers are then performed on the contralateral breast. Before closing the incisions, a critical inspection is made with the patient in a near upright position. The surgeon must assess breast size, symmetry, and mobility of the implant in the pocket. Final adjustments are made, and the wounds are then closed in a layered fashion. The patient is dressed with fluff gauze and a support bra that she will wear for at least 3 weeks. The patient generally requires anywhere from 6 to 12 weeks before resolution of all postoperative edema and scars (Fig. 27-4 and Fig. 27-5).

Complications

Although there is often almost immediate patient satisfaction after breast augmentation, there are several potential complications that may develop over time. Patients must be aware (especially those younger than 40) that they are very likely to require one or more operations during the course of their lifetime because of mechanical complications of breast implants. The most common of these local complications in both silicone gel–filled and saline implants are capsular contracture and rupture/deflation.[9]

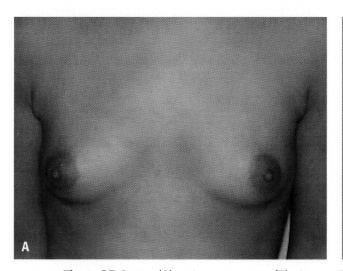
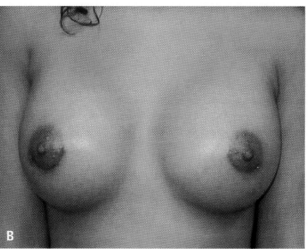

Figure 27-4 Pre- **(A)** and postoperative **(B)** photos of patient who received periareolar, submuscular breast augmentation.

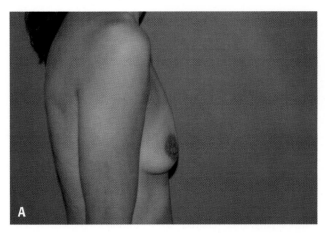
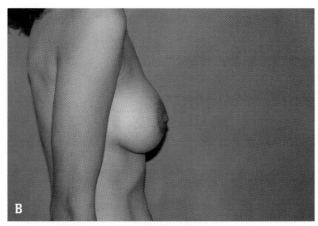

Figure 27-5 Lateral images of 32-year-old Asian woman pre- **(A)** and postoperative **(B)** breast augmentation. (Courtesy of Arthur Jensen, MD.)

Capsular contracture is the development of scar tissue between the implant and the native breast tissue. The etiology of capsular contracture is not completely understood; however, it has been established that higher rates of this undesirable occurrence follow hematoma and/or infection. There are four grades of capsular contracture known as Baker grades (Table 27-1).[10]

For patients with the more severe forms of capsular contracture, treatment often involves reoperation to remove or release the capsule. The implants may be left in place, replaced, and/or moved to a different plane (i.e., subglandular to submuscular) (Fig. 27-6).

Implant rupture and/or deflation occurs at a reported rate of 8% after 11 years.[11] It may be iatrogenic from excessive or rough handling during the initial procedure or, alternatively, from compression or external stresses during the day-to-day life of the patient. Critics of the TUBA attribute this method of insertion to a higher rate of deflation because of the increased manipulation of the implant required for proper positioning. The patient will often note this event by visualizing an acute decrease in the size of her breast. Appropriate treatment involves reoperation to remove and replace the implant.

SUMMARY

Breast reduction and augmentation are some of the most common cosmetic procedures performed in ethnic groups. Reduction mammaplasty is often more than simply a cosmetic procedure, as many patients with breast hypertrophy have significant functional and psychosocial limitations. For these reasons, in patients undergoing breast reduction surgery, there is a great deal of patient satisfaction.

Many plastic surgeons are observing a significant increase in the number of ethnic patients presenting for breast enhancement. The importance of preoperative counseling cannot be overstated, as it is the key to achieving surgical success and patient expectations. Important

Table 27-1	
Baker grades of capsular contracture	

Grade	Sign
Grade I	Breast is normally soft and looks natural
Grade II	Breast is a little firm but looks normal
Grade III	Breast is firm and looks abnormal
Grade IV	Breast is hard, painful, and looks abnormal

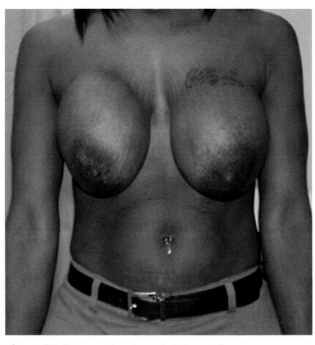

Figure 27-6 Patient with grade IV capsular contracture on the right and grade III capsular contracture on the left.

technical details include the incision site, the size and style of the implants that are to be used, and the tissue plane in which the implant will be placed. Patients must understand the risks of the procedure, including implant-related complications that may require reoperation.

REFERENCES

1. Courtiss EH, Goldwyn RM. Reduction mammaplasty by the inferior pedicle technique. *Plast Reconstr Surg* 1977;59: 500–507.
2. Gradinger GP. Reduction mammaplasty with nipple graft. In: Goldwyn RM, ed. *Reduction Mammaplasty*. Boston: Little, Brown;1990:513–529.
3. Ariyan S. Reduction mammaplasty with the nipple-areola carried on a single, narrow inferior pedicle. *Ann Plast Surg* 1980;5:167.
4. Bostwick J III. Reduction mammaplasty. In Bostwick J III, ed. *Plastic and Reconstructive Breast Surgery*. 2nd ed. St. Louis: Quality Medical Publishing;2000:371–497.
5. Cohen B, Ciaravino ME. Reduction mammaplasty. In: Evans GRD, ed. *Operative Plastic Surgery*. New York: McGraw-Hill;2000:613–630.
6. Lejour M. Vertical mammaplasty and liposuction of the breast. *Plast Reconstr Surg* 1994;94:100–114.
7. Spear SL, Ben Burke J. Augmentation mammaplasty. In: Weinzweig J, ed. *Plastic Surgery Secrets*. Philadelphia: Hanley & Belfus;1999:238–240.
8. Cooper L. Dramatic rise in ethnic plastic surgery in 2005. *Medical News Today*. http://www.medicalnewstoday.com/medicalnews.php?newsid=39814. Accessed August 2006.
9. U.S. Food and Drug Administration, Center for Devices and Radiological Health. Breast implants: potential local complications and reoperations (2004). http://www.fda.gov/cdrh/breastimplants/breast_implant_risks_brochure.html. Accessed December 2005.
10. Spear SL, Baker JL Jr. Classification of capsular contracture after prosthetic breast reconstruction. *Plast Reconstr Surg* 1995;96:1119–1123.
11. Heden P, Nava MB, van Tetering JP. Prevalence of rupture in Inamed silicone breast implants. *Plast Reconstr Surg* 2006; 118:303–308.

28

Body-Contouring Procedures

Luiz S. Toledo

Lipoplasty or liposuction has changed the way aesthetic body-contouring procedures are performed. Before its evolution in the late 1970s and early 1980s, every technique involved long and permanent scars. Liposuction now allows the surgeon to reshape the body through minimal invasion. In Brazil, abdominoplasty is the procedure most commonly associated with lipoplasty: 73% of all procedures. From a historical perspective, liposuction began with descriptions of hollow cannula liposuction by Fischer in 1976.[1] The technique was subsequently refined, improved, and practiced by Illouz and Fournier in the late 1970s and early 1980s.[1]

Body-contour treatments are frequently performed on the breasts, abdomen, thighs, and buttocks, either for reduction, augmentation, or lifting. Today, most reduction procedures of the body involve lipoplasty to some extent, with or without dermolipectomy. Augmentation can be done with autologous fat (except on the breasts) or silicone implants. Choosing the right technique is especially important when treating darker-skinned patients because of the higher possibility of hypertrophic scarring and keloid formation. However, in general, techniques are similar in all skin types and races. Body-contouring procedures are popular among blacks and Hispanics.

CLASSIFICATION AND CONTOURING OF THE ABDOMEN

Although there are several classifications for the abdomen, some of which are outdated, the author prefers to classify the abdomen into six types as a template for optimal selection of lipoplasty and for abdominoplasty procedures.[2] (Fig. 28-1).

A *type I abdomen* has excess fat, with no excess skin and no muscle aponeurotic laxity. The flanks and waist should be treated as an aesthetic unit with the abdomen when indicated. Most of these patients are treated with lipoplasty alone: either deep liposculpture for patients with good skin elasticity or superficial liposculpture (applied only in the areas where retraction is needed) for patients with skin flaccidity. Superficial liposculpture in the abdomen should be performed only by experienced surgeons. Common complications can be irregularities, skin hyperchromia, or even skin necrosis. The abdomen should be treated with the operating table hyperextended to avoid penetration of the abdominal wall.

The *type II abdomen*—with a high umbilicus, with moderate suprapubic excess skin, with or without excess fat, with or without muscle-aponeurotic flaccidity—can be treated with liposuction and suprapubic skin resection. The amount of skin to be resected varies from case to case. The suprapubic incision is usually a Cesarean Pfannenstiel incision with small extension into the inguinal fold.

The *type III abdomen* has a normally placed umbilicus, moderate excess skin in the epigastrium and hypogastrium, but not enough excess to perform a classic abdominoplasty, with or without excess fat and muscle laxity. The excess skin can be resected through a suprapubic incision and the excess fat removed through lipoplasty, thus, freeing the stalk of the umbilicus and suturing it 2 to 3 cm lower. Midline placation can be performed through the same incision, flattening the abdomen and improving the supraumbilical skin excess. If the epigastrium needs skin resection, it can be done through submammary incisions. If necessary, the epigastrium can be suctioned, without dissection, to preserve the perforators.

The *type IV abdomen* has muscle-aponeurotic flaccidity, excess skin, and minimum excess fat. It is treated by abdominoplasty through a suprapubic incision, skin excision, midline dissection, and muscle-aponeurotic placation, with or without umbilical repositioning. It might be necessary to close the old umbilical scar with a small vertical scar and reposition the umbilicus.

The *type V abdomen* has excess skin and fat in the epigastrium and hypogastrium that need muscle-aponeurotic correction. These patients should be treated with the classical abdominoplasty (Callia technique) with umbilical repositioning. The skin and fat flap from the hypogastrium are resected, and excess fat in the epigastrium and flanks is removed through lipoplasty.

The *type VI abdomen* with circumferential skin laxity, muscle laxity, and excess fat should be treated with a complete circumferential abdominoplasty, umbilical repositioning, and flankplasty. If dermolipectomy is continued

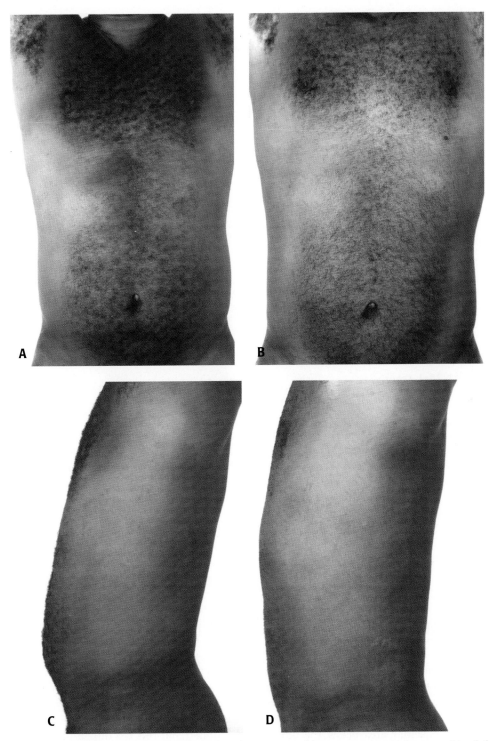

Figure 28-1 **A, C, E:** Preoperative photographs of a 32-year-old man wanting to improve his abdomen and flanks. **B, D, F:** One-year postoperative, showing improvement of the abdominal area and waist, with a 2-inch circumferential reduction after syringe liposculpture with a total removal of 1,200 cc of aspirate.

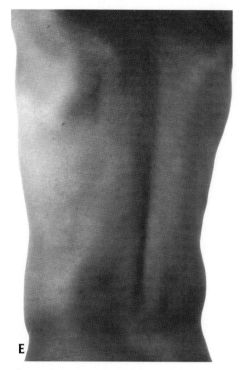
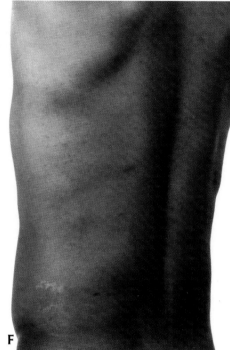

E   F

Figure 28-1 (*continued*)

with lipoplasty, the dissected flap should be sutured to the aponeurosis with a quilting suture to avoid seromas.

Patients with a vertical abdominal scar are better treated using the same scar to remove excess skin combined with lipoplasty, when indicated (*special type I abdomen*). In the author's opinion, the vertical skin excision in a patient with a previous scar can produce a good shape for the waist. Excess skin excision can lead to wide postoperative scars.

THIGH CONTOURING

There are specific treatments for different parts of the thighs. Some areas, like the lateral thighs, are more forgiving than others, and better results with simpler approaches, such as deep liposuction to remove the excess, can be obtained. Others are more difficult to treat, such as the anterior thigh and the posterior area below the gluteal fold, the so-called banana fold. These are areas that have to be treated very cautiously because of the higher possibility of provoking depressions or a "dropped buttock" look.[3] The medial thigh can be a simple area to treat on a younger patient, but very difficult on an older one, with the possibility of creating skin folds that can only be fixed through a thigh lift. Usually the only area of the thighs that needs augmentation through fat grafting is the internal midthigh to correct the "cowboy leg" deformity (Fig. 28-2 and Fig. 28-3).

The thigh lift is often performed through an incision that starts in the pubic area and follows the crease of the thigh back to the gluteal fold. Skin is resected, and the subcutaneous tissue is sutured tightly to the fascia to avoid the descent of the incision below the area covered by underwear.

BUTTOCKS CONTOURING

Buttocks can be reduced, augmented, or lifted. Sometimes a combination of techniques is necessary. Reduction is done by aspiration, respecting the "Bermuda triangle" mentioned by Illouz.[4] To give the illusion of a buttock lift, the author combines the superficial aspiration of the lower third of the buttock with the injection of up to 500 cc of fat per side in the higher two thirds of the buttock.[5] The area below the gluteal fold superficially suctioned, but this is a difficult procedure that should be performed with great care. When the patient does not have enough fat for harvesting, a silicone implant to augment the buttock, inserted through a vertical sacral incision in the intragluteal area, can be used. This augmentation also helps to eliminate some of the ptosis of the buttock without the need for skin resection. When indicated, skin resection can be performed in the gluteal fold or through a V incision on the waist (the angle of the V at the sacral area, where the intergluteal fold begins) (Fig. 28-4).

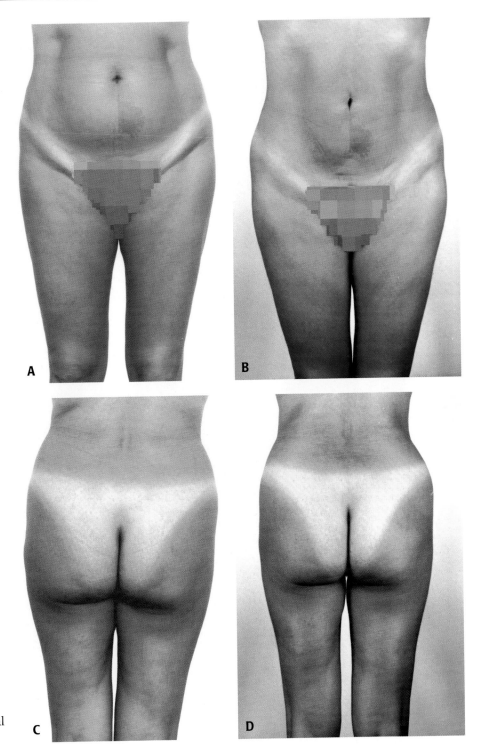

Figure 28-2 A, C: Preoperative photograph of a 42-year-old woman wanting to improve her abdomen and flanks. **B, D:** One-year postoperative, with a reduction of the abdominal area and waist after syringe liposculpture with a total removal of 2,800 cc of aspirate.

TECHNIQUE AND ANESTHESIA

For local anesthesia, the author uses a modification of the Klein tumescent solution, which contains 20 mL of 2% lidocaine, 5 mL of 3% sodium bicarbonate, 1 mL adrenaline 1:1,000, and Ringer's lactate quantitie suffisante pour (qsp) 500 mL. Up to 2 L of this solution at body temperature is injected into the abdominal tissue and suctioning begins after 10 to 15 minutes. Infiltration is performed one area at a time, and only after suctioning this area does the author infiltrate the other side. If the flanks are going to be treated in the same procedure, they should be treated first in the lateral position. Local anesthesia can be combined with oral or intravenous sedation. Combination procedures require epidural or general anesthesia. Oral sedation with midazolam 15 mg is used to remove up to 1 L of aspirate. For larger procedures, intravenous sedation with midazolam, fentanyl, and propofol is preferred. The

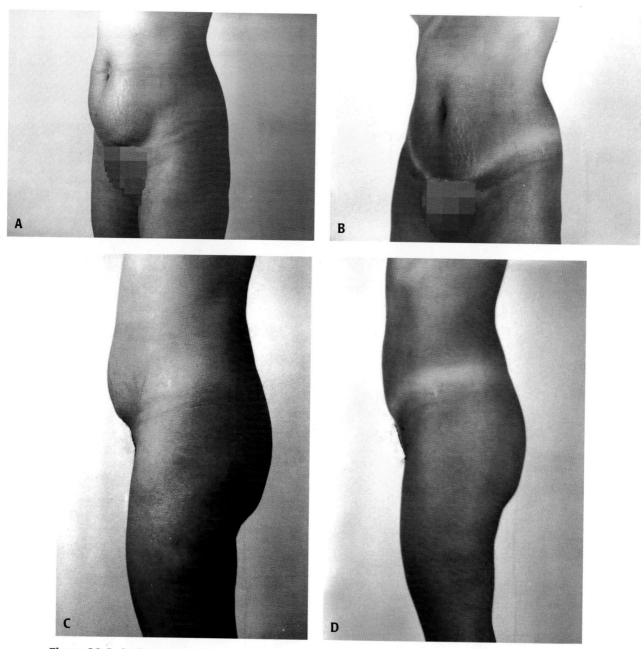

Figure 28-3 A, C: Preoperative photographs of a 42-year-old woman wanting to improve her abdomen. **B, D:** Two-year postoperative, showing improvement of the abdominal area after syringe liposculpture with a total removal of 1,000 cc of aspirate, combined with a suprapubic skin resection and placation of recti muscles.

induction is done with tenoxicam 20 mg, Dramin DL 10 mL, dipyrone 2 mL, dexamethasone 4 mg, and meperidine 1.0 to 1.5 mg/kg. Maintenance is with midazolam 0.1 mg/kg to 0.3 mg/kg, propofol 0.025 mg/kg/min, fentanyl 50 μg, slowly. Cephalexin 2 g is administered intravenously (6 g in 8 hours). The local infiltration solution contains 20 cc 2% lidocaine, 1 cc adrenaline, 500 cc Ringer's lactate, and 5 cc 3% sodium bicarbonate.[6]

This solution is heated to 37°C and injected slowly at a rate of 1:1 to 1.5:1 (injecting 1 cc of fluid per cc of fat is

estimated to aspirate). This proportion avoids pulmonary edema and lidocaine overdose. By warming the solution, hypothermia and shivering is avoided.[7]

SAFETY

Liposuction has been promoted as a safe, easy-to-learn outpatient procedure. Plastic surgeons and dermatologists have developed safety measures to perform the technique, but

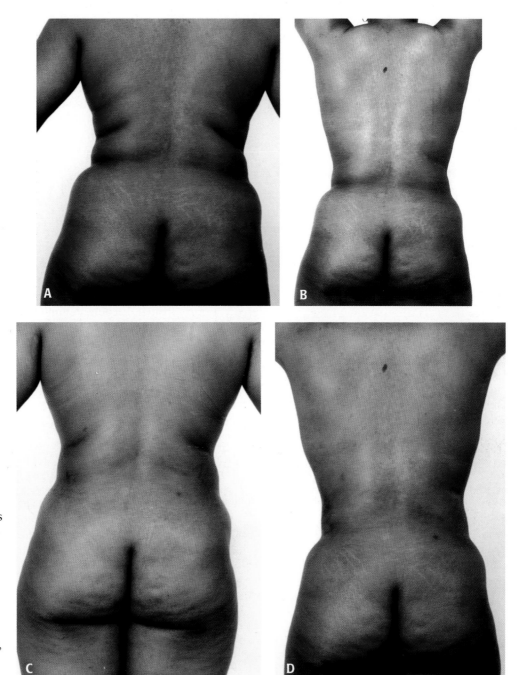

Figure 28-4 A, C: Preoperative photographs of a 28-year-old woman wanting to improve her dorsal region and flanks. **B, D:** Three-weeks postoperative after syringe liposculpture of the scapular, dorsal, flanks, and waist regions, with a total removal of 3,200 cc of aspirate.

there can be serious risks, including death at a rate of 1/5,000 procedures.[8] By 2000, the numbers of liposuction fatalities were 67 for the previous 3 years nationwide related only to board-certified plastic surgeons (not including other doctor groups performing liposuction). The American Society of Plastic Surgery enforced a rule limiting the extracted fat to a 5,000-cc maximum, and the mortalities dropped to zero the next year.[9] Dermatologists, aesthetic medicine practitioners, gynecologists, oral

surgeons, and otolaryngologists also perform liposuction in facilities from hospital to outpatient surgery centers to private offices.

Although the complication rate seems high, according to the French Society of Plastic Reconstructive and Aesthetic Surgery,[10] liposuction is among the techniques for which there are complications in less than 5%. The techniques which produce between 5% and 10% of complications are rhinoplasty, facelift, and breast augmentation.

When more than 1 L of fat is removed, the procedure should be performed in an accredited facility with an anesthesiologist present. The facility will have a cardiac monitor, pulse oximeter, noninvasive blood-pressure monitor, defibrillator, intubation equipment, laryngeal mask, reanimation material, vasoactive drugs, support equipment, infusion pump, a gas central, and an aspirator.

LIFE-THREATENING COMPLICATIONS

The main factors that increase risk in lipoplasty (according to the American Society of Aesthetic Plastic Surgeons Lipoplasty Task Force) are injecting too much fluid and local anesthesia, removing too much fat, performing too many procedures during the same surgical act, having the wrong indication for surgery (health problems, etc.), and inadequate monitoring of megaliposuction patients (Table 28-1).[11]

Safety measures in body-contour procedures should avoid life-threatening complications and aesthetic complications. Life-threatening complications are pulmonary embolism, hemorrhage, perforation, infection, lidocaine and epinephrine toxicity, third-space fluid shifts, and fat embolism syndrome. Pulmonary embolism should be prevented in patients with a higher risk of deep venous thrombosis, either with intraoperative drugs or massaging devices. Hemorrhage can be caused by major vessel perforation, coagulopathy, or simply a bad surgical technique. Extra caution should be used when using vibrating cannulas for power-assisted liposuction and internal ultrasound assisted liposuction.

Treating the abdominal wall without proper planning can cause perforation that is due to bad positioning of the patient during surgery or to misdirection of the cannula. By hyperextending the abdominal region, the cannula

introduced in the pubic area will tend to come up through the skin of the epigastrium rather than perforating the abdomen. Infection can be avoided with total antisepsis and proper antibiotics, intra- and postoperatively. Lidocaine and epinephrine toxicity can occur when performing tumescent anesthesia. Care and caution should be used regarding the amount of lidocaine and epinephrine injected, injecting 1 cc of solution for each cc of aspirate removal. Excessive infiltration of wetting solution, in a proportion of 3:1, can cause lidocaine toxicity, cardiotoxicity, convulsions, drug interaction, and overdose. A patient should not be released too soon after surgery, because the peak of lidocaine absorption happens 8 to 12 hours after the injection. Third-space fluid shifts can occur in megaliposuction procedures when 8 to 10 L of fat or more are removed from a patient in a single procedure. The limit on aspirate should be less than 5% of the body weight, and less than 30% of the body surface should be treated, keeping in mind that it is safer to repeat the procedure to remove more fat. The possibility of hypothermia is reduced by heating every intravenous and subcutaneous fluid to 37° C and by using hot-air blankets pre- and postoperatively. This avoids complications, such as infections, blood loss, heart attacks, and even death. Fat embolism syndrome is very rare after liposuction,[12] and only five cases have been reported.[13]

AESTHETIC COMPLICATIONS

Photographing, weighing, and measuring the patient are important for the surgeon during the surgery and for postoperative comparisons. When a patient does not see any change with the procedure, it is time to show preoperative records. Patients are usually several kilos lighter after the surgery.

The aesthetic complications can be undercorrection (insufficient fat removal), overcorrection (excess fat removal), irregular fat removal with palpable and visible irregularities, edema, and seroma, local infection (because of insufficient sterilization or a patient with low immunity) (Table 28.2). Bad patient selection is a common cause of problems, especially when a patient who needs skin resection is treated with liposuction alone. Cutaneous slough, hyperpigmentation, vasculopathies, hypertrophic scars, and permanent color changes in the skin are some other possible complications. Hypertrophic scars and hyperpigmentation are more common in deeply pigmented skin.

The most common complications of lipoplasty are undercorrection, overcorrection, and irregular fat removal with palpable and/or visible irregularities. The syringe technique allows a precise measurement of the aspirated and injected amount of fat. The aspirator vial is too big to measure the aspirated fat with precision. Using a 60-cc syringe, the exact amount of aspiration can be determined.

Table 28-1
Life-threatening complications
Pulmonary embolism
Hemorrhage
Perforation
Lidocaine toxicity
Epinephrine toxicity
Third-space fluid shifts
Fat embolism syndrome

Table 28-2

Aesthetic complications

Undercorrections (insufficient fat removal)

Overcorrection (excess fat removal)

Irregularities (irregular fat removal)

Hyperpigmentation

Cutaneous slough

Hypertrophic scars

To treat undercorrection, additional fat has to be aspirated. Overcorrection is treated with fat injection. Irregularities can be treated with fat suction, fat injection, subcision, fat shifting or mobilization, and, finally, skin resection. Depressions are addressed by first freeing the fibrous adherences with the V-tip Toledo cannula and injecting fat to obtain a 40% to 50% improvement on the irregularities.

CONCLUSION

Lipoplasty can be a safe outpatient procedure. There are serious risks involved, including a death rate of 1/5,000 procedures. Surgeons should limit procedures to the safety limits of their surgical skills, always keeping in mind that the safety of the patient comes first. When complications occur, surgeons should be prepared to treat them.

REFERENCES

1. Fischer G. Liposculpture: the correct history of liposuction, part I. *J Dermatol Surg Oncol.* 1990;16:1087–1089.
2. Toledo LS. The overlap of lipoplasty and abdominoplasty: indication, classification and treatment. *Clin Plast Surg* 2004; 31(4):539–553.
3. Toledo LS. Total liposculpture. In: Gasparotti M, Lewis CM, Toledo LS, eds. *Superficial Liposculpture.* New York: Springer Verlag;1993:43:29–51.
4. Illouz YG. Une nouvelle technique pour les lipodistrophies localizes. *Rev Chir Est Lang Franç* 1980;619.
5. Toledo LS. Syringe liposculpture. *Clin Plast Surg* 1996;23: 683.
6. Toledo LS. Superficial syringe liposculpture. In: Annals of the II Symposium "Recent Advances in Plastic Surgery-RAPS/90," São Paulo, Marques-Saraiva, 28–30 March 1990, pg. 446.
7. Toledo LS, Regatieri FLF, Carneiro JDA. The effect of hypothermia on coagulation and its implications for infiltration in lipoplasty: a review. *Aesthetic Surgery Journal* 2001; 21(1):40–44.
8. Lehnhardt M, Homann HH, Druecke D, et al. No problem with liposuction? *Chirurg* 2003;74(9):808–814.
9. Gorney M. Personal communication, July 2004.
10. Knipper P, Jauffret JL. Aesthetic snapshot: study about cosmetic surgical procedures and complications. *Ann Chir Plast Esthet* 2003;48(5):299–306.
11. ASAPS Lipoplasty Task Force Jan 1998. http://www.plasticsurgery.org/medical_professionals/publications/PSNews_Bulletin-1-26-1998.cfm.
12. Fourme T, Vieillard-Baron A, Loubieres Y, et al. Early fat embolism after liposuction. *Anesthesiology* 1998;89(3): 782–784.
13. Boezaart AP, Clinton CW, Braun S, et al. Fulminant adult respiratory distress syndrome after suction lipectomy. *S Afr Med J* 1990;78(11):693–695.

Vascular Surgery in Darker Racial Ethnic Groups

Parrish Sadeghi

This chapter will focus on modalities used to treat visible lower-extremity venous diseases, such as spider veins and varicose veins. There is an absolute paucity of published data regarding the treatment of spider veins and varicosities in darker racial ethnic groups. Treatment modalities using sclerosing agents are similar in lighter and darker skin types.

Venous disease of the legs encompasses a variety of conditions affecting the veins, including visible disease—such as spider veins, varicose veins, trophic changes, or edema—and functional disease—such as reflux, obstruction, phlebitis, or thrombosis. Venous disease in the legs occurs very commonly in the general population of industrialized countries and is a substantial source of morbidity in the United States and the Western world.[1,2] Many patients seek leg vein treatment for symptomatic relief, whereas others find varicose veins cosmetically unsightly and seek treatment for that reason. According to a 2005 survey by the American Society of Dermatologic Surgery, the eradication of leg veins was one of the most commonly reported procedures by dermasurgeons in the United States.[3]

EPIDEMIOLOGY AND RISK FACTORS

Estimates of the prevalence of venous disease are varied. Although it is difficult to estimate the overall prevalence of venous disease worldwide, a large U.S. survey, the Framingham study, reported that 27% of the American adult population had some form of venous disease in their legs.[4] There is evidence that geographic location and race can influence susceptibility to superficial venous disease. People living in North American and Western European countries seem to be at a greater risk for venous disease as compared with those who live in South America, India, the Far East, or Africa.[1] Venous disease is less prevalent in African Americans, Hispanics, and Asians.[5] It has been suggested that the low prevalence of varicose veins in Africans (1%–2%) may be associated with the higher number of venous valves in their lower extremities as compared with Caucasians.[6]

To date, most studies have investigated factors that influence susceptibility to superficial venous disease. The data suggest that female sex,[7] increased age,[8] pregnancy,[9] and oral contraceptive use[10] are risk factors for varicose veins. There are also reports that chronic venous disease is higher in those whose job involves prolonged standing and those working under conditions of high temperature and humidity.[11,12] Although some studies have suggested that obesity is associated with varicose veins, a number of studies have not confirmed this finding.[1,13] There is no evidence that there is a strong genetic component to these disorders.[14]

CLINICAL PRESENTATION

The clinical presentation of patients with venous disease of the lower extremities can be variable. Visible venous disease can manifest as telangiectasias or varicose veins, whereas functional disease involves reflux or obstruction of the veins. Leg swelling has been shown to be the most specific predictor of visible and functional leg vein disease.[15] Ankle edema is usually the first manifestation of chronic venous insufficiency (CVI) and can lead to venous stasis. Stasis dermatitis and pigmentary changes, resulting from extravasation of erythrocytes and hemosiderin deposition, are common sequelae of long-standing venous stasis. Recurrent or chronic cellulitis, ulceration, scarring, and malignant degeneration are more serious complications of leg vein disease.[16]

Many patients with visible venous disease have minimal to no symptoms, whereas others may report localized pain, burning, itching, or more generalized leg fatigue, aching, and swelling. Symptomatic varicose veins occur in approximately 15% of men and 25% of women;[1] women are more likely to report symptoms than men.[15,17,18]

ANATOMY

In the leg there are two systems of veins: the deep and the superficial. The deep venous system consists of veins that lie within the muscular system. The superficial venous

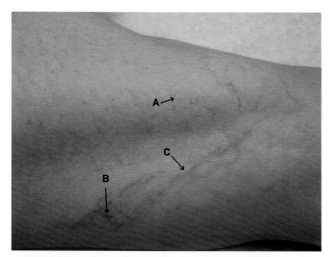

Figure 29-1 Telangiectasia (**A**), venulectasias (**B**), reticular veins (**C**), and varicose veins of the lower extremities.

system has two main veins: the greater saphenous vein (also known as the long saphenous vein) and the lesser saphenous vein (also referred to as the short saphenous vein). The greater saphenous vein (GSV) originates at the medial side of the foot and runs superiorly along the medial aspect of the leg to empty into the femoral vein at the saphenofemoral junction. The lesser saphenous vein starts at the lateral aspect of the foot and runs along the back of the calf and typically joins the popliteal vein at the saphenopopliteal junction. The deep and superficial veins are connected via perforator veins. Veins in the same fascial plane are often interconnected by a complex of communicating veins.

Venous valves are a significant part of the venous system, maintaining the blood's upward flow. Valves are present between the superficial and deep systems at the saphenofemoral and saphenopopliteal junctions. More valves are located below the knee than above. Elevated venous pressure is most often the result of venous insufficiency with reflux through incompetent valves in the deep or superficial veins. Telangiectasias, venulectasias, reticular veins, and varicose veins represent the undesirable pathways by which venous blood refluxes back into the congested extremity (Fig. 29-1). Although most large varices arise from tributaries of incompetent truncal vessels, failed perforating veins or connecting veins can also give rise to independent varices in the greater saphenous distribution without involving the saphenous system itself.

APPROACH TO A PATIENT WITH VARICOSE VEINS

History and physical examination are important in the evaluation of patients with venous disease. Risk factors such as prior pregnancies, use of oral contraceptives, and

history of superficial thrombophlebitis or deep venous thrombosis should be noted. A careful physical examination should be done to determine the nature, extent, and location of varicose veins. Photographs of the affected areas are helpful for tracking disease progression and response to treatment. Laboratory workup to evaluate hypercoagulability or bleeding risks may be appropriate if indicated by the patient's history.

Extensive diagnostic imaging is often unnecessary before treating spider veins and venulectasias, however, for largely dilated (>4 mm) vessels or for more severe cases, imaging modalities are available and should be used to evaluate and determine the extent of the venous disease. Duplex ultrasound has become the most widely used mode of investigation for both arterial and venous disease. This noninvasive and inexpensive technique enables the physician to evaluate competence of the deep and superficial venous valves as well as the competence of the saphenofemoral and saphenopopliteal junctions. Photoplethysmography can be used to measure venous refilling time and distinguish between deep and superficial venous insufficiency.

COMPRESSION THERAPY

Graded compression stockings are often prescribed for patients with varicose veins as a method of relieving symptoms. They may be prescribed either as a definitive treatment or temporarily after varicose vein treatment.[19] Compression stockings are designed to provide a pressure gradient that is greatest at the ankle and decreases proximally, mimicking the normal hydrostatic pressures of the lower extremity.[20] Therapy with compression stockings has been shown to improve venolymphatic drainage substantially in both healthy patients and those suffering from CVI.[21] Most clinicians advocate the use of compression stockings after sclerotherapy; however, there are variations in the suggested duration of use, ranging from 48 hours to several weeks.

SCLEROTHERAPY

For treatment of leg veins less than 4 mm in diameter, sclerotherapy has been considered to be the gold standard.[22] Sclerotherapy involves the direct injection of a sclerosing agent into a visible vein or telangiectasia. The solutions are designed to either irritate, dehydrate, change the surface tension of, or completely destroy the venous endothelial cells, thereby creating a thrombus. Ultimately, the vein is permanently occluded as the thrombus is replaced by fibrosis. There are three types of sclerosant agents: osmotic agents, detergents, and chemical irritants. The most commonly used sclerosants in the United States are hypertonic saline, sodium tetradecyl sulfate, and polidocanol.

Osmotic agents

Osmotic agents, such as hypertonic saline or hypertonic saline with dextrose, cause thrombus formation through dehydration and disruption of the cell walls of endothelial cells and erythrocytes. Osmotic agents are best for treatment of smaller vessels and for low-flow vessels, because rapid dilution can diminish the efficacy of the sclerosant.[23] Severe muscle cramping as a result of transient hyperosmolality induced by hypertonic saline may be experienced.[23] A more serious potential complication—cutaneous ulceration and necrosis—can arise if these agents extravasate into surrounding tissue. One advantage of these agents is that there is a very low risk of allergenicity.

Hypertonic saline is used as a 23.4% solution of sodium chloride, and at this concentration, it can be directly injected into reticular veins and larger vessels.[24] For treatment of smaller vessels, it can be diluted with either normal saline or bacteriostatic water to achieve a concentration of 11.7% solution.[25] In very fine vessels or in vessels near the ankle, a solution of approximately 6% sodium chloride may be more appropriate.[26]

A solution composed of 10% saline, 5% dextrose, propylene glycol, and phenethyl alcohol is manufactured under the brand name Sclerodex. This product is not FDA approved in the United States, although it is approved in Canada. It has limited use because it can only be used in very small vessels (<1 mm in diameter).[26] It is associated with a decreased incidence of muscle cramping, presumably because of the lower percentage of saline, but has an increased risk of pigmentation, allergenicity, and necrosis. The manufacturer recommends a maximum volume of 1 cc at any injection site, with a total per session of no more than 10 cc.

Detergents

Detergent sclerosants produce vascular injury by interfering with cell surface lipids and altering the surface tension around endothelial cells. This results in irritation of the vein intimal endothelium, endothelial cell death,[27] and subsequent thrombus formation and vein fibrosis.

Sodium tetradecyl sulfate (STS), a long-chain fatty acid salt with strong detergent properties, is FDA approved for the treatment of varicose veins. Concentrations of 0.1% to 0.3% are commonly used for the treatment of telangiectatic veins from 0.2 to 1.0 mm in diameter, 0.5% to 1% for treatment of uncomplicated varicose veins that are 2 to 4 mm in diameter, and 1.5% to 3% for the treatment of larger varicose veins.[28] At high concentrations, it is associated with an increased incidence of postsclerosing hyperpigmentation and cutaneous necrosis. Allergic reactions to STS have been reported and include generalized urticaria, bronchospasm, and anaphylactic shock.[29]

Polidocanol (POL), a synthetic fatty alcohol with detergent activity, is currently not FDA approved for use in the United States, but is used extensively in Australia and Europe. In a 2-year Australian study of the efficacy and safety of POL, POL appeared to be superior to STS and hypertonic saline in terms of efficacy and had fewer associated side effects.[30] Other studies have shown comparable results between POL and STS[28,31] or POL and hypertonic saline.[32] POL has been used as an anesthetic and is therefore painless upon injection and well tolerated by patients for that reason.[27] In a double-blind, placebo-controlled study, POL 0.25% was found to have fewer adverse reactions and afforded the greatest patient comfort when compared with STS 0.5%.[33]

Fitzpatrick skin types V and VI treated with POL appear to have less incidence of postsclerosis pigmentary change than skin types I and II.[34] Liquid POL is associated with decreased incidence of ulceration and urticaria,[28] however, its negative features include slower fading of treated vessels and risk of allergic reaction. Because of this latter risk, a test dose of 0.5% solution should be injected into a vessel before a treatment session.[26] The solutions should be diluted appropriately as follows: 0.25% to 0.75% for telangiectasias, 1% for vessels of 1 to 2 mm, and 2% solution for vessels of 2 to 4 mm. There are total daily dose limitations with polidocanol based on body weight (2 mg/kg/d).

Chemical irritants

Chemical irritants injure cells by acting as corrosives. Chromated glycerin has been used in Europe but is not approved for use by the FDA. It can be used for telangiectasias and has a low potential of hyperpigmentation. Only a total of a 0.1 cc prediluted solution should be used in a single session.[26] Chromated glycerin can be painful upon injection and should be avoided in patients with chronic renal insufficiency.[35]

Polyiodinated iodine is one of the strongest currently available sclerosing solutions worldwide. It is mainly indicated as a last resort for treatment of saphenofemoral and saphenopopliteal junction-related vein abnormalities.[23] It is contraindicated in patients with hyperthyroidism.

FOAM SCLEROTHERAPY

Foam sclerotherapy has become an increasingly popular modality in the treatment of varicose veins. In foam sclerotherapy, a sclerosing solution is mixed with oxygen to produce foam. This technique was first described in 1939,[36] and since then, various methods of producing foam agents have been described.[37–40] Foam sclerotherapy is considered to be more effective by some clinicians because a smaller quantity of sclerosant is needed to treat a greater surface area. The most popular agents used for foam sclerotherapy worldwide are STS and POL.

Studies comparing foamed and liquid POL and STS found both agents to be safe and effective sclerosing agents

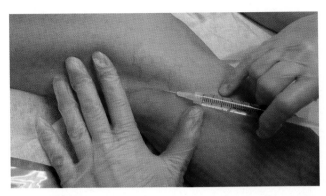

Figure 29-2 Sclerotherapy technique. The needle is placed parallel to the skin with a 1- or 3-mL Luer-Lok syringe firmly held into place between the thumb and index finger and supported by the other fingers. The needle is then carefully inserted into the vessel while using slow and steady injection with light pressure.

in the treatment of varicose and telangiectatic leg veins.[31] In addition to potential adverse effects of liquid detergent sclerotherapy, when treating larger veins, foam detergent sclerotherapy has been associated with transient visual disturbances, such as scotomas[37,41] and phlebitis.[41]

A recent study demonstrated that for the same given concentration of POL, the foam preparation has greater sclerosant efficacy compared with the liquid form in the treatment of reticular and postoperative varices not involving the saphenofemoral junction.[34] However, minor adverse effects, such as pain, inflammation, and skin pigmentation, are more frequent with foam POL.[42]

SCLEROTHERAPY TECHNIQUE

As before any procedure, the patient must be appropriately evaluated, the affected areas photographed, and informed consent obtained. The patient is positioned in either the supine or prone position. The area to be treated is liberally cleansed with 70% isopropyl alcohol, which reduces light reflection and allows for better visualization of the vessels. A 30-gauge needle is bent to an angle that is comfortable for the practitioner, usually between 10° to 30° with the bevel facing upward. The needle is placed parallel to the skin with a 1- or 3-mL Luer-Lok syringe firmly held into place between the thumb and index finger and supported by the other fingers (Fig. 29-2). The needle is then carefully inserted into the vessel while using slow and steady injection with light pressure. A small bolus of air may be injected into telangiectasias to ensure proper cannulation of the vessel. For reticular veins, the plunger may slightly be drawn to ensure a return of blood before injection. The first treatment session is usually limited to a few areas to observe for any adverse reactions, primarily being allergic. Because most telangiectasias arise from reticular veins, these feeding veins should be treated before injecting the

telangiectasias.[16] It is advised that no more than 0.5 cc of sclerosant be injected at each site. After the treatment session, pressure is applied to the area with the use of an elastic bandage, compression stocking, or both. The patient is encouraged to wear the stocking or bandage during the daytime for several days and is permitted to resume normal activity immediately after treatment (Fig. 29-3A,B).

COMPLICATIONS OF SCLEROTHERAPY

Common side effects of sclerotherapy include pain, postinjection urticaria, skin necrosis with ulceration, telangiectatic matting, and hyperpigmentation. The use of compression stockings postsclerotherapy has been shown to decrease the incidence of hyperpigmentation.[43] Postsclerotherapy hyperpigmentation is the most common side effect of sclerotherapy in darker skin types, occurring in the majority of patients. It is caused by hemosiderin and melanin deposition. Topical bleaching agents containing hydroquinone and retinoids often expedite resolution of postsclerotherapy hyperpigmentation. In addition, ankle and calf edema is lessened if a graduated compression stocking is worn immediately after sclerotherapy.[43] If sclerosant flow to small end arterioles, as evidenced by persistent blanching of all the tissues in a roughly circular area, is suspected, application of topical nitroglycerin may prevent or mitigate ulceration.[44] Injection of hyaluronidase or tumescing the skin with lidocaine or normal saline may also prevent or decrease ulceration associated with sclerosant extravasation.[45] Postsclerotherapy telangiectatic matting (TM), which appears as new, fine, red blushlike telangiectasias, occurs in up to 24% of individuals treated with sclerotherapy and may occur from 2 to 3 days to months following sclerotherapy.[46] Thighs, medial ankles, and medial and lateral calves are common locations for appearance of posttreatment TM.[47] A small percentage of patients (10%–20%) will have spontaneous resolution of TM within 3 months.[48] However, another 10% to 20% may experience persistence of such vessels[49] (Fig. 29-4).

CONTRAINDICATIONS TO SCLEROTHERAPY

Sclerotherapy is contraindicated in pregnancy, breast-feeding, and in patients with allergy to the sclerosant, lack of mobility, significant deep-vein incompetence, or a history of thrombophilia.[50]

LASER AND LIGHT MODALITIES

Although lasers have successfully been used to treat many vascular lesions and facial telangiectasias, this modality

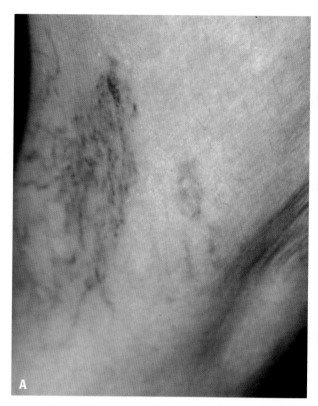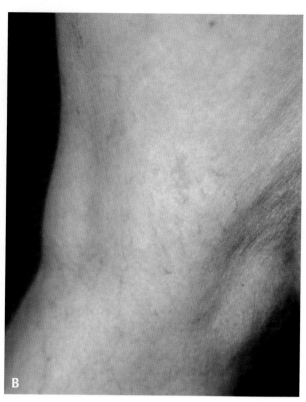

Figure 29-3 Before **(A)** and after **(B)** sclerotherapy. These photographs present results obtained following one injection. (Courtesy of David Duffy, MD.)

has had limited use in the treatment of leg veins. Laser leg vein treatment appears to be most beneficial in special circumstances, such as patients with hard-to-cannulate small vessels (0.1–0.3 mm), TM, needle phobia, or sclerosant allergy.[51,52] Laser therapy more commonly is used adjunctively with sclerotherapy techniques.[23,53] Combination approaches of sclerotherapy plus laser treatments performed during the same treatment session may produce synergistic results in selected individuals.[54] In general, laser therapies should be used with care and extreme caution in darker skin types to avoid hyperpigmentation, hypopigmentation, and scarring.

Lasers have been shown to induce endothelial cell injury.[55] The extended-pulse, longer-wavelength technologies, such as 1,064-nm Nd:YAG laser, have allowed the treatment of individuals with darker skin as well as treatment of deep blue reticular veins that are up to 3 mm in diameter.[54] The 1,064-nm Nd:YAG allows darker skin types to be treated with minimal risk to the epidermis because of decreased interaction with melanin, thus minimizing the potential for irregularities in epidermal contour and pigmentation.[56] Hyperpigmentation is most commonly observed with larger veins and appears to be primarily related to hemosiderin deposition.

The 755-nm alexandrite laser at fluences of 60 to 70 J/cm², 3-msec pulse width, and an 8-mm spot can be effective for larger leg veins, but the inflammatory response, purpura, and long-term pigmentary alterations limit its

usefulness.[57] The KTP (532 nm) laser has been shown to be effective for treating spider leg veins with a vascular diameter under 0.7 mm.[58] Pulsed diode laser therapy (810 nm) is another treatment option for spider leg veins,[59] but results can be unpredictable.[60]

A bimodal wavelength approach of short and long wavelengths using an intense pulsed light source (550-nm cut-off filter), and the 1,064-nm Nd:YAG laser has been also shown to be effective in treating variably colored 0.1- to 4-mm telangiectasias and venulectasias.[61]

In summary, for leg vein treatment, the 1,064-nm wavelength is very safe for Fitzpatrick skin type V skin, the 810-nm wavelength at superlong pulse widths of 400 to 1,000 msec is very safe for type IV and marginal for type V skin, and the 755-nm wavelength is limited to non-tanned type I to III skin.[60]

MINIMALLY INVASIVE PROCEDURES

For varicosities greater than 4 mm, GSV reflux, or sapheno-femoral incompetence, minimally invasive treatments, such as endovascular modalities, are alternatives to surgical treatment. Following the procedure, a compression stocking is worn for 5 to 7 days. Patients are able to walk immediately after the procedure, and most individuals are able to return to work the next day. There are three types of endovenous procedures: ultrasound-guided scle-

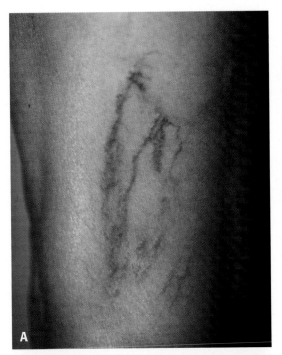

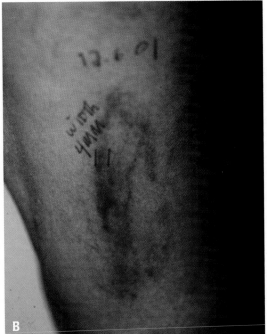

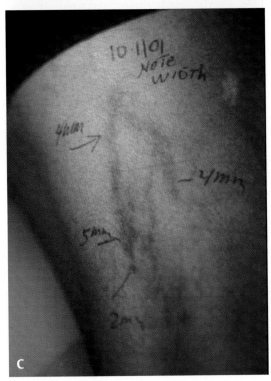

Figure 29-4 Before **(A)** and after **(B,C)** sclerotherapy. Note excellent response but some residual hyperpigmentation. (Courtesy of David Duffy, MD.)

rotherapy, endovenous laser treatment, and endovenous radiofrequency ablation.

Ultrasound-guided sclerotherapy

With this technique, ultrasound equipment is used to both map the veins and guide the physician during the injection of the sclerosing agent. The map provides the physician with the location of the veins and the valves,

the size of each vein, the point of reflux, and the presence of thrombosis. Using the map, the physician determines the locations to be injected as well as the amount and type of sclerosant that is required. The ultrasound device is used to guide the injections to the precise locations.[22] Possible complications of ultrasound-guided sclerotherapy include transient visual disturbances and deep vein thrombosis.[41,62]

Endovenous laser treatment

Endovenous laser treatment is an alternative to surgical stripping of the GSV. Instead of removing the saphenous vein, it is ablated from within by resistive heating. The skin on the inside of the knee is anesthetized, and under ultrasound guidance, a laser fiber is inserted into the saphenous vein. The laser is fired, and as the fiber is withdrawn, the vein collapses and seals shut.[63] Endovenous laser treatment is FDA approved. Possible complications of endovenous laser treatment are thermal skin burns and transient numbness.

Endovenous radiofrequency ablation

Endovenous radiofrequency ablation (closure procedure) is another minimally invasive, FDA-approved, in-office treatment alternative to surgical stripping. The procedure is similar to endovenous laser treatment, except that instead of a laser fiber, a radiofrequency catheter is used. Postprocedure care is similar to other endovenous procedures. Possible complications of endovenous radiofrequency ablation are deep vein thrombosis, thermal skin burns, and transient numbness.[64–66]

SURGERY

There are several surgical options for varicose veins: traditional ligation and stripping, Perforate Invaginate (PIN) stripping, and ambulatory phlebectomy.

Vein stripping and ligation

Traditional surgical ligation and stripping of the GSV is done under general anesthesia and usually performed in an outpatient surgical center or in a hospital operating room. PIN stripping is an updated method of vein stripping. A small incision is made in the leg, and the PIN stripper is inserted and advanced through the vein. The tip of the PIN stripper is sewn to the end of the vein, and as the PIN stripper is withdrawn, the vein is pulled on itself and is stripped out.[67] This procedure can be done under local anesthesia with intravenous sedation or general anesthesia and is thought to achieve better cosmesis than traditional stripping.[68]

Ambulatory phlebectomy

Ambulatory phlebectomy is an in-office procedure that can be performed using local tumescent anesthesia. It allows for complete removal of affected veins by hook avulsion below the saphenofemoral and saphenopopliteal junctions. The area surrounding the varicose veins is tumesced with anesthetic fluid. A needle is then used to make a puncture near the varicose vein, a small hook is inserted into the needle hole, and the vein is grasped and removed.

CONCLUSION

Venous disease of the legs is a common cosmetic and medical problem. Fortunately, the clinician now has a sizable armamentarium for treating these affected vessels (Fig. 29-5).

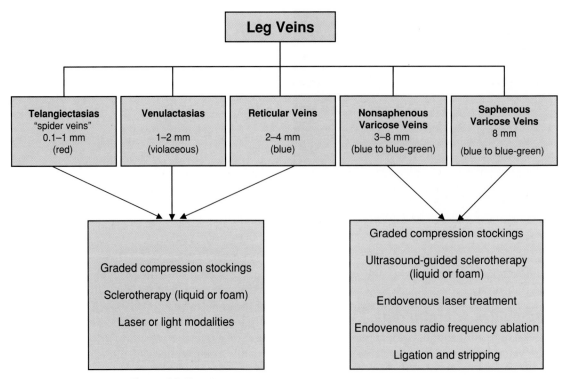

Figure 29-5 Leg vein classification and treatment options.

Sclerotherapy remains the gold standard for treatment of telangiectasias and small veins. New and emerging lasers and light sources can be used as adjuvant treatment. For larger veins, endovenous procedures are available as less-invasive alternatives to traditional surgical vein stripping and ligation.

REFERENCES

1. Callam MJ. Epidemiology of varicose veins. *Br J Surg* 1994;81(2):167–173.
2. Evans CJ, Fowkes FGR, Hajivassiliou CA, et al. Epidemiology of varicose veins: a review. *Int Angiol* 1994;13(3): 263–270.
3. American Society for Dermatologic Surgery. 2005 Procedural Survey.
4. Brand FN, Dannenberg AL, Abbott RD, et al. The epidemiology of varicose veins: the Framingham Study. *Am J Prev Med* 1988;4(2):96–101.
5. Criqui MH, Jamosmos M, Fronek A, et al. Chronic venous disease in an ethnically diverse population: the San Diego Population Study. *Am J Epidemiol* 2003;158(5):448–456.
6. Banjo AO. Comparative study of the distribution of venous valves in the lower extremities of black Africans and Caucasians: pathogenetic correlates of prevalence of primary varicose veins in the two races. *Anat Rec* 1987;217(4):407–412.
7. Ahumada M, Vioque J. [Prevalence and risk factors of varicose veins in adults]. *Med Clin (Barc)* 2004;123(17): 647–651.
8. Laurikka J, Sisto T, Auvinen O, et al. Varicose veins in a Finnish population aged 40–60. *J Epidemiol Community Health* 1993;47(5):355–357.
9. Dindelli M, Parazzini F, Basellini A, et al. Risk factors for varicose disease before and during pregnancy. *Angiology* 1993;44(5):361–367.
10. Vin F, Allaert FA, Levardon M. Influence of estrogens and progesterone on the venous system of the lower limbs in women. *J Dermatol Surg Oncol* 1992;18(10):888–892.
11. Tomei F, Baccolo TP, Tomao E, et al. Chronic venous disorders and occupation. *Am J Ind Med* 1999;36(6):653–665.
12. Ziegler S, Eckhardt G, Stoger R, et al. High prevalence of chronic venous disease in hospital employees. *Wien Klin Wochenschr* 2003;115 (15–16):575–579.
13. Berard A, Abenhaim L, Pla HR, et al. Risk factors for the first-time development of venous ulcers of the lower limbs: the influence of heredity and physical activity. *Angiology* 2002;53(6):647–657.
14. Beebe-Dimmer JL, Pfeifer JR, Engle JS, et al. The epidemiology of chronic venous insufficiency and varicose veins. *Ann Epidemiol* 2005;15(3): 175–184.
15. Langer RD, Ho E, Denenberg JO, et al. Relationships between symptoms and venous disease: the San Diego population study. *Arch Intern Med* 2005;165(12):1420–1424.
16. Goldman MP, Bergan JJ. *Sclerotherapy: Treatment of Varicose and Telangiectatic Leg Veins.* 3rd ed. St. Louis: Mosby; 2001:xxii,401.
17. Kroger K, Ose C, Rudofsky G, et al. Symptoms in individuals with small cutaneous veins. *Vasc Med* 2002;7(1):13–17.
18. Bradbury A, Evans C, Allan PL, et al. What are the symptoms of varicose veins? Edinburgh vein study cross sectional population survey. *BMJ* 1999;318(7180):353–356.
19. Shami SK, Cheatle TR, Fegan G. *Fegan's Compression Sclerotherapy for Varicose Veins.* New York: Springer;2003:xvi, 100, xii of plates.
20. Sadick NS. *Manual of Sclerotherapy.* Philadelphia: Lippincott Williams & Wilkins; 2000:xiii, 272.
21. Hauer G, Staubesand J, Li Y et al. [Chronic venous insufficiency]. *Chirurg* 1996;67(5):505–514.
22. Sadick NS. Advances in the treatment of varicose veins: ambulatory phlebectomy, foam sclerotherapy, endovascular laser, and radiofrequency closure. *Dermatol Clin* 2005;23(3): 443–455, vi.
23. Weiss RA, Feied C, Weiss MA. *Vein Diagnosis and Treatment: a Comprehensive Approach.* New York: McGraw-Hill Medical Publishing Division;2001: xv, 304.
24. Sadick NS. Sclerotherapy of varicose and telangiectatic leg veins: minimal sclerosant concentration of hypertonic saline and its relationship to vessel diameter. *J Dermatol Surg Oncol* 1991;17(1):65–70.
25. Sadick NS, Farber B. A microbiologic study of diluted sclerotherapy solutions [see comment]. *J Dermatol Surg Oncol* 1993;19(5):450–454.
26. Parsons ME. Sclerotherapy basics. *Dermatol Clin* 2004; 22(4):501–508.
27. Noel B. Polidocanol or chromated glycerin for sclerotherapy of telangiectatic leg veins? With reply from Dr. Kern et al. [comment]. *Dermatol Surg* 2004;30(9):1272; author reply 1272–1273.
28. Goldman MP. Treatment of varicose and telangiectatic leg veins: double-blind prospective comparative trial between aethoxysclerol and Sotradecol. *Dermatol Surg* 2002;28(1): 52–55.
29. Fronek H, Fronek A, Saltzberg G. Allergic reactions to Sotradecol. *J Dermatol Surg Oncol* 1989;15(6):684.
30. Conrad P, Malouf GM, Stacey MC. The Australian polidocanol (aethoxysclerol) study: results at 2 years. *Dermatol Surg* 1995;21(4) 334–336; discussion 337–338.
31. Rao J, Wildemore JK, Goldman MP. Double-blind prospective comparative trial between foamed and liquid polidocanol and sodium tetradecyl sulfate in the treatment of varicose and telangiectatic leg veins. *Dermatol Surg* 2005;31(6): 631–635; discussion 635.
32. Sadick NS. Hyperosmolar versus detergent sclerosing agents in sclerotherapy: effect on distal vessel obliteration. *J Dermatol Surg Oncol* 1994;20(5):313–316.
33. Carlin MC, Ratz JL. Treatment of telangiectasia: comparison of sclerosing agents. *J Dermatol Surg Oncol* 1987;13(11): 1181–1184.
34. Alos J, Carreno P, Lopez JA, et al. Efficacy and safety of sclerotherapy using polidocanol foam: a controlled clinical trial. *Eur J Vasc Endovasc Surg* 2006;31(1):101–107.
35. Guex JJ, Allaert FA, Gillet JL, et al. Immediate and midterm complications of sclerotherapy: report of a prospective multicenter registry of 12,173 sclerotherapy sessions. *Dermatol Surg* 2005;31(2): 123–128; discussion 128.
36. McAusland S. The modern treatment of varicose veins. *Med Press Circular* 1939;201:404–410.
37. Tessari L, Cavezzi A, Frullini A. Preliminary experience with a new sclerosing foam in the treatment of varicose veins. *Dermatol Surg* 2001;27(1):58–60.
38. Frullini A. New technique in producing sclerosing foam in a disposable syringe. *Dermatol Surg* 2000;26(7):705–706.

39. Cabrera J, Cabrera J Jr., Garcia-Olmedo MA. Sclerosants in microfoam: a new approach in angiology. *Int Angiol* 2001; 20(4):322–329.

40. Wollmann JC. The history of sclerosing foams. *Dermatol Surg* 2004;30(5):694–703; discussion 703.

41. Frullini A, Cavezzi A. Sclerosing foam in the treatment of varicose veins and telangiectases: history and analysis of safety and complications. *Dermatol Surg* 2002;28(1):11–15.

42. Kervinen H, Kaartinen M, Makynen H, et al. Serum tryptase levels in acute coronary syndromes. *Int J Cardiol* 2005;104(2): 138–143.

43. Goldman MP, Beaudoing P, Marley W, et al. Compression in the treatment of leg telangiectasia: a preliminary report. *J Dermatol Surg Oncol* 1990;16(4):322–325.

44. Weiss RA, Goldman MP. Advances in sclerotherapy. *Dermatol Clin* 1995;13(2):431–445.

45. Zimmet SE. The prevention of cutaneous necrosis following extravasation of hypertonic saline and sodium tetradecyl sulfate. *J Dermatol Surg Oncol* 1993;19(7):641–646.

46. Duffy DM. Small vessel sclerotherapy: an overview. *Adv Dermatol* 1988;3:221–242.

47. Davis LT, Duffy DM. Determination of incidence and risk factors for postsclerotherapy telangiectatic matting of the lower extremity: a retrospective analysis. *J Dermatol Surg Oncol* 1990;16(4):327–330.

48. Sadick NS, Urmacher C. Estrogen and progesterone receptors: their role in postsclerotherapy angiogenesis telangiectatic matting (TM). *Dermatol Surg* 1999;25(7):539–543.

49. Goldman MP, Sadick NS, Weiss RA. Cutaneous necrosis, telangiectatic matting, and hyperpigmentation following sclerotherapy: etiology, prevention, and treatment. *Dermatol Surg* 1995;21(1):19–29; quiz 31–32.

50. Barrett JM, Allen B, Ockelford A, et al. Microfoam ultrasound-guided sclerotherapy of varicose veins in 100 legs. *Dermatol Surg* 2004;30(1): 6–12.

51. Ross EV, Domankevitz Y. Laser treatment of leg veins: physical mechanisms and theoretical considerations. *Lasers Surg Med* 2005;36(2):105–116.

52. Lupton JR, Alster TS, Romero P. Clinical comparison of sclerotherapy versus long-pulsed Nd:YAG laser treatment for lower extremity telangiectases. *Dermatol Surg* 2002;28(8):694–697.

53. Levy JL, Elbahr C, Jouve E, et al. Comparison and sequential study of long pulsed Nd:YAG 1,064 nm laser and sclerotherapy in leg telangiectasias treatment. *Lasers Surg Med* 2004;34(3): 273–276.

54. Sadick NS. Laser treatment of leg veins. *Skin Therapy Lett* 2004;9(9):6–9.

55. Sadick NS, Prietro VG, Shea CR, et al. Clinical and pathophysiologic correlates of 1064-nm Nd:YAG laser treatment of reticular veins and venulectasias. *Arch Dermatol* 2001; 137(5):613–617.

56. Weiss RA, Weiss MA. Early clinical results with a multiple synchronized pulse 1064 nm laser for leg telangiectasias and reticular veins. *Dermatol Surg* 1999;25(5):399–402.

57. McDaniel DH, Ash K, Lord J, et al. Laser therapy of spider leg veins: clinical evaluation of a new long pulsed alexandrite laser. *Dermatol Surg* 1999;25(1):52–58.

58. Spendel S, Prandl EC, Schintler MV, et al. Treatment of spider leg veins with the KTP (532 nm) laser—a prospective study. *Lasers Surg Med* 2002; 31(3):194–201.

59. Wollina U, Konrad H, Schmidt WD, et al., Response of spider leg veins to pulsed diode laser (810 nm): a clinical, histological and remission spectroscopy study. *J Cosmet Laser Ther* 2003;5(3–4):154–162.

60. Eremia S, Li C, Umar SH. A side-by-side comparative study of 1064 nm Nd:YAG, 810 nm diode and 755 nm alexandrite lasers for treatment of 0.3–3 mm leg veins. *Dermatol Surg* 2002;28(3):224–230.

61. Sadick NS. A dual wavelength approach for laser/intense pulsed light source treatment of lower extremity veins. *J Am Acad Dermatol* 2002;46(1):66–72.

62. Guex JJ. [Contraindications of sclerotherapy, update 2005]. *J Mal Vasc* 2005;30(3):144–149.

63. Beale RJ, Gough MJ. Treatment options for primary varicose veins—a review. *Eur J Vasc Endovasc Surg* 2005;30(1):83–95.

64. Merchant RF, DePalma RG, Kabnick LS. Endovascular obliteration of saphenous reflux: a multicenter study. *J Vasc Surg* 2002;35(6):1190–1196.

65. Rautio T, Ohinmaa A, Perala J, et al. Endovenous obliteration versus conventional stripping operation in the treatment of primary varicose veins: a randomized controlled trial with comparison of the costs. *J Vasc Surg* 2002;35(5):958–965.

66. Sybrandy JE, Wittens CH. Initial experiences in endovenous treatment of saphenous vein reflux. *J Vasc Surg* 2002;36(6): 1207–1212.

67. Wigger P. [Surgical therapy of primary varicose veins]. *Schweiz Med Wochenschr* 1998;128(45):1781–1788.

68. Durkin MT, Turton EP, Scott DJ et al. A prospective randomised trial of PIN versus conventional stripping in varicose vein surgery. *Ann R Coll Surg Engl* 1999;81(3):171–174.

Surgical Approaches for Hair Disorders

22. Grimes PE, Davis LT. Cosmetics in blacks. *Dermatol Clin* 1991;9:53–68.

23. Scott DA. Disorders of the hair and scalp in blacks. *Dermatol Clin* 1988;6:387–395.

24. Earles RM. Surgical correction of traumatic alopecia marginalis or traction alopecia in black women. *J Dermatol Surg Oncol* 1986;12:1:78–82.

25. Sperling LC. Traction alopecia. In: Sperling LC, ed.. *An Atlas of Hair Pathology with Clinical Correlations.* New York: Parthenon Publishing Group;2003:51–57.

26. Wilborn WS. Disorders of hair growth in African-Americans. In: Olsen EA. *Disorders of Hair Growth: Diagnosis and Treatment* 2nd ed. New York: McGraw-Hill;2003:389–407.

27. Callender VD. Hair transplantation for pigmented skins. In: Halder RM. *Dermatology and Dermatological Therapy of Pigmented Skins.* Boca Raton, FL: Taylor & Francis;2006: 245–257.

28. Lopresti P, Papa CM, Kligman AM. Hot comb alopecia. *Arch Dermatol* 1968;98:234–238.

29. Dawber R. What is pseudopelade? *Clin Exp Dermatol* 1992;17:305–306.

30. Nicholson AG, Harland CC, Bull RH, et al. Chemically induced cosmetic alopecia. *Br J Dermatol* 1993;128: 537–541.

31. Sperling LC, Sau P. The follicular degeneration syndrome in black patients: "hot comb alopecia" revisited and revised. *Arch Dermatol* 1992;128:68–74.

32. Sperling LC. A new look at scarring alopecia. *Arch Dermatol* 2000;136:235–242.

33. Olsen EA, Bergfeld WF, Cotsarelis G, et al. Summary of North America Hair Research Society (NAHRS)–sponsored workshop on cicatricial alopecia, Duke University Medical Center, February 10 and 11, 2001. *J Am Acad Dermatol* 2003;48:103–110.

34. Sperling LC. Central centrifugal scarring alopecia. In: Sperling LC, ed. *An Atlas of Hair Pathology with Clinical Correlations.* New York: The Parthenon Publishing Group;2003: 91–100.

35. Tan E, Martinka M, Ball N, et al. Primary cicatricial alopecias: clinicopathology of 112 cases. *J Am Acad Dermatol* 2004;50:25–32.

36. McMichael AJ. Scalp and hair diseases in the black patient. In: Johnson BL, Moy RL, White GM, eds. *Ethnic Skin.* St. Loius: Mosby;1998:214–230.

37. International Society of Hair Restoration Surgery. 2005 Practice Census. www.ishrs.org. Accessed March 2006.

38. Orentreich N. Autographs in alopecias and other selected dermatological conditions. *Ann N Y Acad Sci* 1959;83: 463–479.

39. Bernstein RM, Rassman WR, Szaniawski W, et al: Follicular transplantation. *Int J Aesthet Rest Surg* 1995;3:119–132.

40. Bernstein RM, Rassman WR. The aesthetics of follicular transplantation. *Dermatol Surg* 1997;23(9):785–799.

41. Headington JT. Transverse microscopic anatomy of the human scalp. *Arch Dermatol* 1984;120:449–456.

42. Pierce HE. The uniqueness of hair transplantation in black patients. *J Dermatol Surg Oncol* 1977;3:533–535.

43. Rook A. Hair II: racial and other genetic variations in hair form. *Br J Dermatol* 1975;92:599–600.

44. Lindelof B, Forslind B, Hedblad MA, et al. Human hair form. *Arch Dermatol* 1988;124:1359–1363.

45. Sperling LC. Hair density in African-Americans. *Arch Dermatol* 1999;135:656–658.

46. Cooley JE. Hair transplantation in blacks. In: Haber RS, Stough DB, eds. *Procedures in Cosmetic Dermatology: Hair Transplantation.* Philadelphia: Elsevier;2005:143–147.

47. Brown MD, Johnson T, Swanson NA. Extensive keloids following hair transplantation. *J Dermatol Surg Oncol* 1990;16: 867–869.

48. Unger WP. Hair transplantation in Blacks. In: Unger WP, Shapiro R, eds. *Hair Transplantation.* 3rd ed. New York: Marcel Dekker, Inc;1995:281–285.

49. Dinehart SM, Tanner L, Mallory SB, et al. Acne keloidalis in women. *Cutis* 1989;44:250–252.

50. Callender VD, Young CM, Haverstock CL, et al. An open label study of clobetasol propionate 0.05% and betamethasone valerate 0.12% foams in the treatment of mild to moderate acne keloidalis. *Cutis* 2005;75:317–321.

51. McMichael AJ, Callender VD. Hair and scalp disorders in pigmented skins. In: Halder RM. *Dermatology and Dermatological Therapy of Pigmented Skins.* Boca Raton, FL: Taylor & Francis;2006:63–90.

52. Fox H. Observations on skin diseases in the negro. *J Cutan Dis* 1908;26:67–79.

53. George AO, Akanji AO, Nduka EU, et al. Clinical, biochemical and morphologic features of acne keloidalis in a black population. *Int J Dermatol* 1993;32:714–716.

54. Child FJ, Fuller LC, Higgins EM, et al. A study of the spectrum of skin disease occurring in a black population in south-east London. *Br J Dermatol* 1999;141:512–517.

55. Sperling L, Homoky C, Pratt L, et al. Acne keloidalis is a form of primary scarring alopecia. *Arch Dermatol* 2000;136: 479–484.

56. Macquire HC Jr. Treatment of keloids with triamcinolone acetonide injected intralesionally. *JAMA* 1965;192:325–326.

57. Layton AM, Yip J, Cunliffe WJ. A comparison of intralesional triamcinolone and cryosurgery in the treatment of acne keloids. *Br J Dermatol* 1994;130:498–501.

58. Glenn MJ, Bennett RG, Kelly AP. Acne keloidalis nuchae: treatment with excision and second-intention healing. *J Am Acad Dermatol* 1995;33:243–246.

59. Gloster HM Jr. The surgical management of extreme cases of acne keloidalis nuchae. *Arch Dermatol* 2000;136:1376–1379.

60. Kantor GR, Ratz JL, Wheeland RG. Treatment of acne keloidalis nuchae with carbon dioxide laser. *J Am Acad Dermatol* 1986;14:263–267.

61. Seager DJ, Simmons C. Local anesthesia in hair transplantation. *Dermatol Surg* 2000;28:320–328.

62. Stough DB, Berger RA, Orentrich N. Surgical improvement of cicatricial alopecia of diverse etiology. *Arch Dermatol* 1968;97:331–334.

63. Rose PT, Shapiro R. Transplanting into scar tissue and areas of cicatricial alopecia. In: Unger WP, Shapiro R. *Hair Transplantation.* 4th ed. New York: Marcel Dekker;2004:606–610.

31

Hair Transplantation for Men

Marc R. Avram

The goal of hair transplantation is to establish an aesthetically appropriate frontal hairline to frame the face. From the 1960s into the late 1990s, ten to twenty-five 3- to 4-mm hair grafts were the mainstay of hair transplantation, despite the fact that hair naturally grows in the scalp in bundles of 1 to 4 hair follicles. The 10 to 25 hair grafts looked unnatural because they *were* unnatural. Today, surgeons and their surgical assistants meticulously harvest the natural 1–4 hair-follicular groupings from donor hair and implant them in the recipient region. This technique consistently creates natural-appearing hair (Fig. 31-1A,B). Contemporary hair transplantation requires a highly skilled transplant team. A skilled team is created by having enthusiastic, dedicated members train more than 6 to 12 months to develop skills necessary to create grafts and place them in recipient sites. The surgeon and team work together to accurately and efficiently harvest the donor hair, create a large number of natural 1–4 grafts, create recipient sites, and place the grafts into these sites. This chapter will provide an overview of appropriate candidate selection, the role of medication with surgery, donor harvesting techniques, graft creation, hairline design, and graft placement for consistently natural transplanted hair in men. Hair transplantation procedures are indeed performed in men of darker racial ethnic groups, including Asians, Hispanics, Africans, and African Americans. Techniques are similar for Asians, Hispanics, and Caucasians. However, the unique morphological features of Afrocentric hair require special considerations for hair transplantation, as discussed in this chapter and in Chapter 30.

THE CONSULT

Male pattern hair loss is an *involuntary* change in a man's appearance. It affects 50% of men by age 50.[1] The involuntary change in physical appearance is a source of stress for many men. Unfortunately, many believe there is nothing that can be done to halt or reverse their hair loss. In fact, the vast majority of men could halt or reverse their hair loss via safe medical and/or surgical options. A consultation for

male pattern hair loss is vital to create the appropriate treatment plan for each individual.

MEDICAL THERAPY

The introduction of minoxidil and finasteride as effective treatment options for hair loss have provided physicians with new tools to treat hair loss[2,3] (Table 31-1). Both medications are more effective for patients with earlier stages of hair loss and are an excellent treatment option for patients losing hair but who are not candidates for surgery. For patients who are candidates for surgery, continuing medical treatment will often help increase the density of transplanted hair by slowing down the rate of loss of existing hair and increasing the caliber of existing and transplanted hair. In addition, these medications may help reduce a postsurgical telogen effluvium and maintain donor density.[4]

There are a variety of supplements and products advertised on the Internet and television that purport to stop and reverse male pattern hair loss. The majority are herbal and vitamin supplements. Good nutrition is important for hair growth. The vast majority of men receive more-than-adequate nutrition for normal hair growth, and supplements are not needed. The problem is a genetic, not a nutritional, one. Some men, in their zeal to treat their hair loss, take megadoses of vitamins that have a counterproductive effect and promote further hair loss. Minoxidil and finasteride are the only two medications that have demonstrated through studies to have a consistently positive impact on male pattern hair loss.

SURGERY

A hair transplant is an outpatient procedure performed under local anesthesia. The average procedure takes 3 to 4 hours. The majority of the time is used to create an average of 1,000 to 1,500 1–4 hair grafts, produce recipient sites, and place the grafts. Patients resume normal activities immediately, with a restriction on heavy exercise for 3 to 7 days after surgery. If there is pain after the procedure, it occurs during

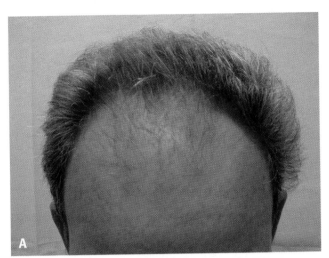 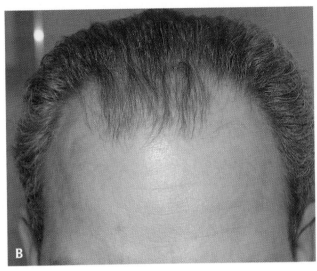

Figure 31-1 Before hair transplant **(A)** and after 800 1–3 hair grafts **(B)**.

the day of the procedure, and a mild pain medication is adequate for relief. The day after the procedure, patients should feel no discomfort. Typically, the only physical evidence of the procedure is the perifollicular crusting that remains 6 to 8 days and in some patients edema in the forehead for 2 to 3 days. Most patients return to work 2 to 3 days after the procedure without any negative cosmetic impact.

All patients undergoing hair transplantation should expect natural-appearing transplanted hair. During the consult, realistic expectations need to be created for short- and long-term density from a hair transplant. All skin types and hair colors are candidates for surgery. The phys-

ical exam includes evaluating the donor density and caliber of the hair follicle which will help determine the expected density from the procedure. Patients with below-average donor density and fine-caliber hair will have natural but thin transplanted hair. Those with above-average density with wide-caliber hair follicles can expect greater perceived density. The density of transplanted hair will be affected by the rate of hair loss and/or postsurgery telogen effluvium. Patients with a lot of remaining hair but rapid loss of hair may even have less hair 12 months after surgery. The extent and rate of hair loss varies from person to person. During the consult, the surgeon must emphasize

Table 31-1

FDA-approved medical therapy: comparison of the only two FDA approved medications for male pattern hair loss

	Finasteride	Minoxidil
Mechanism of action	5-alpha reductase type II inhibitor Blocks the conversion of testosterone to dihydrotestosterone	Unknown
Key to success	Emphasize maintenance over regrowth of hair Compliance for at least 6–8 months to see a benefit	Emphasize maintenance over regrowth of hair Compliance 6–8 months to see a benefit
Side effects	2% of men experience sexual dysfunction. Reversible within days if discontinued. No allergic reactions, blood monitoring, or drug interactions. Women should never handle or take medication.	Dryness and pruritus of the scalp. Rare allergic reaction.
Clinical onset of action	6–8 months	6–8 months
Dose	1 mg once daily with or without food	2–4 drops 1–2 times daily to frontal and vertex of scalp

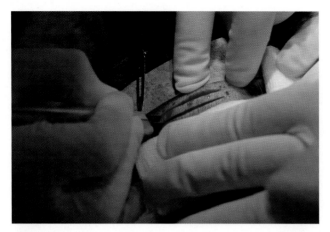

Figure 31-2 Donor ellipse harvesting.

the ongoing nature of hair loss with or without surgery. Despite recent 5-year studies confirming the long-term benefit from these medications, it is vital that surgeons still apply the same criteria for candidate selection and hairline design in patients with successful medical treatment.

Patients should be aware of a permanent scar in the donor region from the harvesting of hair for the transplant. For the majority of patients, the scar does not create any physical or cosmetic concern. Some patients that may shave their hair or wear it closely cropped to the scalp should be aware the scar will be visible before the procedure is performed. Explaining the ongoing loss of hair with or without transplantation, role of medications, permanent donor scar, realistic density based on hair caliber, and long-term hair loss will help create realistic expectations for patients. If a patient does not have a realistic expectation for what a transplant can and cannot achieve in the short and long term, the surgery should not be performed.

DONOR REGION

The limiting factor in hair transplantation is the amount of hair available in the donor scalp of patients. From the 1960s into the 1990s, steel punches measuring from 3 to 4 mm in diameter were used to harvest donor tissue from the posterior scalp. This resulted in extensive scarring over the posterior scalp and an inefficient use of valuable donor hair. In the mid-1990s, multibladed knives were popularized as an easy method to obtain elliptical strips that were easily dissected into smaller follicular units.[5] Although efficient for creating grafts, the transection rate of follicles was higher because of the multiple blades through the tissue. The clinical significance in the yield of transected hair is unclear, but minimizing trauma to hair follicles is a goal of all hair-transplant surgery teams. The single-blade donor ellipse does reduce transection of follicles and has become the most popular method for donor harvesting (Fig. 31-2).

The donor region is trimmed with a moustache trimmer. The patient is placed in the prone position and the area anesthetized with 1% lidocaine with 1:200,000 epinephrine. Saline is added to the donor region. The saline helps with hemostasis and through increased turgor reduces the transection of hair follicles. The donor ellipse is created using No. 10 blades on a surgical handle with 0.8- to 1.0-cm spacers between the blades. The length of the donor strip is determined by the number of grafts required for the surgery. The average patient has 60 to 85 follicular groupings per cm^2.[6] For example, a donor strip 12 to 14 cm long and 1 cm wide will create approximately 800 to 1,200 grafts.

Recently, the idea of harvesting donor hair using 1- to 1.3-mm punches has been advocated to minimize a visible scar in the donor region.[7] Follicular unit extraction does leave less visible scarring for most patients. Despite this, follicular unit extraction has a limited role in hair transplantation. Its chief advantages are for patients with shaved hair or closely cropped hair and patients with severely depleted donor hair from multiple previous hair transplants. The disadvantages of this method include (a) less hair harvested for each session, resulting in less density from each procedure; (b) a higher transection rate of hair than with elliptical donor harvesting; and (c) longer operative time (Table 31-2).

Table 31-2		
Advantages and disadvantages of donor harvesting techniques		
	Ellipse	Follicular unit extraction
Minimal transection of donor hair	Yes	No
Number of 1–4 grafts safely harvested per procedure	1,500–2,000	200–400
Time to harvest donor hair	15–20 minutes	1–2 hours
Visible donor scar with hair length >1 cm long	No	No
Visible donor scar with hair <0.5 cm long	Yes	Likely not
Overall percentage of cases used	>95%	<5%

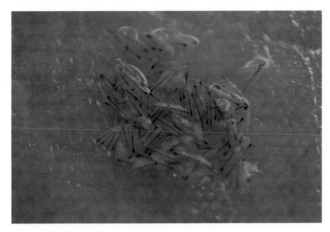

Figure 31-3 A 1–4 hair-follicular grouping in saline.

GRAFT SIZE

Hair naturally grows in bundles of 1–4 hair units. In nature, hair is randomly, yet evenly, distributed throughout the scalp. In traditional methods of hair transplantation, plugs contained 15 to 25 hairs per graft. They were placed into 3- to 4-mm recipient punch sites and grew 6 months after surgery. This technique produced the "pluggy" unnatural appearance of transplanted hair because, our eyes are used to seeing thousands of 1–4 hair bundles of hair on the scalp. Transplanting unnaturally large bundles of 15–25 hair together inevitably resulted in their "pluggy" appearance. The exclusive use of 1–4 hair grafts allows for consistently natural-appearing transplanted hair for men. Terms such as *follicular units* and *micrografts* have been used to describe these grafts.[8,9] Today, surgical teams carefully separate 500 to 2,000 natural bundles of hair from the donor strip (Fig. 31-3). The 1–4 hair grafts are produced by a variety of methods. Cutting instruments include no. 11 and no. 15 blades and no. 10 prep blades. Good lighting, comfortable chairs, and well-designed instruments are prerequisites to produce thousands of high-quality grafts (Fig. 31-4). Some surgeons believe microscopic dissection of 1–4 hair grafts from donor tissue is essential for the highest-quality grafts.[10] Data regarding microscopically dissected donor tissue and subsequent yield of transplanted hair are still inconclusive. What is not debated is the need to create intact, minimally traumatized, follicular groupings and place the transplanted hair as efficiently and quickly as possible into the recipient sites to optimize the survival of hair and produce the greatest density possible.

HAIRLINE DESIGN AND RECIPIENT SITE CREATION FOR MEN

The hairline is what defines the cosmetic success of a hair transplant. As with hair-graft creation, the trend in hairline design has been toward mimicking as closely as possible

what occurs in nature. The goal of a hairline is to frame the face in an undetectable manner. Hairlines do not exist, but a natural transition zone of gradually increasing density from skin to terminal hair–bearing skin occurs. This ill-defined "feathering zone" is created by randomly placing, in an irregular pattern, one to three hair grafts along the newly created hairline.[11] The level at which the hairline is created varies from individual to individual. It is important for a surgeon to look at each patient in a global, 360-degree view before deciding where to place the hairline. Androgenetic alopecia is progressive, but transplanted hair will grow long term. Therefore, when viewing patients, surgeons must assume all patients will progress to complete hair loss with only transplanted hair remaining. This assumption allows transplanted hair to look equally natural 1 year and 20 years after surgery. Hard-and-fast rules of how many centimeters a hairline should be placed above the glabella are generally not followed, but the shape of a patient's forehead and level of temporal hairline recession will determine the ideal aesthetic placement of grafts to produce a natural frontal hairline.

The posterior hairline should mimic the natural semicircle that expands as hair loss progresses in the vertex of the scalp. It should, as with the frontal hairline, appear to be designed anticipating ongoing hair loss in the future. To avoid future aesthetic complications, the posterior hairline should be placed on the same plane as the frontal hairline. This will avoid "chasing" the ever-expanding ring of hair loss on the vertex of the scalp with valuable donor grafts. Recipient sites should mimic the natural 30- to 45-degree angle of hair growth on the scalp. There are a variety of needles that are used to make sites large enough to place the 1–4 hair-follicle grafts. Some of the most popular needles to make sites include no. 18 and no. 19 needles and CAG needles. When making recipient sites, surgeons must be careful not to transect existing hair follicles. Magnification for making recipient sites has recently been advocated

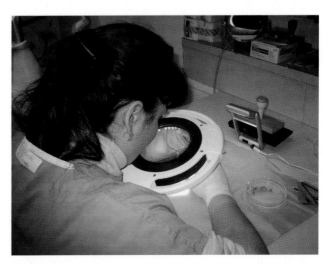

Figure 31-4 Surgical assistant producing 1–4 hair grafts.

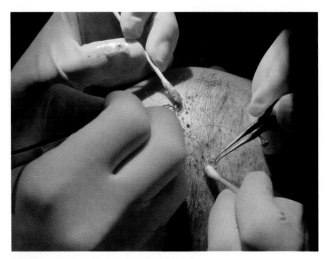

Figure 31-5 Placement of grafts using microvascular forceps.

to limit any loss of existing hair during surgery.[12] The key to success is to create recipient sites in a random, highly irregular pattern with 10 to 30 sites per cm², depending on the density of existing hair on the scalp.

GRAFT PLACEMENT AND POSTOPERATIVE COURSE

The grafts are placed by two to three surgical assistants using microvascular forceps (Fig. 31-5 and Fig. 31-6). The forceps pick up the 1–4 hair grafts by their perifollicular tissue, avoiding trauma to the hair follicles. Regular surgical forceps will not work. The placement of grafts into recipient sites is often the most challenging part of the procedure for novice and experienced hair-transplant teams. The chief challenges are hemostasis and "popping" of grafts from sites after they are placed. Hemostasis is achieved via dermal infiltration of 1:100,000 epinephrine 5 to 10 minutes before placing the grafts. The "popping" of grafts is unpredictable from patient to patient. "Popping" of grafts is overcome by placing light pressure over a paced graft and holding it for 10 to 20 seconds with a moist, saline-soaked, cotton-tip applicator before placing the next graft.

Once all the grafts are placed, a dressing is placed overnight. The dressing helps protect the grafts from any unintended trauma as they heal overnight. All patients are given a mild pain medication, which the majority of patients take the afternoon of surgery. The next day, the dressing is removed, and patients may shower but are told not to pick or rub off the perifollicular crusting that occurs around some grafts and lasts for 6 to 8 days. Patients may resume regular activities immediately, light exercise 3 to 4 days postoperatively and full exercise 7 days after surgery once the donor sutures are removed. The transplanted hair

does not begin to grow for 3 to 6 months after the surgery and does not achieve its full cosmetic impact for 9 to 12 months (Fig. 31-7A,B and Fig. 31-8A,B).

HAIR TRANSPLANTATION FOR MEN OF AFRICAN ANCESTRY

The hair transplant process is essentially a *peg-in-a-hole* surgery. Straight hairs are nursed into small recipient site holes. Of all global racial ethnic groups, only the tightly coiled hair of individuals of African ancestry make the peg-in-a-hole metaphor difficult to implement. There are some differences in hair transplantation that are unique to the coarse. First, the overall hair density is substantially less than other ethnic groups (1.3 hairs/mm² for Africans, 1.6 hairs/mm² for Asians, and 2.1 hairs/mm² for Caucasians), so that the overall supply of the donor hairs is less for Afrocentric hair. Second, the grouping of hair follicles in the follicular unit is higher in Afrocentric hair. For instance, there are more three hair follicular units in individuals of African ancestry than in other racial ethnic groups. The higher number of hairs per follicular unit and the lower density means that the number of follicular units per square mm is substantially more disproportional than with other racial groups. The implications of this are such that Africans or African Americans do not have enough hair to produce adequate cover for extensive balding, but as the hair "wants" to mat together, the value of each hair is higher than the straight hair of, for example, Asians. Thirdly, the Afrocentric hair shaft curls in the fatty dermis, and once the follicular unit is severed from its fibrous attachment, the curly nature of the follicles tends to dominate its shape outside the body. These follicular units have a wide splay in their natural home in the deep dermis, and the splay becomes even wider when they are

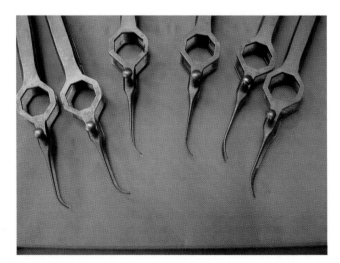

Figure 31-6 Microvascular forceps for planting grafts.

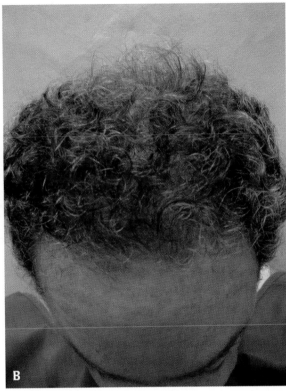

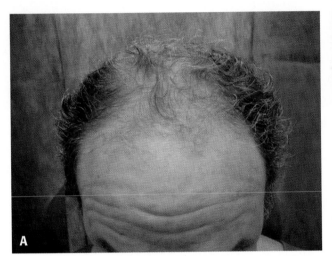

Figure 31-7 Before hair transplant **(A)** and after 1,000 1–4 hair grafts **(B)**.

out of the body. Making the hair graft behave according to the above peg-in-a-hole metaphor requires a very experienced technician who must know how to coerce the graft into the hole in the recipient site. It is not uncommon that recipient sites may have to be slightly larger to accommodate the larger bulk of the coarse hair and its corkscrew shape outside of the body. Less dense packing is also advisable for Afrocentric hair because the supply and the numbers of available grafts are more limited. Still, in experienced

hands, follicular unit transplants can be performed to the exact same quality as those that better fit the peg-in-a-hole metaphor. Despite inherent difficulties in the transplantation process of Afrocentric hair, excellent results can indeed be achieved. So if there is a problem with African hair, it is not in the quality arena [13,14] (Fig. 31-9). Keloids and hypertrophic scars can indeed occur at the donor site, requiring treatment with intralesional and or topical steroids (see Chapter 34).

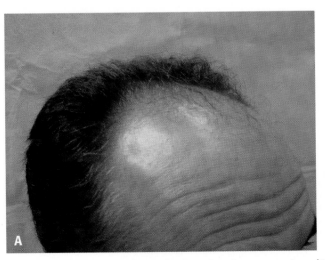

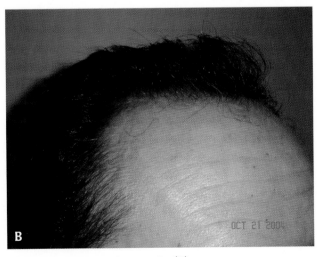

Figure 31-8 Before hair transplant **(A)** and after 1,450 1–3 hair grafts **(B)**.

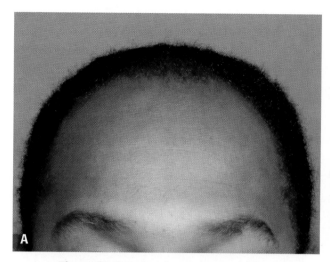
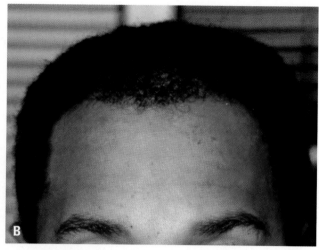

Figure 31-9 Before hair transplant **(A)** and after hair transplant in African American patient **(B)**. (Courtesy of William Rassman, MD.)

THE FUTURE

The public image of hair transplantation remains the "corn row" and plug. Hundreds of thousands of patients have benefited from the revolutionary changes in technique and are in the position of voluntarily—not involuntarily—informing friends or the public of their surgery. The next leap will be cloning hair follicles. In the early 21st century, the claims on Web sites regarding cloning hair are far more optimistic than the actual scientific progress. The amount of research in the area should allow hair to be cloned in the next several years. Future refinements with lasers and robotics will also allow an even more efficient procedure for patients and physicians.

REFERENCES

1. Ellis JA, Sinclair R, Harrap SB. Androgenetic alopecia: pathogenesis and potential for therapy. *Expert Rev Mol Med* 2002;19:2002:1–11.
2. Price VH, Menefee E, Sanchez M, et al. Changes in hair weight in men with androgenetic alopecia after treatment with finasteride (1 mg daily): 3- and 4-year results. *J Am Acad Dermatol* 2006;5(1):71–74.
3. Roenigk HH, Berman MD. Topical 2% minoxidil with hair transplantation. *Face* 1993;4:213–216.
4. Avram MR, Cole JP, Gandelman M, et al. The potential role of minoxidil in the hair transplantation setting. *Dermatol Surg* 2002;28:894–900.
5. Bisaccia E, Scarborough D. Hair transplant by incisional strip harvesting. *J Dermatol Surg Oncol* 1994;20(7):443–448.
6. Jimenez F, Ruifernandez JM. Distribution of human hair in follicular units: a mathematical model for estimating the donor size in follicular unit transplantation. *Dermatol Surg* 1999;25(4):294–298.
7. Rassman WR, Bernstein RM, McClellan R, et al. Follicular unit extraction: minimally invasive surgery for hair transplantation. *Dermatol Surg* 2002;28:720–728.
8. Lucas MW. The use of minigrafts in hair transplantation surgery. *J Dermatol Surg Oncol* 1988;14:1389–1392.
9. Nordstrom RE. Micrografting for improvement of frontal hairline. *Aesthetic Plast Surg* 1981;5:97.
10. Limmer BL. Elliptical donor stereoscopically assisted micrografting as an approach to further refinement in hair transplantation. *J Dermatol Surg Oncol* 1994;20:789–793.
11. Stough DB. Hair transplantation by the feathering zone technique. *Am J Cosmet Surg* 1993;10:243–248.
12. Avram MR. Polarized light-emitting diode for optimal recipient site creation during hair transplant. *Dermatol Surg* 2005;31:1124–1127.
13. Callender VD. Hair transplantation for pigmented skins. In: Halder RM, ed. *Dermatology and Dermatological Therapy of Pigmented Skins.* Boca Raton, FL: Taylor & Francis;2006:245–257.
14. Cooley JE. Hair transplantation in blacks. In: Haber RS, Stough DB eds. *Procedures in Cosmetic Dermatology: Hair Transplantation.* Philadelphia: Elsevier;2006:143–147.

32

Laser Hair Removal in Darker Racial Ethnic Groups

Teresa Soriano, David Beynet, and Dafnis C. Carranza

Laser-assisted hair removal (LHR) is a commonly performed cosmetic procedure today. Initially, LHR was reserved for patients with lighter skin types (Fitzpatrick I–III) because of the increased incidence of adverse effects in patients with darker skin. Over the last decade, with the advent of lasers with longer wavelengths, longer pulse durations, and improved cooling mechanisms, LHR can be safely performed in all skin types, including Fitzpatrick types IV to VI. It has the ability to significantly reduce the number of hairs and their rate of growth while maintaining a low incidence of side effects.[1–3]

LHR is of special importance in ethnic skin types for several reasons. Darker-skinned patients often have darker, coarser, and thus more noticeable hair than lighter-skinned patients. This may lead to increased cosmetic concern of unwanted hair in darker-skinned patients. In addition, certain diseases that are more prevalent in patients of color—such as hirsutism, pseudofolliculitis barbae, and acne keloidalis—can be improved with laser therapy.[4]

LASER CHOICES

The mechanism of LHR is based on the theory of selective photothermolysis. In selective photothermolysis, heat is released by a target chromophore, which has absorbed photons from the laser. This heat destroys neighboring structures, causing permanent damage.[5] In LHR, the target chromophore is melanin, which is primarily found in the hair bulb and hair shaft. After photon absorption, heat is released by the hair shaft and hair bulb, causing permanent thermal destruction of the surrounding follicular structures.

The higher concentration of melanin in the epidermis of darker skin types presents a challenge in LHR treatment of this population compared with lighter skin types. There are two unwanted outcomes. The first is that less photons ultimately reach their intended site, the follicular structures, which results in decreased efficacy. The second is that there is increased heating of the epidermis.[6] This can lead to side effects, such as hyperpigmentation, hypopigmentation, blistering, and scarring.

The melanin absorption spectrum ranges from approximately 300 to 1,200 nm, with absorption decreasing as wavelength increases. Follicular structures are located to a depth of 2 to 4 mm within the dermis. The ideal laser thus should have a wavelength that can provide adequate photon absorption by melanin, as well as penetration into the dermis. Wavelengths between 600 and 1100 nm are capable of this.[7]

In addition to wavelength, pulse duration is an important consideration in LHR. Relatively long pulse durations are necessary. Long pulse duration results in slow heating of the follicular unit and greater diffusion of heat from the hair shaft and bulb during the pulse. This allows for destruction of the entire follicular unit, not only the pigmented components.[8]

There has been a marked increase in the number of lasers for LHR since the first lasers were approved in 1996.[9] LHR has primarily been done with the following light sources: the ruby laser (694 nm), the alexandrite laser (755 nm), the diode laser (810 nm), the neodymium:yttruium-aluminum-garnet laser (Nd:YAG) (1,064 nm), intense pulsed light (IPL), and IPL with radiofrequency (IPL/RF) (Table 32-1). The ruby laser is the most selective for melanin absorption but has short penetration depth and a higher incidence of side effects. The Nd:YAG laser has the deepest penetration but the least specificity for absorption by melanin.[8] This may result in decreased efficacy; however, it lends itself to fewer adverse effects. The alexandrite and the diode lasers have benefits of both of these extremes. IPL works by using noncoherent light with wavelengths ranging from 515 to 1,200 nm. By using different cutoff filters, treatment parameters can be adjusted to allow safer treatment for patients with different skin types. In addition, devices combining radiofrequency with an intense pulsed light have been used for LHR. It has been proposed that lower fluences can achieve hair reduction in these devices, thus making IPL/RF a safe alternative of LHR for darker-skinned patients.[10]

Table 32-1

Lasers and light sources for hair removal

Ruby laser (694 nm)

Alexandrite laser (755 nm)

Diode laser (810 nm)

Neodymium:yttrium-aluminum-garnet laser
(Nd:YAG) (1,064 nm)

Intense pulsed light (IPL)

IPL with radiofrequency (IPL/RF)

Table 32-2

Optimal lasers for darker racial ethnic groups

Types	Features
Diode laser (810 nm)	Longer wavelength, Longer pulse duration, Optimal cooling
Neodymium:yttrium-aluminum-garnet laser (Nd:YAG) (1,064 nm)	FDA approved for darker skin types

In ethnic skin, the safest lasers are those with longer wavelengths, longer pulse durations, and optimal cooling devices. The longer wavelength diode and Nd:YAG are the preferred devices to safely perform LHR in ethnic skin. (Table 32-2) (Figs. 32-1 and 32-2).[3,11] The increased wavelength allows for decreased epidermal melanin absorption and increased penetration depth. The long pulse duration causes slower heating and results in a lower incidence of dyspigmentation. Between the two laser systems, the longer-wavelength 1,064-nm Nd:YAG laser is generally safer, particularly for very dark skin types, however, the diode laser may be more effective because of greater melanin absorption.[9] A mean hair reduction ranging from 58% to 62% on facial sites and 66% to 69% on nonfacial sites has been reported after three treatments with the long-pulsed Nd:YAG compared with 74% to 84% hair reduction with the diode laser 6 months after the final laser treatment.[8] Both long-pulsed Nd:YAG and diode devices are FDA approved for LHR in darker skin types.

Efficient cooling devices provide added benefit for LHR, especially in ethnic skin. Cooling devices function to cool the epidermis and prevent laser-induced thermal damage. Epidermal thermal damage can result in dyspigmentation, scarring, and blistering, especially in darker skin types. Cooling devices also have the added benefit of

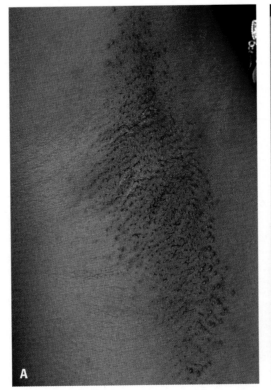
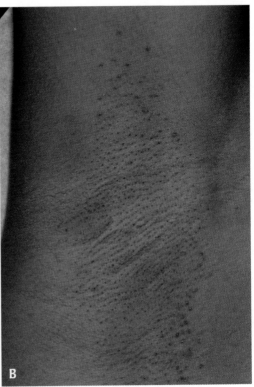

Figure 32-1 Axillary hair, skin type V: baseline **(A)**, after five long-pulsed 1064 nm Nd:YAG treatments **(B)**. (Courtesy of Pearl E. Grimes, MD.)

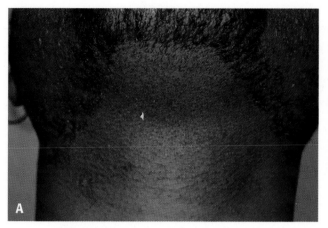 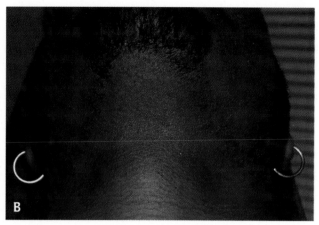

Figure 32-2 Unwanted facial hair, skin type V: baseline (**A**), after four long-pulsed 1064 nm Nd:YAG treatments (**B**). (Courtesy of Pearl E. Grimes, MD.)

decreasing pain associated with the procedure. Current cooling devices use both evaporative and conductive mechanisms. These tend to provide more efficient epidermal cooling than older techniques of using ice or water-based gel. Dynamic cooling devices function by using a cryogen spray immediately before the laser pulse, which evaporates and instantaneously cools the epidermis.[12] Conductive cooling devices include cooled sapphire laser windows, which cool the epidermis by conductive heat transfer. Conductive devices also lead to dermal compression, which has two benefits: It brings follicular structures closer to the area of maximal dermal laser penetration, and it compresses blood vessels, thereby decreasing the concentration of the hemoglobin.[6]

PRACTICAL ASPECTS

The ideal patient for laser-assisted hair removal is one with dark hair and light skin. Gray or light hair absorbs insufficient energy to cause permanent follicular destruction with current hair-removal systems. Darker skin carries a higher risk of epidermal melanin absorption, which can potentially lead to adverse side effects. Performing test spots, initiating treatments at lower fluences, and accepting the likelihood that the patient may require an increased number of treatments compared with lighter-skinned patients are all especially important for LHR in ethnic skin.

Patients should be instructed to avoid suntanning, self-tanning products, plucking, and waxing for at least 2 weeks before treatments. Plucking and waxing removes the hair shaft, leaving the laser energy without a target, thus potentially making treatment less effective. Regular shaving or trimming of hair before and in between laser treatments is acceptable. The use of 2% to 4% hydroquinone cream for 2 to 4 weeks before treatment may reduce the incidence of posttreatment hyperpigmention.[2]

Test spots should be done in a representative area that closely resembles the treated area. For example, the posterior auricular or submental area is commonly used as a test spot for LHR of the upper lip. Patients should be seen approximately 2 weeks after the test spot and evaluated for side effects. If no pigmentary change is noted, a full treatment can be done at that visit.

Some level of discomfort is expected during the procedure. A topical anesthetic, such as eutectic mixture of local anesthetics (EMLA, lidocaine 2.5% and prilocaine 2.5%) or topical lidocaine (LMX, 4% or 5%) can help decrease pain. A recent study showed no statistical significance between EMLA and LMX (5%) for pain control in laser hair removal.[13] EMLA has been associated with rare cases of methemoglobinemia in selected patient populations.[14] The amount of topical anesthesia applied should be limited to the recommended quantities, as toxicity may result from increased systemic absorption. The use of compounded high-dosage topical lidocaine preparations over large body surface areas can also have serious and life-threatening toxicities. In addition to preoperative topical anesthesia, the use of ice packs or air-cooling devices peri- and postoperatively can provide some additional pain relief.

Before laser treatments, the hair should be shaved or clipped to skin level. All makeup should be removed. Everyone in the room should wear proper eye protection. Fluence and pulse duration is determined based on test-spot parameters. With lasers that use contact cooling, care should be taken to ensure that the handpiece is in direct contact with the skin. This allows for maximum benefit of the cooling tips. In addition, burned debris that may accumulate on the tips of some devices should be cleaned to avoid suboptimal contact cooling. When treating the upper lip, some have advocated covering the teeth with a gauze pad to protect the enamel.[15]

Perifollicular erythema and edema lasting several hours after treatment typically occurs immediately after treatment.[6] Icing the area immediately after the treatment may reduce this erythema and discomfort. A topical steroid can be applied for prolonged irritation, erythema, and edema. Careful sun avoidance and the regular use of a broad-spectrum sunscreen are recommended during laser treatments.

COMPLICATIONS AND CONTRAINDICATIONS

The most common complications of laser hair removal include hyperpigmentation, hypopigmentation, blistering, and scarring (Table 32-3). Thermal damage after unwanted partial epidermal absorption of laser energy accounts for these adverse reactions. Darker ethnic skin and tanned skin are at higher risk for adverse events because of the increased epidermal melanin that acts as a competitive chromophore for melanin in the hair follicle. Some perifollicular erythema and edema for several hours are expected responses immediately after LHR treatments. However, if more severe epidermal injury occurs, long-lasting side effects may result. Blistering, scabbing, and persistent erythema may lead to hypopigmentation, hyperpigmentation, and scarring. Studies have demonstrated that the longer wavelength lasers with appropriate cooling devices are safer for darker skin types.[16] In a study from the United Kingdom of 109 patients with skin types IV to VI, the highest incidence of side effects was seen in patients with darker skin treated with the long-pulsed ruby laser. The overall incidence of blistering and dyspigmentation was 9.4% with the Nd:YAG laser and 29.9% with the ruby laser.[16] Hyperpigmentation often resolves with time and can be treated with bleaching agents and topical retinoids. Hypopigmentation is often also transient, but may be permanent because of thermally induced destruction of melanocytes (Figs. 32-3 and 32-4).

A phenomenon termed *hair induction* has been reported in which patients develop terminal hairs in areas not present before laser and IPL treatment.[17] It has been seen most

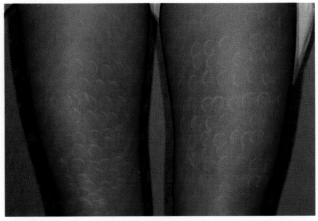

Figure 32-3 Long-term hypopigmentation following laser hair removal treatment of the lower extremities with alexandrite laser. (Courtesy of Pearl E. Grimes, MD.)

commonly after laser hair removal of the face and neck of women of Mediterranean ancestry with darker skin types.[18] This may suggest a greater tendency of hair-follicle transformation from vellus to terminal hair in this population. In a retrospective Greek study, hair induction occurred after at least three treatments and on an average of 7 months after the first treatment. Most of the increased hair growth developed at the edges of the treated areas. Some have advocated that continuation of laser treatment in these cases results in decreased hair growth.[18] Stopping treatments, re-evaluating to rule out an underlying endocrine abnormality, and resuming laser treatment to small test areas to evaluate response is recommended. If hair reduction is noted after multiple laser treatments to the test areas, then one may proceed cautiously to treat the entire face and neck.

Acneform reactions have been reported to occur after laser hair removal.[19] The exact mechanism for the formation of acneform lesions is unknown. A possible explanation may be related to secondary follicular inflammation and blockage to the sebaceous gland following disruption of the pilosebaceous unit. The perioperative use of soothing creams and topical steroids may also be a contributing factor in certain cases. In a prospective multicenter study in the United Kingdom, 26 out of 411 patients (6%) developed acneform reactions following LHR.[19] The reactions tend to be mild, with a mean duration of 9.6 days. History of polycystic ovarian disease and number of prior treatments did not seem to affect the incidence of acneform reactions. It occurred most frequently on the face in young women with skin type V undergoing long pulsed Nd:YAG laser treatment.

There are few contraindications for laser hair removal. Photosensitizing medication is considered a relative contraindication. LHR is generally contraindicated for approximately 6 months after oral isotretinoin therapy because of the potential for delayed wound healing and increased risk of scarring associated with oral retinoids. Although there

Table 32-3
Complications of laser hair removal
Blistering
Scabbing/crusting
Persistent erythema
Hyperpigmentation
Hypopigmentation
Scarring

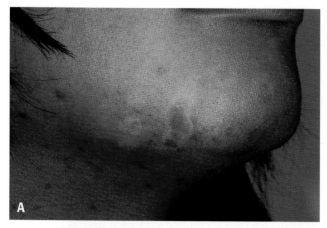 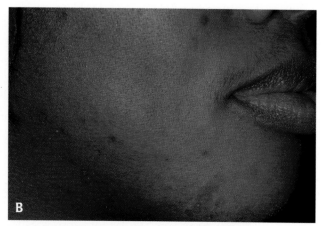

Figure 32-4 Transient hypopigmentation following blistering after laser hair removal of the perioral area with long-pulsed Nd:YAG treatments **(A)**, with clearing after 2 weeks, without treatment **(B)**. (Courtesy of Pearl E. Grimes, MD.)

are no large clinical studies demonstrating an increased incidence of laser hair removal associated adverse effects on individuals who are on or have recently been on isotretinoin, there have been isolated reports of bullae and keloid formation after LHR in patients on isotretinoin.[20,21] Individuals with a history of keloids or hypertrophic scars should also be treated cautiously. Lastly, patients with a history of herpetic infections, especially if they erupt in or around the treatment area, should have prophylactic treatment with an antiviral agent.[1]

SPECIFIC CLINICAL APPLICATIONS

Pseudofolliculitis barbae

Pseudofolliculitis barbae (PFB) is a chronic inflammatory disease caused by tightly curled hairs that re-enter the skin approximately 1 to 2 mm from the respective follicular orifices. It is most common in the beard and neck area of men but may occur in other shaved areas. Papules and pustules develop at the site of re-entry and may lead to hyperpigmentation and keloidal scarring. Although PFB may be seen in patients of any ethnic background, it is more common in patients of African descent, with the prevalence approaching 80% in certain populations.[4] Allowing the hair to grow out typically improves the condition, however, individuals often find this socially or cosmetically unacceptable. LHR has become an effective treatment option for PFB. With removal of the hair, improvement of the lesions and subsequent postinflammatory dyspigmentation can be achieved (Fig. 32-5).

LHR, particularly using the long-pulsed diode and YAG lasers, can safely and effectively improve pseudofolliculitis barbae.[22,23] In a side-by-side study using a long-pulsed Nd:YAG laser on 37 patients (skin types IV–VI)

with PFB, Ross et al.[22] reported a decreased mean papule count on the treated side compared with the untreated side (1 versus 6.95) at 90 days posttreatment. Similarly, another study of 20 patients with skin types V to VI had significant reduction of lesions and hair growth 3 months after two treatments with a long-pulsed Nd:YAG laser.[24] Side effects included transient dyspigmentation, itching, and erythema. A study using the 810-nm diode laser demonstrated a greater than 50% improvement in signs of PFB after three treatments.[25] However, in very dark-skinned patients, blistering and crusting with subsequent dyspigmentation was observed. Epidermal damage in very dark-skinned patients can be decreased by reducing the total energies delivered.

Acne keloidalis nuchae

Acne keloidalis nuchae is a chronic inflammatory disease in which patients develop papules, pustules, and keloidal scarring in the posterior neck and scalp region, usually following a chronic folliculitis. It is commonly seen in men of African descent. Although its exact etiology is not characterized, shaved or short haircuts, pseudofolliculitis, low-grade bacterial infection, and chronic irritation from shirt collars have been proposed as possible contributing factors. Histologically, early lesions demonstrate a perifollicular infiltrate in the upper portion of the hair follicle, whereas older lesions display a granulomatous infiltrate around broken hair fragments and scarring.

Treatment of acne keloidalis nuchae can be challenging. Therapies have included topical and oral antibiotics, retinoids, intralesional steroid injections, and surgical and laser excision. LHR has been used as an adjunctive therapy with some anecdotal benefit for the papular and pustular lesion, however, it has no known effect on already-formed keloids. In two patients with recalcitrant papules, Shah[26] reported a 90% to 95% clearance after

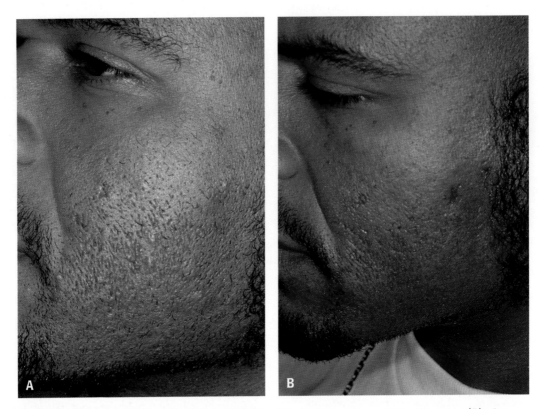

Figure 32-5 Marked improvement of pseudofolliculitis barbae, skin type V at baseline **(A)** after seven long-pulsed 1,064 nm Nd:YAG treatments **(B)**. (Courtesy of Pearl E. Grimes, MD.)

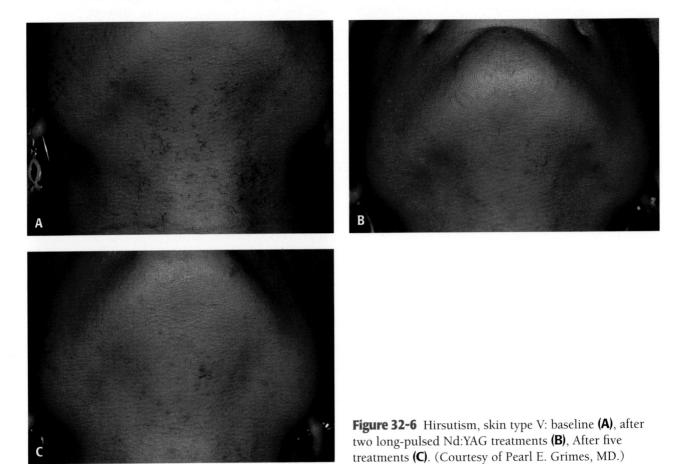

Figure 32-6 Hirsutism, skin type V: baseline **(A)**, after two long-pulsed Nd:YAG treatments **(B)**, After five treatments **(C)**. (Courtesy of Pearl E. Grimes, MD.)

four diode laser treatment sessions at 4- to 6-week intervals used in conjunction with a daily retinoid and topical steroid cream. The patients had regrowth of thinner hair and no recurrent papules or pigmentary changes at 6 month follow-up.

Hypertrichosis and hirsutism

Hypertrichosis is an increased amount of hair in a normal physiologic pattern. Hirsutism is defined as excessive male pattern hair growth in women. A wide range of etiologies, including repeated trauma, genodermatoses, endocrine diseases, and medications can lead to increased hair growth. Hirsutism is more common in certain ethnicities, such as women of Middle Eastern descent, and may be considered a normal variant. Regardless of the cause, hirsutism and hypertrichosis can result in significant psychological morbidity in women.[27] LHR is an effective and safe treatment option (Fig. 32-6). In a study by Levy et al.,[28] 29 women with hypertrichosis (skin types I–VI) were treated with a long-pulsed Nd:YAG laser. The average reduction in hair counts after three treatments at 1-month intervals was 46% at 9 months after treatment. No significant complications were observed. Unlike traditional treatments to remove hair, such as waxing, plucking, shaving, and depilatory creams, LHR can offer long-lasting hair removal.

REFERENCES

1. Battle EF Jr., Hobbs LM. Laser-assisted hair removal for darker skin types. *Dermatol Ther* 2004;17(2):177–183.

2. Garcia C, Alamoudi H, Nakib M, et al. Alexandrite laser hair removal is safe for Fitzpatrick skin types IV–VI. *Dermatol Surg* 2000;26(2):130–134.

3. Greppi I. Diode laser hair removal of the black patient. *Lasers Surg Med* 2001;28(2):150–155.

4. Bridgeman-Shah S. The medical and surgical therapy of pseudofolliculitis barbae. *Dermatol Ther* 2004;17(2):158–163.

5. Anderson RR, Margolis RJ, Watenabe S, et al. Selective photothermolysis of cutaneous pigmentation by Q-switched Nd:YAG laser pulses at 1064, 532, and 355 nm. *J Invest Dermatol* 1989;93(1):28–32.

6. Baugh WP, Trafeli JP, Barnette DJ Jr., et al. Hair reduction using a scanning 800 nm diode laser. *Dermatol Surg* 2001;27(4):358–364.

7. Anderson RR, Parrish JA. The optics of human skin. *J Invest Dermatol* 1981;77(1):13–19.

8. Tanzi EL, Alster TS. Long-pulsed 1064-nm Nd:YAG laser-assisted hair removal in all skin types. *Dermatol Surg* 2004;30(1):13–17.

9. Galadari I. Comparative evaluation of different hair removal lasers in skin types IV, V, and VI. *Int J Dermatol* 2003;42(1):68–70.

10. Yaghmai D, Garden JM, Bakus AD, et al. Hair removal using a combination radio-frequency and intense pulsed light source. *J Cosmet Laser Ther* 2004;6(4):201–207.

11. Alster TS, Bryan H, Williams CM. Long-pulsed Nd:YAG laser-assisted hair removal in pigmented skin: a clinical and histological evaluation. *Arch Dermatol* 2001;137(7):885–889.

12. Nahm WK, Tsoukas MM, Falanga V, et al. Preliminary study of fine changes in the duration of dynamic cooling during 755-nm laser hair removal on pain and epidermal damage in patients with skin types III–V. *Lasers Surg Med* 2002;31(4):247–251.

13. Guardiano RA, Norwood CW. Direct comparison of EMLA versus lidocaine for pain control in Nd:YAG 1,064 nm laser hair removal. *Dermatol Surg* 2005;31(4):396–398.

14. Hahn IH, Hoffman RS, Nelson LS. EMLA-induced methemoglobinemia and systemic topical anesthetic toxicity. *J Emerg Med* 2004;26(1):85–88.

15. Yee S. Laser hair removal in Fitzpatrick type IV to VI patients. *Facial Plast Surg* 2005;21(2):139–144.

16. Lanigan SW. Incidence of side effects after laser hair removal. *J Am Acad Dermatol* 2003;49(5):882–886.

17. Kontoes P M-AG, Castelo-Branco C, Ferrando J. Paradoxical effect after IPL photoepilation. *Dermatol Surg* 2002;28:1013–1016.

18. Kontoes P, Vlachos S, Konstantinos M, et al. Hair induction after laser-assisted hair removal and its treatment. *J Am Acad Dermatol* 2006;54(1):64–67.

19. Carter JJ, Lanigan SW. Incidence of acneform reactions after laser hair removal. *Lasers Med Sci* 2006;21(2):82–85.

20. Khatri KA. Diode laser hair removal in patients undergoing isotretinoin therapy. *Dermatol Surg* 2004;30(9):1205–1207; discussion 1207.

21. Bernstein LJ, Geronemus RG. Keloid formation with the 585-nm pulsed dye laser during isotretinoin treatment. *Arch Dermatol* 1997;133(1):111–112.

22. Ross EV, Cooke LM, Timko AL, et al. Treatment of pseudofolliculitis barbae in skin types IV, V, and VI with a long-pulsed neodymium:yttrium aluminum garnet laser. *J Am Acad Dermatol* 2002;47(2):263–270.

23. Yamauchi PS, Kelly AP, Lask GP. Treatment of pseudofolliculitis barbae with diode laser. *J Cutan Laser Ther* 1999;1:109–111.

24. Weaver SM, Sagaral EC. Treatment of pseudofolliculitis barbae using the long pulsed NC:YAG laser on skin types V and VI. *Dermatol Surg* 2003;29:1187–1191.

25. Kauvar AN. Treatment of pseudofolliculitis with a pulsed infrared laser. *Arch Dermatol* 2000;136(11):1343–1346.

26. Shah GK. Efficacy of diode laser for treating acne keloidalis nuchae. *Indian J Dermatol Venereol Leprol* 2005;71(1):31–34.

27. Clayton WJ, Lipton M, Elford J, et al. A randomized controlled trial of laser treatment among hirsute women with polycystic ovary syndrome. *Br J Dermatol* 2005;152(5):986–992.

28. Levy JL, Trelles MA, de Ramecourt A. Epilation with a long-pulse 1064 nm Nd:YAG laser in facial hirsutism. *J Cosmet Laser Ther* 2001;3(4):175–179.

Tumors

33

The Pathogenesis of Keloids

Heather Woolery–Lloyd

Darker racial ethnic groups have unique wound-healing characteristics to be considered when performing cosmetic procedures. The main concern with surgical procedures in patients with skin of color is the occurrence of keloids and hypertrophic scars. Keloids and hypertrophic scars are most common in darker racial ethnic groups and are most prevalent in African American, Hispanic, and Asian populations (Fig. 33-1 and Fig. 33-2). Statistics on the incidence of keloids in specific populations vary greatly; however, an incidence of 4.5% to 16% has been reported in black and Hispanic populations. Keloids are least common in Caucasians and albinos.[1]

Patients with keloids usually present in the second or third decade. There is an equal risk between women and men. Although most keloids occur sporadically, familial cases have been described. These cases appear to have an autosomal dominant pattern with incomplete penetrance and variable expression.[2]

Commonly affected sites for keloids include earlobes, shoulders, upper back, and chest. Postsurgically, they appear to be most common in areas of highest tension. Unlike hypertrophic scars, keloids rarely regress spontaneously. Once excised, they tend to recur. Common symptoms include pruritus and tenderness at the site of the keloid. These symptoms are most severe in new scars and tend to diminish with time.

Histopathology of keloidal tissue reveals a thickened dermis consisting of hypereosinophilic, hyalinized collagen (Fig. 33-3). Few adnexal structures or elastic fibers are observed. Hypertrophic scars are more cellular than keloids, and hyalinized collagen is less prominent (Fig. 33-4).[3]

The mechanism behind keloid formation has not yet been elucidated; however, abnormal fibroblast metabolism and enhanced response to growth factors have been suggested. Other theories include aberrant apoptosis and abnormal epidermal-dermal interaction during wound healing. In this chapter, the many proposed mechanisms behind keloid formation will be explored. (Table 33-1).

There has been much discussion on the relationship between keloids and hypertrophic scars. Older studies often grouped these two entities and studied them together. More recently, an effort has been made to study these scars separately as two distinct disease entities. Keloid pathogenesis will be the main focus of this chapter to maximize clarity of the discussion.

ALTERED GROWTH FACTORS/CYTOKINES

Transforming growth factor beta

Transforming growth factor beta (TGF-beta) has been closely implicated in scar formation. Its role in keloid biology has been extensively studied, and it has been found to be profibrotic in wound healing. There are three isoforms of TGF-beta: TGF-beta1, TGF-beta2, and TGF-beta3. Of the three isoforms, TGF-beta1 is most abundant in all tissues and in wound fluid. In vitro studies demonstrate that TGF-beta1 and TGF-beta2 are profibrotic isoforms and promote scar formation.[4] Interestingly, some studies suggest TGF-beta3 may have the opposite effect and may, in fact, reduce scar formation.[5] Other data suggests that the ratio between TGF-beta3 and TGF-beta1 most affects scar formation.[6]

During wound healing, TGF-beta is first released by degranulating platelets. Other major cells involved in

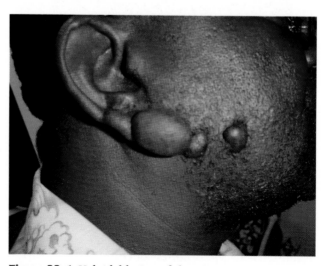

Figure 33-1 Keloidal lesion of the ear.

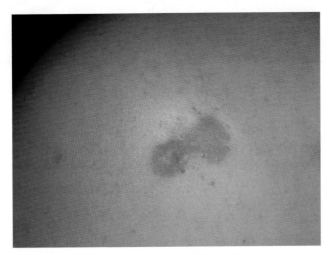

Figure 33-2 Hypertrophic scar of the back.

wound healing that secrete TGF-beta include lymphocytes, macrophages, endothelial cells, epithelial cells, and fibroblasts. Once released, TGF-beta is involved in chemotaxis, angiogenesis, and extracellular matrix formation. It also stimulates dermal fibroblast proliferation and migration.[4]

Because of its clearly profibrotic role in wound healing, TGF-beta has been extensively studied in keloid formation. In vitro studies have shown that TGF-beta1 stimulates synthesis of keloid-derived fibroblasts more than it stimulates

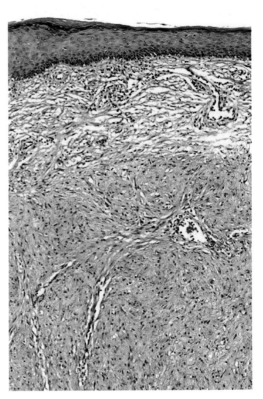

Figure 33-4 Hematoxylin, eosin stain of a hypertrophic scar. Note greater cellularity compared with keloid, and hyalinized collagen is less prominent. (Courtesy of Pearl E. Grimes, MD and Jag Bhawan, MD)

normal fibroblasts. TGF-beta also increases collagen synthesis in keloid fibroblasts more than in normal fibroblasts. These results suggest that keloid fibroblasts may have increased sensitivity to the effects of TGF-beta compared with normal fibroblasts.[7]

In addition to increased fibroblast and collagen synthesis, TGF-beta may also inhibit collagen degradation. Matrix metalloproteinases (MMPs) and plasminogen activator are the two main enzymes involved in breakdown of the extracellular matrix. Plasminogen activator is inhibited by plasminogen activator inhibitor 1 (PAI-1). MMP is inhibited by tissue inhibitor of metalloproteinase-1 (TIMP). TGF-beta up-regulates both PAI-1 and TIMP and, thus, may inhibit collagen degradation.[8,9]

Most studies clearly demonstrate the profibrotic role that TGF-beta plays in wound healing. Accordingly, multiple studies have examined the effect of anti-TGF antibodies on wound healing. Not unexpectedly, inhibition of TGF-beta with anti-TGF-beta antibodies in animal studies reduces scar formation.[5,10]

One study specifically examined the temporal effect of TGF-beta1, 2, and 3 on wound healing. In this study, anti-TGF-beta1, 2, and 3 were applied to rabbit ear wounds at different periods in wound healing. Anti-TGF-beta actually delayed wound healing when applied early to the wounds. Additionally, anti-TGF-beta applied early did not improve

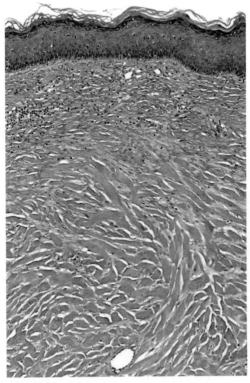

Figure 33-3 Hematoxylin, eosin stain of a keloid. Thickened dermis with hypereosinophilic and hyalinized collagen. (Courtesy of Pearl E. Grimes, MD and Jag Bhawan, MD)

the scar compared with untreated controls. This implies that TGF-beta is important and necessary for optimal wound healing in the first week after injury. However, anti-TGF-beta applied 1 week or more after injury resulted in reduced scar hypertrophy. Thus, early in wound healing, TGF-beta is necessary for optimal healing. However, after 1 week, the presence of TGF-beta may contribute to hypertrophic scar formation.[11]

TGF-beta clearly appears to be involved in abnormal scar formation; however, it does not appear to be the sole causative agent in keloids and hypertrophic scars. In fact, plasma levels of TGF-beta are no different in patients with keloids and controls. Additionally, common polymorphisms of the TGF-beta 1 gene are not associated with a risk of keloid disease.[12] Although it appears that TGF-beta is important in understanding keloid biology, it does not appear to be the sole factor in keloid pathogenesis.

Platelet-derived growth factor

Platelet-derived growth factor (PDGF) is another profibrotic growth factor that has been implicated in keloid pathogenesis. In wound healing, PDGF acts both as a chemoattractant and as a mitogen for fibroblasts. Interestingly, in fetal (nonscarring) wounds, this growth factor disappears quickly. In scarring wounds there is prolonged expression of PDGF.[13] Keloid fibroblasts also appear to be more responsive to PDGF's profibrotic effects than normal fibroblasts. The enhanced PDGF response of keloid fibroblasts may be influenced by increased levels of PDGF alpha receptors on keloid fibroblasts.[14]

Connective tissue–derived growth factor

Connective tissue–derived growth factor (CTGF) is another tissue growth factor that has been implicated in

Table 33-1		
Research and theories in keloid biology		
Area of research	Role and significance in keloid biology	
TGF-beta	Profibrotic	• Increases collagen production • Inhibits collagen degradation • Causes hypertrophic scars in animal studies
PDGF	Profibrotic	• Enhanced PDGF response in keloid fibroblasts
CTGF	Profibrotic	• Up-regulated in hypertrophic scars
IL-6	Profibrotic	• Enhanced expression in keloid fibroblasts • Increased production seen in peripheral blood mononuclear cells of keloid patients
IFN	Antifibrotic	• Suppresses collagen synthesis • Used with varied success as a keloid therapy
Apoptosis	Altered	• Multiple studies demonstrate increased and decreased apoptosis • Clearly altered in keloids
TNF	Antifibrotic	• Keloid fibroblasts less sensitive to the inhibitory effects of TNF on collagen synthesis
Epidermal-dermal interaction	Significant	• Keratinocyte paracrine function appears to regulate fibroblasts
Sebum	Profibrotic	• Sebum induces an immune reaction in susceptible patients resulting in keloids
Hypoxia	Profibrotic	• Tissue hypoxia stimulates excessive collagen production
Tension	Profibrotic	• Stress tension on fibroblasts induces excessive collagen production

CTGF, connective tissue–derived growth factor; IFN, interferon; IL-6, interleukin-6; PDGF, platelet-derived growth factor; TGF-beta, transforming growth factor beta; TNF, tumor necrosis factor.

fibroproliferative disorders.[15] CTGF is important for skeletal development, angiogenesis, cell adhesion, and cell migration.[16] CTGF is also a downstream mediator of TGF-beta activity and is secreted by fibroblasts after activation by TGF-beta.[17] In one study, CTGF expression was up-regulated in hypertrophic scar fibroblasts at baseline and after TGF-beta stimulation. In this study, a trend toward increased CTGF expression was also seen in keloid fibroblasts; however, this increased expression did not reach statistical significance.[18] CTGF represents yet another growth factor, which may play a role in keloids and hypertrophic scars.

Interleukin-6

Cytokines such as interleukin-6, interferon-gamma, and interferon-alpha have all been implicated in fibrosis and keloids. Interleukin-6 (IL-6) is a profibrotic cytokine that stimulates monocyte chemotaxis.[19,20] Wounding stimulates IL-6 production. Elevated IL-6 persists in adult wounds but disappears in the fetus.[19] Interestingly, addition of IL-6 to fetal wounds results in early scarring.[19]

Enhanced expression of IL-6 has been demonstrated in keloid fibroblasts.[21] Increased IL-6 production has also been demonstrated in peripheral blood mononuclear cells of keloid patients.[22] In another study examining the effect of electron-beam radiation on keloids, researchers found the IL-6 pathway was primarily involved in the electron-beam irradiation response.[23] Thus, it appears that IL-6 may not only be important in keloid pathogenesis but may also play a crucial role in the mechanism behind certain keloid therapies.

Interferon

Interferons have been studied in keloids because of their antifibrotic activity. Interferons (IFN)-alpha, -beta, and -gamma suppress collagen synthesis.[24] Interestingly, decreased IFN-alpha and IFN-gamma production has been demonstrated in peripheral blood mononuclear cells of keloid patients.[22]

Intralesional IFN-gamma and IFN-alpha2b have both been evaluated as keloid therapies. A few studies have demonstrated decreased size of keloids after IFN-gamma injections.[25,26] Other studies have shown that monotherapy of keloids with intralesional IFN-alpha2b is not effective.[27–29] Intralesional IFN-alpha2b postexcision has been found to have minimal to no efficacy.[30,31] Although in vitro studies of interferon suggest that it may be a novel treatment for keloids, clinically, interferon does not appear to be a highly efficacious treatment alternative. (See Chapter 34)

Apoptosis
Increased apoptosis

There are varied reports on the role of apoptosis in keloids. Caspase plays an important role in apoptosis and has been studied in keloids. The caspase family is a group of proapoptotic proteases, which cleave proteins at aspartic

acid residues. The sequential activation of one caspase by another leads to a mounting cascade of proteolytic activity and eventual cell death. One study examined the expression of activated caspase-9 and caspase-3 in keloid fibroblasts. Immunohistochemistry showed that fibroblasts positive for activated caspase-9 or caspase-3 was greater in keloid tissues than in normal scar tissues.[32] Another study examined caspase-3 staining in surgically resected normal scars and in hypertrophic or keloid scars. This study found that caspase-3 staining was significantly higher in the hypertrophic scar/keloid group. The authors suggested that there is increased cell death and reduced cell survival in hypertrophic scars and keloids.[33]

Decreased apoptosis

In contrast, other studies suggest that keloids and keloid fibroblasts may have lower rates of apoptosis than normal fibroblasts. Researchers have demonstrated resistance of keloid-derived fibroblasts to both ceramide-induced apoptosis and Fas-mediated apoptosis.[34,35] Keloid fibroblasts also appear to exhibit decreased expression of apoptosis-related genes compared with normal scars.[36]

p53 is a tumor suppressor gene. Expression of p53 results in either cell cycle arrest or apoptosis.[37] Focal mutations in p53 have been demonstrated in patients with keloids. These mutations may result in increased cell proliferation and decreased cell death in patients with keloids.[38]

The role of apoptosis in common keloid treatments has also been examined. Following stimulation by hydrocortisone, gamma-interferon, and hypoxia, keloid fibroblasts display enhanced apoptosis compared with normal fibroblasts.[39] This data suggests that apoptosis may, in fact, be decreased in keloids, and treatment with intralesional steroids or interferon may enhance or normalize apoptosis. This could be one mechanism to explain the improvement of keloids that is observed clinically with these treatments.

Tumor necrosis factor and apoptosis

The tumor necrosis factor (TNF) superfamily includes both the TNF ligand and the TNF receptor family. TNF can activate both cell-survival and cell-death mechanisms. This complex group of transmembrane proteins is an important regulator of homeostasis. Keloid fibroblasts are less responsive to the inhibitory effects of TNF-alpha on collagen synthesis.[40] Additionally, compared with normal fibroblasts, keloid fibroblasts showed decreased expression of apoptosis-associated genes when exposed to TNF-alpha.[41] TNF may represent yet another cytokine important in understanding keloid biology.

It appears that apoptosis does play a role in keloid pathogenesis, however, the research on apoptosis in keloids is varied. One can conclude that there is aberrant apoptosis in keloids. This role of apoptosis in keloids needs to be further elucidated.

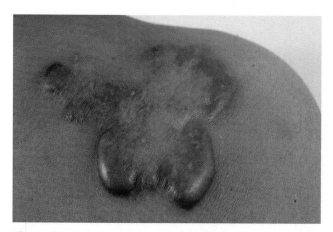

Figure 34-1 Central clearing of Keloid.

Berman and Kaufman[8] evaluated the effects of postoperative imiquimod 5% on the recurrence of excised keloids. Imiquimod cream was applied to the postoperative site daily for 8 weeks, starting immediately after surgery. Those who experienced marked irritation had to discontinue the medication for 3 to 7 days and then resume therapy. Patients with large excisions, wounds under tension, or wounds closed with flaps or grafts are advised not to use imiquimod for 4 to 6 weeks after excision because the postoperative site may splay or dehisce. Approximately half of the patients treated with imiquimod developed hyperpigmentation. Berman and Kaufman[8] also demonstrated that postoperative imiquimod cream reduced recurrence of keloids. The expression of genes associated with apoptosis is significantly altered in keloidal tissue treated with imiquimod.

5-FLUOROURACIL THERAPY

Intralesional 5-fluorouracil (5-FU) can also be used for treatment of hypertrophic scars and keloids. 5-FU is an antimetabolite that blocks DNA synthesis by blocking thymidylate synthetase. It decreases collagen synthesis in proliferating fibroblasts. It can be used alone or in conjunction with triamcinolone.[9] Better results are achieved when used in combination with triamcinolone. The standard dosage is 5-FU 50 mg/mL, 0.9 mL, and 0.1 mL of triamcinolone acetonide 10 mg/mL. Lesions are injected 1 to 3 times a week for 10 to 12 weeks.

OTHER THERAPIES

The use of pentoxifylline (Trental) 400 mg three times a day has been suggested as a useful antifibrotic agent but had limited success in preventing recurrence of excised keloids.[10] A recent publication provides a rationale for

postoperative use of tacrolimus in the prevention of postexcision keloid recurrence.[11] It was demonstrated that *gli*-1 protein is highly expressed in keloidal tissues but not in scar or normal-skin fibroblast. During the course of a clinical trial, it was noted that a patient on topical tacrolimus noted clearing of a keloid after treatment, and *gli*-1 has been shown to be a target of tacrolimus.

An old and somewhat abandoned adjuvant therapy to prevent postexcision recurrence is the use of methotrexate, 15 to 20 mg every 4 days, starting 1 week before surgery and continuing for 3 to 4 months. Postoperative use of colchicine is another old and somewhat successful therapy.

ADJUNCT MEDICAL THERAPIES

Pressure garments, starting 1 week after suture removal, combined with a topical class-1 steroid helps prevent recurrence (Fig. 34-4). Silicone gel sheeting, flurandrenolide tape, or Curad Scar Therapy cosmetic pad used postoperatively, starting 1 week after suture removal, will also help prevent recurrence.

EXCISIONAL SURGERY

Surgical methods differ according to the size and location of lesions. Excisional surgery as a monotherapy is usually not recommended because the likelihood of recurrence is greater than 50%. The best results are achieved when excision is combined with other modalities.[1] The first rule of keloid excision is withholding elective cosmetic surgery from known keloid formers (those with only earlobe lesions should not be considered keloid formers). All surgical wounds should be closed with as little tension as possible, incisions should not cross joint spaces, midchest incisions should be avoided, and excisions should follow

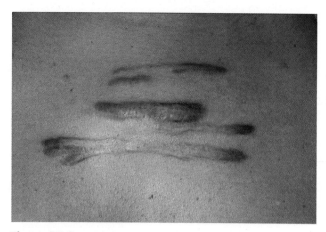

Figure 34-2 Keloid with erythematous border.

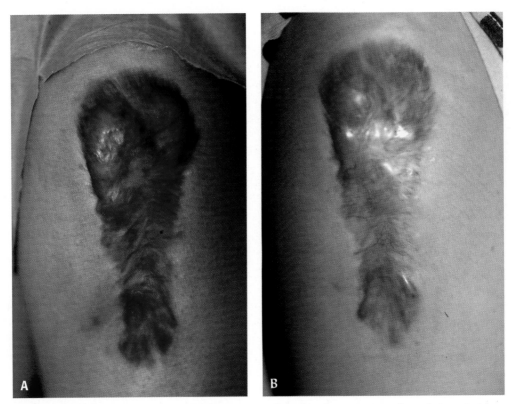

Figure 34-3 A: Keloid, left shoulder. **B:** Same keloid 8 weeks after triamcinolone (40 mg/mL) injection every 2 weeks and topical clobetasol cream daily.

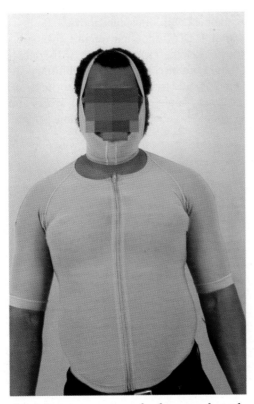

Figure 34-4 Pressure garment for face, trunk, and arms.

the skin creases. During the history section of the examination, the patient should be asked if he/she has a family history of keloids, or if the keloid developed secondary to a chemical or thermal burn or surgical procedure. Also, ascertain if the operative site is infected. If any of these answers is yes, the patients will have a greater risk of keloid recurrence.

The patient should be informed that the risk for postexcision recurrence is approximately 50% if surgery is used as a monotherapy. For keloids with narrow bases (less than 1–2 cm), a simple elliptical excision followed by undermining the base and closing with interrupted sutures will suffice.

For posterior pedunculated earlobe keloids, shaving followed by pressure hemostasis is a simple and efficient method. Once the postoperative site heals, daily use of a pressure earring with a silicone backing helps prevent keloid recurrence.

For large nonpedunculated earlobe keloids and keloids with wide bases on other parts of the body, removal is more complex. First, a tonguelike incision approximately one fifth the size of the lesion is made from one border onto the part of the keloid with the smoothest and flattest-looking surface. The remaining part of the keloid is then excised, and the tongue of keloid tissue is used like a flap to close the postoperative site (Figs. 34-5, 34-6, and 34-7). In some cases, when the skin of the keloid is not smooth, a tissue expander

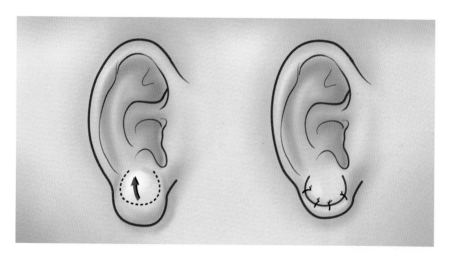

Figure 34-5 Drawing to illustrate keloid surgery using some of the overlying skin as an autograph.

may be inserted so the keloid can be excised and closed primarily several months later.

CRYOSURGERY

Cryosurgery can be used alone or in conjunction with intralesional steroids. When used alone, two 15- to 20-second freeze-thaw cycles are used at each visit every 3 weeks. Freezing more than 20 seconds may produce hypopigmentation, which lasts longer than a year; freezing less than 20 seconds may cause hyperpigmentation, which may last 6 to 12 weeks. Freezing can also cause mild edema of the tissue, enabling easier intralesional triamcinolone injections.

In a double-blind study, Layton et al.[12] compared the efficacy of intralesional triamcinolone and cryosurgery in the treatment of acne keloids. Data demonstrated an 85% improvement in flattening when treated early and in particular vascular lesions. Treatment with intralesional

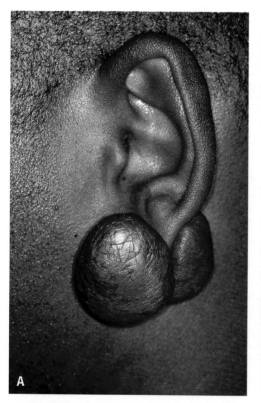
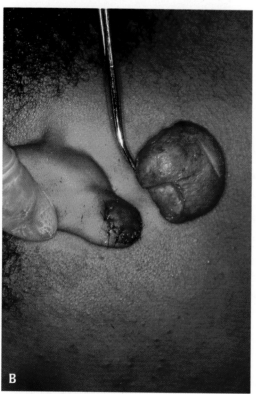

Figure 34-6 A: Keloids of right anterior and posterior lobe. **B:** Posterior keloid removed 4 weeks after anterior lobe keloid removal.

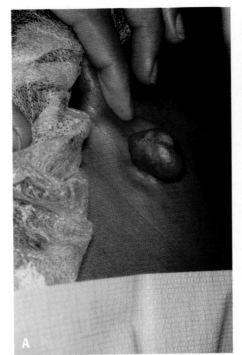

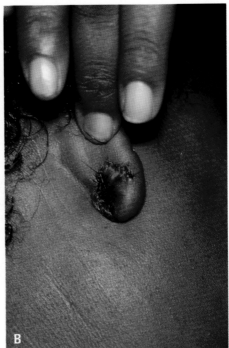

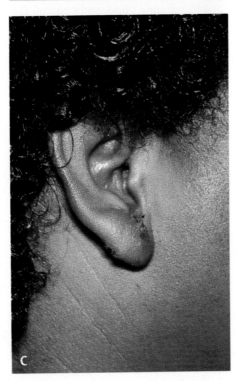

Figure 34-7 A: Right posterior earlobe keloid. **B:** Same patient as A, showing excision with excellent earlobe contour. **C:** Anterior view of the right earlobe showing preservation of anterior earlobe contour.

triamcinolone was also beneficial, but the response to cryosurgery was significantly better in early vascular lesions.[12]

LASER SURGERY

There seems to be a laser for each dermatosis, but the jury is still out on laser success for keloid therapy. Laser treatment of keloidal scars includes argon, CO_2, Nd:YAG laser, and 585-nm flashlamp-pumped pulsed-dye laser.[13,14] Favorable preliminary findings were reported using argon lasers. However, subsequent studies failed to confirm these results.[15] The carbon dioxide laser can be used to soften and flatten large lesions, but when used as monotherapy, the recurrence rate is often more than 70%.[16,17] Sherman and Rosenfield[14] reported improvement in 16 out of 17 patients treated with Nd:YAG 1,064-nm laser. The study, however, was lacking

Table 34-1

Therapeutic alternatives

Surgical	Medical-injectable	Medical	Physical	Medical-topical
Excision with 1-degree closure	IL steroids	Imiquimod	Pressure earrings	Steroids
Excision with second-intention healing	IL bleomycin	Verapamil	Pressure garments	Flurandrenolide tape
Excision with grafting	IL 5-FU	Colchicine	UVA-1	Silicone gel
Cryosurgery	Interferon alfa-2b	D-penicillamine		Curad scar therapy
Laser surgery		Tacrolimus		

5-FU, 5-fluorouracil; IL, interleukin; UVA, ultraviolet A.

in outcome definitions and adequate follow-up. The 585-nm flashlamp-pumped pulsed-dye laser has had some success in treating sternotomy scars.[18] Therapy was more successful if intralesional triamcinolone was used in conjunction with a pulsed-dye laser every 3 weeks.

A comparison study evaluated the clinical response of keloidal and hypertrophic scars after treatment with intralesional corticosteroid alone or combined with 5-FU, 5-FU alone, and the 585-nm flashlamp-pumped pulsed-dye laser. Significant clinical improvement was noted in all treated segments; however, no significant difference in treatment outcome versus method of treatment was observed.[19]

A recent study assessed the efficacy of a combination treatment of triamcinolone, 5-FU, and pulsed-dye laser for treatment of keloids and hypertrophic scars in a 12-week study of 69 patients. Patients were randomly assigned to one of three arms: triamcinolone alone; triamcinolone and 5-FU; or the triple-combination therapy. Overall efficacy was best in the triamcinolone + 5-FU group and the triple-combination groups. However, the triple combination of triamcinolone, 5-FU, and pulsed-dye laser was more acceptable to patients.[20]

RADIATION

Radiation therapy as a monotherapeutic modality for keloid removal is not very effective unless large doses of radiation are used; however, large doses may result in squamous cell carcinoma at the treated sites 15 or more years later (Fig. 34-7). Radiation is more successful when given within the first 2 weeks after excision, when the fibroblasts are proliferating. The usual doses are 300 rads (3Gy) five times a day or 500 rads (5Gy) three times every other day, starting immediately after surgery. Postoperative interstitial radiotherapy with iridium 192 has lowered the

keloid recurrence rate by 20% to 30%[5]. Ragoowansi et al.[21] found that extralesional excision of keloid followed by early postoperative single fraction radiotherapy is both simple and effective in preventing recurrence of excision sites in high-risk keloids that have failed prior treatment.

CONCLUSION

Keloids are medically benign but often psychologically and socially malignant fibrous growths that result from an abnormal connective tissue response in predisposed individuals. They occur more often in blacks than whites, with the incidence in Asians and Hispanics falling between the two extremes. They may be pruritic and painful and occur most often on the earlobes, chest, upper back, and shoulders. They pose a tremendous challenge to the treating physician because of the high incidence of recurrence. The multiplicity of therapeutic modalities illustrates that there is not one that is universally efficacious (Table 34-1). Surgery as a monotherapy usually has a high recurrence rate; however, when used in conjunction with some medical, physical, or radiation therapy, the recurrence rate is lower. All patients undergoing keloid excision should be advised that postoperation compliance is the most important part of surgical therapy.

REFERENCES

1. Kelly PA. Medical and surgical therapies for keloids. *Dermatol Ther* 2004;17(2):212–218.
2. Kelly AP, Zheng P, Johnson BL. Mast cells and keloid formation. *J Invest Dermatol* 1996;106:838.
3. McCoy BJ, Dieglemann RI, Cohen JK. In vitro inhibition of cell growth, collagen synthesis and prolyl hydroxylase activity

by triamcinolone acetonide. *Proc Soc Exp Biol Med* 1980;163: 216–222.

4. Chowdri NA, Maserat M, Mattoo A, et al. Keloids and hypertrophic scars: results with intraoperative and serial postoperative corticosteroids injection therapy. *Aust N Z J Surg* 1999;69(9):655–659.

5. Berman B, Flores F. Recurrence rates of excised keloids treated with post operative triamcinolone injections or interferon alfa-2b injections. *J Am Acad Dermatol* 1997;137:755–757.

6. Niessen FB, Spauwen PH, Chalkwijk J, et al. On the nature of hypertrophic scars and keloids: a review. *Plast Reconstr Surg* 1999;104(5):1435–1458.

7. Mustoe TA, Cooter RD, Gold MD, et al. International clinical recommendations on scar management. *Plast Reconstr Surg* 2002;110(2):56–71.

8. Berman B, Kaufman J. Pilot study of the effects of postoperative imiquimod 5% cream on the recurrence rate of excised keloids. *J Am Acad Dermatol* 2002;47(Suppl):S209–S211.

9. Fitzpatrick RE. Treatment of inflamed hypertrophic scars using intralesional 5-FU. *Dermatol Surg* 1999;25:224–232.

10. Berman B, Duncan MR. Pentoxifylline inhibits the proliferation of human fibroblasts derived from keloid, scleroderma and morphoea skin and their production of collagen, glycosaminoglycans and fibronectin. *Br J Dermatol* 1990;123(3):339–346.

11. Kim A, DiCarlo J, Cohen C, et al. Are keloids really *gli*-loids? High level expression of *gli*-1 oncogene in keloids. *J Am Acad Dermatol* 2000;25:707–711.

12. Layton AM, Yip J, Cunliffe WJ. A comparison of intralesional triamcinolone and cryosurgery in the treatment of acne keloids. *Br J Dermatol* 1994;130:498–501.

13. Apfelberg DB, Maser MR, Lash H, et al. Preliminary results on argon and carbon dioxide laser excision of keloids. *Lasers Surg Med* 1984;4:283.

14. Sherman R, Rosenfield H. Experience with the Nd:YAG laser in the treatment of keloidal scars. *Ann Plast Surg* 1988;21: 231–235.

15. Apfelberg DM, Maser MR, White DN, et al. Failure of carbon dioxide laser excision of keloids. *Lasers Surg Med* 1989;9:382.

16. McCraw JB, McCraw JA, McMellin A, et al. Prevention of unfavorable scars using early pulsed dye laser treatments: a preliminary report. *Ann Plast Surg* 1999;42:7–14.

17. Stern JC, Lucente FT. Carbon dioxide laser excursion of earlobe keloids: a prospective study and critical analysis of existing data. *Arch Otolaryngol Head Neck Surg* 1989;115: 1107–1111.

18. Alster TS, Williams CM. Treatment of keloid sternostomy scars with 585 nm flashlamp-pumped pulsed dye-laser. *Lancet* 1995;345:1998–2000.

19. Manuskiatti W, Fitzpatrick RE. Treatment response of keloidal and hypertrophic sternotomy scars: comparison among intralesional corticosteroids, 5-fluorouracil, and 585 nm flashlamp-pumped pulsed dye laser treatments. *Arch Dermatol* 2002;138:1149–1155.

20. Asilian A, Daroughen A, Shariati F. New combination of triamcinolone, 5-fluoracil, and pulsed dye laser for treatment of keloid and hypertrophic scars. *Dermatol Surg* 2006;7: 907–915.

21. Ragoowansi R, Corns PGS, Moss Al, et al. Treatment of keloids by surgical excision and immediate postoperative single-fraction radiotherapy. *Plast Reconstr Surg* 2003;111: 1853–1858.

Cosmetic Aspects of Common Benign Tumors

Doris M. Hexsel and Mariana Soirefmann

Benign tumors are frequent in all skin types. The diagnosis of benign skin tumors may need careful dermatologic exam; patient history and familial history; physical exam, including gross visualization; dermoscopy; and biopsy to confirm it is truly benign and to rule out malignancies.

Benign tumors are mainly located on the face, interfering with the appearance not only by fact of the lesions themselves but also because some are numerous.

All benign skin tumors may affect darker racial ethnic groups, but some are more frequent. This chapter will discuss the diagnosis and treatment of the most frequently benign skin tumors, including dermatosis papulosa nigra, dermatofibromas, acrochordons (skin tags), syringomas, trichoepitheliomas, and sebaceous hyperplasia.

DERMATOSIS PAPULOSA NIGRA

General features

Dermatosis papulosa nigra (DPN) is a pigmented eruption of the face and neck caused by a nevoid development defect of the pilosebaceous follicles, with histology resembling seborrhoeic keratosis.[1,2] The condition occurs almost exclusively in darker racial ethnic groups and is more frequent in women than in men.[3,4]

DPN is probably genetically determined.[1] It begins to appear in adolescence or early adulthood and progresses with age.[3,5] Incidence in darker racial ethnic groups rises from about 5% in the first decade to more than 40% by the third decade.[1] It has been estimated that lesions of DPN occur in about 50% of dark-skinned patients.[3] Dunwell and Rose studied 1,000 Afro-Caribbean patients and found DPN a notable common diagnoses.[6] Babapour et al. reported a case of DPN in a 3-year-old dark-skinned boy.[7] Grimes et al. studied 82 dark-skinned patients and reported predominance in women of almost 2:1. Fifty-four percent of these patients reported that other members of their families were also affected.[8] Some authors believe DPN to be a variant of seborrheic keratosis, whereas others consider both lesions as variants of epidermal nevus

with delayed onset. A few regard DPN as a variant of acrochordon.[3]

Individual lesions are black or dark brown, flattened or cupuliform papules 1 to 5 mm in diameter[1,3] and can be elevated from 1 to 3 mm above the skin.[4] Older lesions can become very long and pedunculated or filiform. Growth rate and size usually slow during the fifth or sixth decade.[4] They are more common on the face and neck, especially on the upper cheek area, although they may form on almost any area of the body. Any one individual can have hundreds, even thousands, of these lesions.[1,4] DPNs are benign epidermal tumors that do not spontaneously regress.[3] There have been no reports of malignant degeneration, and the lesions are not associated with any systemic diseases or syndromes.[3,4] They are usually free of pain and itching, although these can develop if the lesions become large and are irritated by friction from clothing. Although lesions may hang over the eyelids and obstruct vision, most patients are more concerned with the cosmetic effects of the lesions than with health effects.[4] The epidermis occasionally has a gently lobulated configuration, similar to that seen in a fibroepithelial polyp. The keratinocytes are basaloid, and horned pseudocysts may be present, resembling seborrheic keratosis.[3]

The clinical differential diagnosis of DPN is relatively small, as these lesions have a classic appearance. Lesions that might be considered in the differential diagnosis include multiple seborrheic keratoses or verrucae, fibroepithelial polyps, syringomas, and trichoepitheliomas. Multiple pigmented melanocytic nevi might rarely be mistaken for DPN.[3]

Treatment

DPNs can cause significant cosmetic and functional impairment when they occur in a frequent location, such as head and neck area. Multiple methods of treatment—including surgery, cryosurgery, curettage, and superficial chemical peeling—have been reported in the literature (Table 35-1).[3] However, it is important to inform the patient that any treatment is likely to cause more cosmetic disturbance than the lesions themselves.[5]

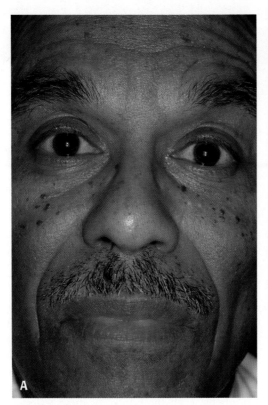 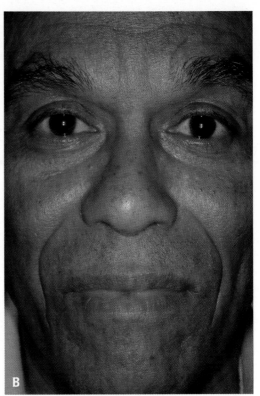

Figure 35-1 A: Dermatosis papulosa nigra: baseline. **B:** Dermatosis papulosa nigra after epilation of multiple lesions. (Courtesy of Pearl E. Grimes, MD.)

Treatment is usually surgical. Electrodesiccation and curettage is a common and accepted technique for removing DPN lesions[5] (Fig. 35-1A,B and Fig. 35-2A,B). Electrodesiccation is also routinely performed for destruction of benign skin lesions, including DPN.[9] Results are normally successful when the procedure is done by an experienced practitioner and follow-up care is given.[4] Kauh et al. reported success on the use of curettage with a small, sharp curette without anesthesia. There was little bleeding and no postoperative scarring or significant pigmentary change in several hundred patients, mostly African Americans, who were followed for 10 years.[10] Moreover, electrofulguration is ideal for very superficial benign lesions, such as DPN. This procedure carbonizes the surface of the lesion, protecting deeper tissue from additional fulguration, so healing is rapid and scarring rare.[11] Chemical peeling using alpha hydroxyl acids will soften and flatten these lesions and does seem to prevent some new lesions. Daily use of lactic acid or other alpha hydroxyl acid–containing lotion or creams is also useful.[3] Cryosurgery results in variable pigmentation and is not considered the treatment of choice for DPN.[3]

Complications

Some degree of hypopigmentation or hyperpigmentation can be expected from surgical procedures. Postinflammatory hyperpigmentation may occur in dark-skinned patients, and it is more frequent than hypopigmentation changes in such patients. Cryosurgery should be undertaken with caution because of the potential for hypopigmentation in black skin,[4] as the melanocytes are very sensitive to this surgical treatment modality. Electrodesiccation is successful, but may also result in hyperpigmentation.[3]

DERMATOFIBROMAS

General features

Dermatofibroma (DF) (also called *benign fibrous histiocytoma, sclerosing hemangioma,* or *histiocytoma cutis*) is a benign dermal and often superficial subcutaneous proliferation of oval cells resembling histiocytes and spindle-shaped cells resembling fibroblasts and myofibroblasts.[12] The etiology of DF is unknown, but recent cytogenetic studies demonstrating clonality favor these lesions being neoplastic.[12] The previous theory that DF is a dermal response to injury, such as an insect bite, trauma, or vaccination, has been challenged.[12] DF is the most frequent fibrohistiocytic skin tumor. Occurrence is more frequent in women than men, and it appears most often in middle age.[13] Child et al., in a study of prevalence of skin disease in a dark-skinned population in southeast London, showed that dermatofibroma is sufficiently common in this population. It was the ninth (2.7%) dermatological diagnostic

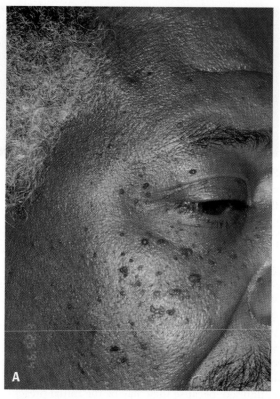 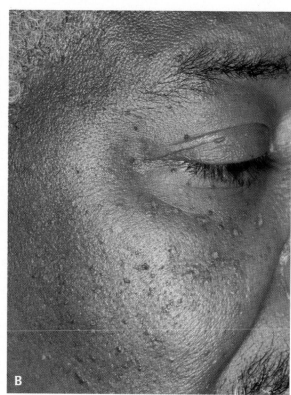

Figure 35-2 A: Dematosis papulosa nigra: baseline. **B:** Dermatosis papulosa nigra after epilation and iris scissor excision of multiple facial lesions. (Courtesy of Pearl E. Grimes, MD.)

most common in 274 consecutive dark-skinned patients.[14] Another more recent article that revised the more common cutaneous alterations of ethnic skin did not cite dermatofibroma as a frequent dermatosis in darker racial ethnic groups, neither in Asian or Hispanic racial groups.[15]

DFs usually appear in adults as a single or multiple firm pigmented papules or nodules that grow slowly and can develop anywhere in the body surface, with predilection for the lower limbs. Their size ranges from a few millimeters to 2 cm, and their color varies from light brown to dark brown, yellow-red, brown-red, or black. They are commonly asymptomatic and rarely can be associated with mild symptoms on palpation. Lateral compression frequently causes dimpling of the skin (Fitzpatrick's sign), although it is not pathognomic.[16] A number of clinicopathological variants of DF have been described. Cellular DFs are larger lesions, more commonly found in men and on the limbs, and represent less than 5% of all DFs. Aneurismal DFs are rapidly growing lesions that mimic a vascular tumor. Atypical DFs are more common in young men, with a predilection for lower limbs. Epithelioid DFs resembles a nonulcerated pyogenic granuloma and present on the lower limbs of young women.[12] Atrophic DF occurs more in women, on the upper trunk, and represent approximately 2% of all DFs.[17] Occasionally, DF is associated with immature follicular structures, which may be confused with basal cell carcinoma.[18]

Dermoscopy can assist in the recognition of DF, mainly to differentiate the DF diagnosis with the diagnosis of melanocytic diseases. There seem to be three standards of DF: (a) isolated pigment network, (b) peripheral pigment network with dark brown globules and dots or with scale crust in the central area, and (c) peripheral pigment network with a central white area.[16]

Treatment

DFs can be treated with surgical excision, cryosurgery, and intralesional injection of corticoid with variable results. All these therapeutic modalities are related with scars and dyschromias, which are more evident in dark-skinned patients. Wang and Lee reported that pulsed-dye laser is a safe and effective treatment of these lesions.[19]

Complications

Cellular, aneurysmal, and atypical variants should be completely removed because of the risk of local recurrence and distant metastases.[12]

ACROCHORDONS (SKIN TAGS)
General features

Acrochordons or skin tags (ST) (also called soft warts) are a common benign, cosmetically disfiguring lesion composed of loose fibrous tissue and occurring mainly on the neck and major flexures as a small soft pedunculated protrusion. They are frequently found together with seborrhoeic keratoses.[1] These lesions are very common, particularly in women at the menopause or later.[1] They are derived from ectoderm and mesoderm and represent a hyperplastic epidermis.[20] STs are found in 25% of all people and increase in number with age.[20] Obesity is a predisposing factor.[18,20] Multiple lesions may appear in the latter trimesters of pregnancy, and as they often resolve postdelivery, it has been suggested that they are probably due to hormonal factors.[21] Multiple acrochordons can be found as part of syndromes, such as Birt-Hogg-Dubé syndrome[22] (fibrofolliculomas, trichodiscomas, and acrochordons) and Bannayan-Riley-Ruvalcaba syndrome[23] (macrocephaly, genital lentiginosis, intestinal polyposis, vascular malformations, lipomatosis, speckled lentiginosis of the penis or vulva, facial verrucae-like or acanthosis nigranslike lesions, and multiple acrochordons). Acrochordons can also be a manifestation of diabetes[24] and diseases associated with atherosclerosis.[25]

The lesions are usually attached to the skin by a thin stalk (pedunculated) but also can be sessile.[1,20] They vary in size and are about 2 mm in diameter on average. They are round, soft, and inelastic. The color may be unchanged (skin colored), but they are frequently hyperpigmented.[1] The most common site is on the sides of the neck, where they may be mixed with typical small sessile seborrhoeic keratoses. When more profuse, they can extend onto the face or down to the back and chest. Similar lesions may be found in and around the axillae and groins.[1,20] Lesions are usually found on the flexural aspects of the body,[26] usually points of chronic trauma.[18]

Melanocytic proliferation and naevus cells are not usually seen, and the majority of such lesions probably come within the seborrhoeic keratosis spectrum. However, some STs may be the last remnants of a pre-existing melanocytic naevus.[1]

The clinical differential diagnosis of ST is relatively small. Lesions that might be considered include wart, nevus, neurofibroma, and seborrheic keratosis.[18]

Treatment

STs pose no malignant threat in adults, but treatment is appropriate for cosmesis or because of irritation.[20] Various treatment modalities have been advocated, such as excision and hemostasis, electrosurgery, chemical cautery, or cryosurgery,[18,26] but recurrences are common,[20] and new lesions may appear. Both electro- and cryosurgery with liquid nitrogen are effective,[1] but there is a risk of secondary bacterial infections.[26] Chemical cautery requires multiple sessions and is associated with cosmetic defects.[26] Simple electrocautery scissor excision at the base of the stalk is sufficient in most of the cases.[20] Electrofulguration is ideal for ST, because healing is rapid and scarring is rare.[11] All these procedures can be performed with or without local anesthesia.[2]

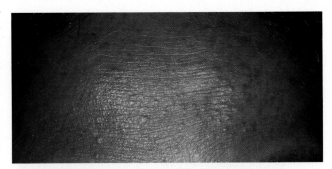

Figure 35-3 Multiple eruptive papules of the forehead consistent with syringomas. (Courtesy of Pearl E. Grimes, MD.)

Mukhtar[26] proposed a method using tissue forceps as a simple and effective instrument for treating STs in the outpatient setting. Five patients with 37 STs were included in the study. The body of the tag was grasped and pulled out gently with a DeBakey's forceps and the base of the pedicle was clamped with a Kocher's forceps for 10 to 15 seconds. None of the patients reported a negative cosmetic effect or recurrence at the site (4 weeks follow-up). Pathologic evaluation is unnecessary unless STs are present in childhood, because they may be the initial presentation of nevoid basal cell carcinoma syndrome.[27]

Complications

All treatments described above should be performed with care in darker racial ethnic groups because of the risks of hyper- or hypopigmentation.

SYRINGOMA
General features

Syringoma (also called *syringoma hidradenoma eruptions, syringocystadenoma,* or *syringocystoma*) is a benign tumor of the skin appendage that is usually multiple and has characteristic histopathologic features.[28] Histochemically, it is a tumor of the eccrine sweat duct. Often it appears at puberty, and lesions continue to develop during adult life but may occur at any age from adolescence onward.[28] There are four clinical variants: localized, familial, associated with Down syndrome, and a generalized form that encompasses multiple and eruptive syringomas.[29] The localized form presents with firm papules and skin colored to yellow on the periorbital region[30] (Fig. 35-3). Familial syringomas affect both sexes equally with a pattern of autosomal inheritance. The incidence of familial syringomas is possibly underestimated.[31] Syringomas are present in patients with Down's syndrome more often than expected.[31] Although Horenstein et al.[32] reported a higher incidence of eruptive syringomas in African Americans, and Sacoor and Medley[33] reported four cases of eruptive syringoma in dark-skinned South African children, these

Table 35-1

Treatment of benign tumors

Tumor	Treatment modality
Dermatosis papulosa nigra	Electrodesiccation Curettage Epilation Iris scissor excision Cryotherapy Superficial chemical peeling
Dermatofibroma	Surgical excision Cryotherapy Intralesional corticosteroid Pulsed-dye laser
Skin tags (acrochordons)	Surgical excision Hemostasis Electrosurgery Chemical cautery Cryosurgery
Syringoma	Intralesional electrodesiccation Electrodesiccation and curettage CO_2 laser and trichloroacetic acid Dermabrasion Q-switched alexandrite laser Iris scissor excision
Trichoepithelioma	Imiquimod Tretinoin Primary excision Dermabrasion Ablative resurfacing Electrocautery
Sebaceous hyperplasia	Isotretinoin Shave excision Trichloroacetic acid (TCA) Bichloroacetic acid (BCA) chemical peeling Electrodesiccation Laser therapy Photodynamic therapy

lesions present mostly in adolescents[31] and tend to be more prevalent in women and whites.[29] Eruptive syringomas have a chronic and persistent course.[33]

The lesions of syringoma are individual skin-colored or yellowish papules with flat-topped or rounded surfaces that vary in size from 1 to 5 mm (usually <3 mm). In general, they are multiple tumors and tend to have a bilateral symmetric distribution.[28] They occur most commonly, on the eyelids and cheeks, but may occur at axillae, abdomen, vulva, scalp, hands, or moustache area.[34] Occasionally, generalized eruptive syringomas develop in a more widespread distribution (eruptive hidradenoma of Darier and Jaquet).[35] The lesions often arise in large numbers and successive crops on the anterior neck, chest, and abdomen.[36] Powell et al. reported a young dark-skinned man with multiple, eruptive, asymptomatic syringomas on his buttocks.[29] The preferential localization of lesions on the ventral area of the body can be explained because this area has more eccrine glands than the dorsal half.[35] Usually, syringoma is asymptomatic, but when located on vulva it can cause pruritus, mainly during menstruation and pregnancy.[37]

A characteristic feature of syringoma is the tail-like strand of cells extending into the stroma, resembling a comma.[28] Syringomas located on the eyelids are typical, histopathologic studies are necessary only if there is diagnostic doubt. Syringoma can be confused with trichoepithelioma when located on the face, but are usually smaller, less superficial, and disposed to the eyelids and cheeks rather than the nasolabial creases. Lesions on eyelids can be mistaken as xanthelasma (but these have an orange characteristic color) or as milium cysts. Those erupting on the trunk may be mistaken for disseminated granuloma annulare.[28]

Treatment

The reason for treatment is cosmetic; the aim is to treat the lesion with minimal scarring to produce an acceptable cosmetic result.[38] Usual treatments aim to remove or flatten the papule produced by each syringoma. All modalities of therapy are ablative and will produce scarring to some degree. There are no studies comparing treatment modalities nor guidelines to follow. Case reports and little series of cases therapies include intralesional electrodesiccation, which consists in the use of a fine electrode into the lesion with the aim of localizing the effect and minimizing the scarring;[39] electrodesiccation and curettage;[40] CO_2 laser and trichloroacetic acid,[40] with good to excellent results; dermabrasion;[40] and temporary tattooing followed by Q-switched alexandrite laser.[41] Surgical excision using iris scissors may also be considered, as it can give cosmetic results.

Complications

All therapeutic modalities may result in cosmetically acceptable scars, and patients should be aware of this. Darker racial ethnic groups may have focal areas of hyperpigmentation that usually clear in 2 to 3 months.[39]

TRICHOEPITHELIOMA

General features

Trichoepithelioma (TE) is a benign cutaneous tumor that originates from hair follicles and occurs either in multiple (autosomal dominant) or solitary (sporadic) lesions.[42–46] It is characterized as a hamartoma of the hair germ composed of immature islands of basaloid cells with focal, primitive follicular differentiation and induction of a cellular stroma.[28] TE is derived from trichogenic epithelium and differentiates toward hair germ, bulb, and infundibulum.[43] It appears predominantly in young adults, and it is most commonly found on the face.[28] Child et al. reviewed the spectrum of skin disease occurring in 461 dark-skinned patients in southeast London and did not find TE as a frequent dermatosis.[14]

Three distinctive forms of TE are recognized, namely solitary, multiple, and desmoplastic.[35] The lesions commonly appear as sporadic solitary lesions or, more rarely, as multiple lesions that are often dominantly inherited.[44]

TE can be confused with basal cell carcinoma, sebaceous hyperplasia, syringoma, and hidrocystoma. The "adenoma sebaceum" of tuberous sclerosis, lesions of which are truly angiofibromas, can also present with many skin-colored papules on the central part of the face. Biopsy is usually required to distinguish TE from basal cell carcinoma. History of a long-standing lesion with little change may be suggestive, but this same history is often obtained with basal cell carcinoma.[43]

Treatment

TEs can cause significant cosmetic and functional impairment when they occur in the head and neck area. Multiple methods of treatment—including plastic surgery, dermabrasion, cryosurgery, and laser surgery—have been reported in the literature. The current treatment of multiple TE is surgical and includes excision, electrocautery, and ablative resurfacing.[45–49] However, Urquhart and Weston used topical imiquimod three times a week for this condition.[47] The patient progressively increased the frequency of application to twice daily and added topical tretinoin gel once daily to her regimen for more resistant lesions. After 3 years of treatment, the patient experienced approximately 80% clearing of lesions without scarring. The advantages of using this nonsurgical treatment are that there is no scarring, it is painless, and there is no need for other invasive procedures, such as injection of local anesthetic.[47] There is a report that documents a case of multiple TEs treated successfully with the argon laser from the face and scalp. The benefits of the argon laser in treatment of multiple TEs include eradication of the lesions without apparent recurrence, restriction of spread of solitary TE into adjacent tumors, and prevention of obstruction of the periorbital region and auditory canal. The treatment may be accomplished as a simple outpatient procedure under local anesthesia with minimal pain or disability.[48]

Complications

Unfortunately, all the treatments described above should be performed with care in darker racial ethnic groups because of the risks of hyper- or hypopigmentation.

SEBACEOUS HYPERPLASIA

General features

Sebaceous hyperplasia (SH) is a benign condition characterized by the proliferation of the sebaceous gland. It is probably the most common of all pilosebaceous tumors and also the one of least significance.[43] Intrinsic and extrinsic aging (photoaging) are causative factors in SH. Reduced androgen levels lead a decreased cellular turnover in aged sebaceous glands of the face, resulting in glandular hyperplasia. Prolonged ultraviolet radiation has been shown to induce marked SH in hair mice. Ultraviolet A penetrates deeper into the dermis to reach the sebaceous gland and is probably the spectrum that causes the sebaceous gland hyperplasia to develop in aging facial skin.[50] SH is also associated with immunosuppressive treatment with cyclosporine in transplant patients,[51] and patients receiving hemodialysis are at increased risk. Although these lesions are common in darker racial ethnic groups, there is no relationship between skin type and the appearance of SH.[52]

SH consists of soft, yellow, dome-shaped papules, some of which are centrally umbilicated. These lesions are commonly found on the forehead, cheeks, lower eyelid, and nose.[52–55] SH also can occur on the vulva.[53] SH is most common in middle-aged and elderly persons. These lesions occur after the age of 30 years in 25% of the population and gradually become more numerous.[2] SH can also occur during the neonatal period by sebaceous hyperactivity caused by androgenic stimulation. In this case, treatment is not necessary because the condition disappears in some weeks.[54] In patients with rare familial forms, SH begins during puberty[55] and has a tendency to worsen with age.

Dermatoscopy of SH shows aggregated white or yellow nodules at the center of the lesion that correspond to hyperplastic sebaceous glands. Sometimes the ostium of these glands is visible as a small crater. The yellowish nodules are surrounded by "cross vessels" that can be defined as a group of orderly winding, scarcely branching, and not arborizing vessels that may extend toward the center but never cross it.[56]

The sebaceous lobules show a proper maturation sequence of the sebocytes with only a single rim of basaloid cells at the periphery and mature sebocytes within the central portions of the lobules.[43]

The differential diagnosis must be with early basal cell carcinomas that are characterized by a mosaic appearance; the surface of SH is generally less uniform than basal cell carcinomas.

Treatment

SH is an asymptomatic condition, but these lesions often represent a cosmetic concern to affected patients, leading them to seek treatment. Treatment options include cauterization or electrodesiccation, shave excision and excision, oral isotretinoin, chemical peelings (bichloracetic acid or trichloroacetic acid), cryosurgery, laser therapy (argon, carbon dioxide, diode, or pulsed-dye laser) and photodynamic therapy (with combined use of 5-aminolevulinic acid [5-ALA] and visible light or lasers).[52] Previous curettage to electrosurgery may also be used. The curetted lesion may be sent to histological evaluation. Previous biopsy is recommended if there is concern that the lesion is a basal cell carcinoma.

In darker racial ethnic groups, complications of nonspecific destructive therapies include considerable risk of postoperative scarring, dyspigmentation, postinflammatory hyperpigmentation, and keloids. Peelings can be used in carefully selected patients, because different ethnicities may respond unpredictably to chemical peeling regardless of skin phenotype.[57] Oral isotretinoin is effective and must be prescribed only for patients without contraindications, but lesions often recur upon discontinuation of therapy.

Photodynamic therapy with topical 5-ALA can achieve safe and effective improvement of SH.[58,59] Alster and Tanzi reported good results from 10 patients with skin types I to IV treated with pulsed-dye laser and 5-ALA (Levulan Keratic, Dusa Pharmaceuticals) with no side effects and without recurrence during the 3 months follow-up.[59] However, Richey mentioned postinflammatory hyperpigmentation and skin discoloration in two patients with skin types IV and V after photodynamic therapy with ALA and 410-nm blue light that cleared with hydroquinone within 10 to 21 days.[60]

CONCLUSIONS

Most of the benign skin tumors that affect darker racial ethnic groups are not specific for this population. Despite the cosmetic effects, most of them do not cause functional impairment. On the other hand, all treatments reported in literature are associated with some degree of dyschromia when performed in darker racial ethnic groups. Scars and keloids also can occur when more invasive procedures are chosen. More studies are necessary to improve the knowledge and safety in treating benign tumors of darker racial ethnic groups as well as to decrease the risks of side effects.

REFERENCES

1. MacKie RM, Quinn AG. Non-melanoma skin cancer and other epidermal skin tumours. In: Burns T, Breathnach S, Cox N, et al., eds. *Rook's Textbook of Dermatology*. 7th ed. Turin: Blackwell Publishing;2004:36.1–36.50.
2. Habif TP, ed. Tumores cutâneos benignos. *Dermatologia Clínica*. 4 ed. Porto Alegre: Artmed;2005:712–737.
3. Smoller BR, Graham G. Benign neoplasms of the epidermis. In: Arndt KA, Leboit PE, Robinson JK, et al., eds. *Cutaneous Medicine and Surgery: An Integrated Program in Dermatology*. Philadelphia: WB Saunders Co.;1996:1441–1449.
4. Thrower A, Gambino H. Black skin conditions and disorders. In: Thrower A, Gambino H. *Black Skin Care for the Practicing Professional*. Clifton Park: Thompson and Delmar Learning;1999:37–67.
5. Schulz EJ. African women. In: Parish LC, Brenner S, Ramos e Silva M, eds. *Women's Dermatology: From Infancy to Maturity*. New York: Parthenon Publishing;2001:429–441.
6. Dunwell P, Rose A. Study of the skin disease spectrum occurring in an Afro-Caribbean population. *Int J Dermatol* 2003; 42(4):287–289.
7. Babapour R, Leach J, Levy H. Dermatosis papulosa nigra in a young child. *Pediatr Dermatol* 1993;10(4):356–358.
8. Grimes PE, Arora S, Minus HR, et al. Dermatosis papulosa nigra. *Cutis* 1983;32(4):385–386,392.
9. Carter E, Coppola CA, Barsanti FA. A randomized, double-blind comparison of two topical anesthetic formulations prior to electrodesiccation of dermatosis papulosa nigra. *Int J Dermatol* 2003;42:287–289.
10. Kauh YC, McDonald JW, Rapaport JA, et al. A surgical approach for dermatosis papulosa nigra. *Int J Dermatol* 1983; 22(10):590–592.
11. Robinson JK, Hruza GJ. Dermatologic surgery: introduction and approach. In: Freedberg IM, Eisen AZ, Wolff K, Austen KF, et al., eds. *Fitzpatrick's Dermatology in General Medicine*. 6th ed. New York: McGraw Hill;2003:2517–2529.
12. Calonje E, Mackie RM. Soft-tissue tumours and tumour-like conditions. In: Burns T, Breathnach S, Cox N, et al., eds. *Rook's Textbook of Dermatology*. 7th ed. Turin: Blackwell Publishing;2004:53.1–53.47.
13. Hügel H. Fibrohistiocystic skin tumors. *J Dtsch Dermatol Ges* 2006;4:544–555.
14. Child FJ, Fuller LC, Higgins EM, et al. A study of the spectrum of skin disease occurring in a black population in south-east London. *Br J Dermatol* 1999;141:512–517.
15. Halder RM, Nootheti PK. Ethnic skin disorders overview. *J Am Acad Dermatol* 2003;48(6):S143–148.
16. Arpaia N, Cassano N, Vena GA. Dermoscopic patterns of dermatofibroma. *Dermatol Surg* 2005;31:1336–1339.
17. Curcó N, Pagerols X, García M, et al. Atrophic dermatofibroma accompanied by aneurysmatic characteristics. *JEAVD* 2006;20:331–333.
18. Shea CR, Prieto VG. Fibrous lesions of dermis and soft tissue. In: Freedberg IM, Eisen AZ, Wolff K, et al, eds. *Fitzpatrick's Dermatology in General Medicine*. 6th ed. New York: McGraw Hill;2003:988–1001.
19. Wang SQ, Lee PK. Treatment of dermatofibroma with a 600nm pulsed dye laser. *Dermatol Surg* 2006;32: 532–535.
20. Luba MC, Bangs SA, Mohler AM, et al. Common benign skin tumors. *Am Fam Physician* 2003;67(4):729–738.
21. Witrowski JA, Parish LC. The girl and the adolescent. In: Parish LC, Brenner S, Ramos e Silva M, eds. *Women's Dermatology: From Infancy to Maturity*. New York: Parthenon Publishing;2001:60–71.
22. Vincent A, Farley M, Chan E, et al. Birt-Hogg-Dubé syndrome: a review of the literature and the differential diagnosis of firm facial papules. *J Am Acad Dermatol* 2003;49(4): 698–705.
23. Erkek E, Hizel S, Sanlý C, et al. Clinical and histopathological findings in Bannayan-Riley-Ruvalcaba syndrome. *J Am Acad Dermatol* 2005;53:639–643.

24. Scheinfeld NS. Obesity and dermatology. *Clin Dermatol* 2004;22(4):303–309.

25. Erdogan BS, Aktan S, Rota S, et al. Skin tags and atherosclerotic risk factors. *J Dermatol* 2005;32(5):371–375.

26. Mukhtar M. Surgical pearl: tissue forceps as a simple and effective instrument for treating skin tags. *Int J Dermatol* 2006;45:577–579.

27. Chiritescu E, Maloney ME. Acrochordons as a presenting sign of nevoid basal cell carcinoma syndrome. *J Am Acad Dermatol* 2001;44(5):789–794.

28. Mackie RM, Calonje E. Tumours of the skin appendages. In: Burns T, Breathnach S, Cox N, et al., ed. *Rook's Textbook of Dermatology.* 7th ed. Turin: Blackwell Publishing;2004: 37.1–37.34.

29. Powell CL, Smith EP, Graham BS. Eruptive syringomas: an unusual presentation on the buttocks. *Cutis* 2005;76:267–269.

30. Hsiung SH. Eruptive syringoma. *Dermatol Online J* 2002;9 (4):14.

31. Draznin M. Hereditary syringomas: a case report. *Dermatol Online J* 2004;10(2):19.

32. Horenstein MG, Shea CR. Syringoma. 2003. Available online at http://www.emedicine.com.derm/topic414.htm. Accessed July 25, 2006.

33. Sacoor MF, Medley P. Eruptive syringoma in four black South African children. *Clin Exp Dermatol* 2004;29:686–687.

34. Nguyen DB, Patterson JW, Wilson BB. Syringoma of the moustache area. *J Am Acad Dermatol* 2003;49(2):337–339.

35. Kadu S, Kerl H. Appendage tumors of the skin. In: Freedberg IM, Eisen AZ, Wolff K, et al., ed. *Fitzpatrick's Dermatology in General Medicine.* 6th ed. New York: McGraw Hill;2003: 785–808.

36. Teixeira M, Ferreira M, Machado S, et al. Eruptive syringomas. *Dermatol Online J* 2005;11(3):34.

37. Bal N, Aslan E, Kayaselcuk F, et al. Vulvar syringoma aggravated by pregnancy. *Pathol Oncol Res* 2003;9(3):196–197.

38. Langtry JAA. Syringomata. In: Lebwohl MG, Heymann WR, Berth-Jones J, et al., eds. *Treatment of Skin Disease: Comprehensive Therapeutic Strategies.* 2nd ed. China: Mosby-Elsevier;2006:644–645.

39. Karma P, Benedetto AV. Intralesional electrodesiccation of syringomas. *Dermatol Surg* 1997;23(10):921–924.

40. Frazier CC, Camacho AP, Cockerell CJ. The treatment of eruptive syringomas in an African American patient with a combination of trichloroacetic acid and CO_2 laser destruction. *Dermatol Surg* 2001;27(5):489–492.

41. Park HJ, Lim SH, Kang HA, et al. Temporary tattooing followed by Q-switched alexandrite laser for treatment of syringomas. *Dermatol Surg* 2001;27(1):28–30.

42. Matt D, Xin H, Vortmeyer AO, et al. Sporadic trichoepithelioma demonstrates deletions at 9q22.3. *Arch Dermatol* 2000;136(5):657–660.

43. Coldiron B, Smoller BR. Neoplasms of the pilosebaceous unit. In: Arndt KA, Leboit PE, Robinson JK, et al., eds. *Cutaneous Medicine and Surgery: An Integrated Program in Dermatology.* Philadelphia: WB Saunders Co.;1996: 1464–1475.

44. Oh DH, Lane AT, Turk AE, et al. A young boy with a large hemifacial plaque with histopathologic features of trichoepithelioma. *J Am Acad Dermatol* 1997;37(5 Pt 2):881–883.

45. Fisher GH, Geronemus RG. Treatment of multiple familial trichoepithelioma with a combination of aspirin and a neutralizing antibody to tumor necrosis factor α: a case report and hypothesis of mechanism. *Arch Dermatol* 2006;142:782–783.

46. Kazakov DV, Soukup R, Mukensnabl P, et al. Brooke-Spiegler syndrome: report of a case with combined lesions containing cylindromatous, spiradenomatous, trichoblastomatous, and sebaceous differentiation. *Am J Dermatopathol* 2005;27(1): 27–33.

47. Urquhart JL, Weston WL. Treatment of multiple trichoepitheliomas with topical imiquimod and tretinoin. *Pediatr Dermatol* 2005;22(1):67–70.

48. Flores JT, Apfelberg DB, Maser MR, et al. Trichoepithelioma: successful treatment with the argon laser. *Plast Reconstr Surg* 1984;74(5):694–698.

49. Rallan D, Harland CC. Brooke-Spiegler syndrome: treatment with laser ablation. *Clin Exp Dermatol* 2005;30(4):355–357.

50. Zoubolius CC, Boschnakow A. Chronological ageing and photoageing of the human sebaceous gland. *Clin Exp Dermatol* 2001;26:600–607.

51. Engel F, Ellero B, Woehl-Jaegle ML, et al. Diffuse sebaceous hyperplasia of the face induced by cyclosporin. *Ann Dermatol Venereol* 2005;132(4):342–345.

52. Martin-Clavijo A, Berth-Jones J. Sebaceous gland hyperplasia. In: Lebwohl MG, Heymann WR, Berth-Jones J, et al., eds. *Treatment of Skin Disease: Comprehensive Therapeutic Strategies.* 2nd ed. China: Mosby-Elsevier;2006:604–605.

53. Malliah R, Gilhooly P, Lambert WC, et al. Sebaceous hyperplasia of the vulva: case report and review of the literature. *J Low Genit Tract Dis* 2006;10(1):55–57.

54. Sampaio SAP, Rivitti EA. Tumores epiteliais benignos. In: Sampaio SAP, Rivitti EA, eds. *Dermatologia.* 2nd ed. São Paulo: Artes Médicas; 1998:822–832.

55. Weisshaar E, Schramm M, Gollnick H. Familial nevoid sebaceous gland hyperplasia affecting three generations of a family. *Eur J Dermatol* 1999;9(8):621–623.

56. Zaballos P, Ara M, Puig S, et al. Dermoscopy of sebaceous hyperplasia. *Arch Dermatol* 2005;141(6):808.

57. Roberts WE. Chemical peeling in ethnic/dark skin. *Dermatol Ther* 2004;17(2):196–205.

58. Gold MH, Bradshaw VL, Boring MM, et al. Treatment of sebaceous gland hyperplasia by photodynamic therapy with 5-aminolevulinic acid and a blue light source or intense light source. *J Drug Dermatol* 2004;3(6):S6–S9.

59. Alster TS, Tanzi EL. Photodynamic therapy with topical aminolevulinic acid and pulsed dye laser irradiation for sebaceous hyperplasia. *J Drugs Dermatol* 2003;2(5):501–504.

60. Richey DF. Treatment of sebaceous hyperplasia with photodynamic therapy. *Cosmetic Dermatol* 2004;17(8):525–529.

Surgical Treatment of Skin Cancers in Darker Racial Ethnic Groups

P. Kim Phillips

Skin cancer is the most common type of cancer in the United States.[1] Important risk factors associated with the development of nonmelanoma skin cancer (NMSC) and melanoma includes Fitzpatrick phototype I skin, Celtic ancestry, fair complexion, and light eyes. Hispanics, African Americans, and Asians, both having darker skin pigmentation than Caucasians, are at lower risk for developing skin cancer.[2–14] Although the incidence of NMSC and melanoma is lower in Hispanics, African Americans, and Asians, tumors in these populations tend to present in more advanced stages and carry a poorer prognosis than those in Caucasians. Skin cancers can cause significant cosmetic disfigurement. Therefore, selection of appropriate excisional modalities is essential for optimizing aesthetic outcomes.

SQUAMOUS CELL CARCINOMA

Squamous cell carcinoma (SCC) is the most common cutaneous malignancy in African Americans. SCC is an invasive epithelial malignancy exhibiting keratinocyte differentiation. When it occurs in African Americans, tumors tend to present in more advanced stages. SCC accounts for about three fourths of the mortality attributable to NMSC in African Americans.[13,14]

Numerous studies have reported that sun exposure does not appear to be an important etiologic factor in the development of SCC in African Americans, as lesions most frequently occur on non–sun-exposed skin. SCCs arising on non–sun-exposed skin tend to be more aggressive and have a greater potential to metastasize. When SCCs do arise on sun-exposed areas of pigmented skin, they are most commonly found on the "midfacial triangle," which includes the forehead, nasal tip and lip. These tumors also occur to a greater degree on the legs, especially in elderly women.

A significant predisposing factor for the development of SCC is the presence of scar tissue arising from a chronic inflammatory process such as discoid lupus erythematosus,

cutaneous horns, chronic leg ulcers, or scrotal ulcers (Fig. 36-1). Further, Hubbell et al. reported that mortality was greater when the lesion arose from a chronic inflammatory process and was highest in perianal tumors.[13]

BASAL CELL CARCINOMA

Basal cell carcinoma (BCC) is the most common skin cancer in the United States, accounting for at least 75% of all NMSCs. However, more than 99% of these cases occur in whites. The rarity of this cancer in darkly pigmented skin is accounted for by the central role of ultraviolet radiation in the development of BCC[13,14]. However, other risk factors have also been reported for BCC, including prior exposure to radiation, trauma, arsenic ingestion, immunosuppression, and the basal cell nevus syndrome.

BCC typically exhibits characteristic nests or cords of small, dark-staining epithelial cells with palisading of the peripheral cells. Tumors may be pigmented or nonpigmented and arise most commonly on the face, head, and neck (Fig. 36-2). However, lesions may also occur on non–sun-exposed skin. BCCs are generally similar in histology and clinical course in both African Americans and Caucasians. Pigmented BCCs are found with increased frequency in blacks.

MALIGNANT MELANOMA

Risk factors for malignant melanoma in darker racial ethnic groups include exposure to ultraviolet light, a history of blistering sunburns, albinism, burn scars, exposure to ionizing radiations, pre-existing pigmented lesions, and history of trauma.[6–12] Interestingly, family history does not appear to be a significant risk factor in the development of melanoma in persons of color.

Individuals with pigmented skin are more likely to develop acral melanoma, both the acral lentiginous and subungual subtypes. Acral lentiginous melanoma is a very

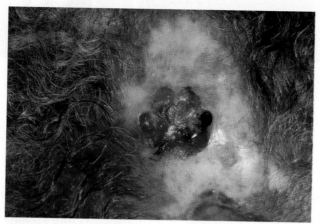

Figure 36-1 Squamous cell carcinoma of the scalp in an African American patient with discoid lupus. (Courtesy of Pearl E. Grimes, MD.)

Overall, the outcome of melanoma is worse for deeply pigmented individuals when compared with white skin. According to the California Cancer Registry, melanoma was diagnosed only after metastasis to a remote site for 12% of black men, compared with only 6% of white men.

When faced with a skin cancer in darker racial ethnic groups, as in all other patient populations, the surgeon's primary focus must be: (a) complete removal of the tumor, (b) preservation of function of key anatomic structures, and (c) restoration of cosmesis. These key principles must be considered in the order presented to achieve high cure rates and prevent tumor recurrence. This chapter will focus on a discussion of common surgical techniques required to manage most cutaneous malignancies as well as reconstruction of postoperative defects to achieve acceptable aesthetic outcomes.

aggressive tumor that commonly occurs on the plantar surface of the feet, palms, and digits and presents as a rapidly spreading, darkly pigmented patch (Fig. 36-3A,B). Subungual melanoma typically arises on the hand, and treatment often requires amputation. Occasionally, these tumors may be amelanotic, which often leads to a delay in the diagnosis. These lesions have a propensity to metastasize to the central nervous system, liver, lungs, bone, and lymph nodes. Prognosis in these cases is poor.

PRIMARY EXCISION

Chief among the surgical procedures performed on skin is the elliptical or fusiform excision. It is used for the therapeutic removal of benign and malignant lesions and is critical to properly diagnose pigmented lesions and inflammatory diseases of the skin. The elliptical excision encompasses all the fundamental elements of more advanced procedures, such as local flaps, skin grafts, and cosmetic procedures. Those elements that must be mastered include knowledge of local anatomy, cosmetic units,

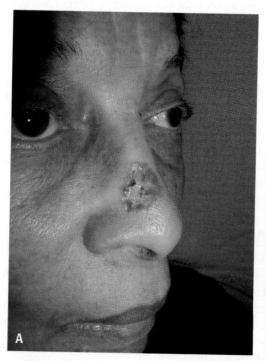
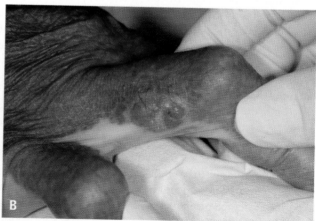

Figure 36-2 A: Basal cell carcinoma of the face in an African American. (Courtesy of Carl Washington, MD.) **B:** Basal squamous cell carcinoma of the finger in a 90-year-old African American male with vitiligo. (Courtesy of Pearl E. Grimes, MD.)

14. Halder RM, Bang KM. Skin cancer in blacks in the United States. *Dermatol Clin* 1988;6:397–405.

15. Mody BR, McCarthy JE, Sengelmann RD. The apical angle: a mathematical analysis of the ellipse. *Dermatol Surg* 2001;27:61–63.

16. Thomas DJ, King AR, Peat BG. Excision margins for non-melanotic skin cancer. *Plast Reconstr Surg* 2003;112:57–69.

17. Brodland DG, Zitelli JA. Surgical margins for excision of primary cutaneous squamous cell carcinoma. *J Am Acad Dermatol* 1992; 27(2 Pt 1):241–248.

18. Boyer JD, Zitelli JA, Brodland DG. Undermining in cutaneous surgery. *Dermatol Surg* 2001;27(1):75–78.

19. Zitelli JA, Moy RL. Buried vertical mattress suture. *J Dermatol Surg Oncol* 1989;15:17–19.

20. Futoryan T, Grande D. Postoperative wound infection rates in dermatologic surgery. *Dermatol Surg* 2005;21:509–514.

21. Cook JL, Perone JB. A prospective evaluation of the incidence of complications associated with Mohs micrographic surgery. *Arch Dermatol* 2003;139:143–152.

22. Hairston BR, Nguyen TH. Innovations in the island pedicle flap for facial reconstruction. *Dermatol Surg* 2003;29:378–385.

23. Whitaker DC, Grande DJ, Johnson SS. Wound infection rates in dermatologic surgery. *J Dermatol Surg Oncol* 1988;14:525–528.

24. Tromovitch T, Stegman S. Microscopic-control of cutaneous tumors: chemosurgery, fresh tissue technique. *Cancer* 1978;41(2):653–658.

Index

Page numbers followed by "*f*" refer to figures; page numbers followed by "*t*" refer to tables.

Abdomen, classification/contouring of, 268–270, 269*f*–270*f*
Acetyl L-carnitine, 98*t*
Acetylcholine (Ach), 211
Ach. *See* Acetylcholine
Ache Indians, 9
Acne
    keloidalis, 291–292
        nuchae, 307–309
    vulgaris, 15, 49, 55–56, 56*f*, 150*f*
        indications of, 84–86, 84*f*, 85*f*
        medications for, 82
Acrochordons, 329–330, 331*t*
Actinic keratoses (AKs), 86
Acyclovir, 157
Adapalene (Differin), 82, 83, 86
Adrenaline, 272
Aesthetic surgery, outcomes in
    assessment of, 37–38
    conclusions on, 40
    good, 38–39, 39*t*
    importance of, 38
    measurement of, 37
    objective measurement tools and, 39–40, 40*t*
Africa, 3, 8, 77
African American(s), 15. *See also* Blacks
    facial features of, 7–9, 8*t*
    women, 12–13, 27, 31*f*, 192–193, 192*f*, 193*f*
Aging
    face, 189
        conclusions on, 34
        in darker racial ethnic groups, 27–35, 28*t*, 29*t*, 30*f*, 31*f*, 32*f*, 33*f*, 34*t*, 35*t*
        Glogau classification of, 27–30, 29*t*, 30*f*, 31*f*, 32*f*
        intrinsic, 31–34, 32*f*, 33*t*
        photodamage and, 27–30, 28*t*, 29*t*, 30*f*, 31*f*, 32*f*
    pigmentation and, 29
    signs of, 27
    theories/antioxidants
        cross-linking, 94
        DNA/genetic, 94
        free-radical, 93
        Hayflick limit, 94
        membrane, 94
        mitochondrial decline, 93–94
        neuroendocrine, 94
AHA. *See* Alpha hydroxy acids
AKs. *See* Actinic keratoses
ALA. *See* Alpha lipoic acids
Aleuts, 15
Allergan, 82
AlloDerm, 231*t*, 234
Aloe barbadensis, 111*t*
Aloesin, 74*t*, 80
Alopecia. *See also specific types*
    androgenetic, 287–294, 288*f*, 288*t*
    hair restoration in, women of color, 287–294, 288*f*, 288*t*, 289*f*, 291*f*, 291*t*, 292*f*, 293*t*
    traction, 288–289, 288*f*, 288*t*
Alpha hydroxy acids (AHAs)
    as antioxidant, 96*t*–97*t*, 99
    as chemical peels, 152
        complications with, 159
        contraindications for, 159

formulations of, 157
    indications for, 157–159, 158*f*, 159*f*, 160*f*
    use of, 22
Alpha lipoic acids (ALA), 96*t*
Aluminum oxide, 152–153
American Academy of Dermatology, 118
American Academy of Facial Plastic Surgery, 257
American Society for Aesthetic and Plastic Surgery, 15
American Society of Dermatologic Surgery, 100, 276
American Society of Plastic Surgeons, 100, 273
Amiodarones, 119
Analgesia, 172
André, Père, 3
Anesthesia, 175, 271–272, 274–275, 275*t*, 305
Anthralinates, 106*t*
Antiandrogens, 288
Antibiotics, 180, 194
Anti-inflammatory agents, 216
Antimalarials, 119
Antioxidant(s)
    aging theories and, 93–94
    AHAs as, 96*t*–97*t*, 101
    benefits of, 100
    free radicals/oxygen reactive species and, 92–93
    process, 93
    skin and, 94–100, 96*t*–97*t*, 100*t*
    surgery and, 100
Aphrodite, 3
Apoptosis, 316
APTOS sutures, 203, 206
Aquaphor, 127
Aramis Erbium: Glass lasers, 198–199
Arbutin, 74*t*, 77–78
Archives of Dermatology, 111
Argon, 324
Arsenics, 119
Ascorbic acid palmitate, 74*t*
Ascorbic acids, 74*t*
Asian(s), 12–13, 15, 86
    eyes, blepharoplasty for, 243–249, 244*f*, 245*f*, 246*f*, 247*f*, 248*f*, 249*f*
    facial features of, 8–9, 9*t*
    photoaging of, 28–29, 34*t*, 86
Aspirin, 193–194
Atharva Veda, 125
Attractiveness, 4
Australia, 12
Australoids, 15
Autologen, 234*t*, 234
Avage. *See* Tazarotene
Avobenzone. *See* Butyl methoxydibenzoyl methane
Azelaic acid, 54, 74*t*, 78, 88

Bacillus botulinus, 211
Balsam of Peru, 110
The Baptism of Pocahontas, 3
Basal cell carcinoma (BCC), 335, 336*f*
BCC. *See* Basal cell carcinoma
BDD. *See* Body dysmorphic disorder

Beauty
    adornment and, 10–11, 12*f*
    changing perceptions of, 11–12
    cultural perceptions of, 9–10
    darker ethnic groups and, 12
    ethnic definition of, 8–9, 8*t*, 9*t*, 10*t*, 11*t*
    Eurocentric standard of, 10
    evolutionary/genetic aspects of, 4–5
    facial aesthetic measurements for, 5–8, 5*t*, 6*f*, 7*f*
    facial characteristics of, 3
    future of, 12–13
    Golden Proportion and, 3, 5*t*, 6*f*
    historical perspectives on
        definitions of, 3
        women as historical icons as, 3–4, 4*f*
Bellamed Microdermabrasion, 151
Benzophenones, 106*t*
Beta-blockers, 216
Beta-carotene, 95, 96*t*–97*t*
Beta-hydroxy acids, 96*t*
Beta-lipohydroxyacid, 96*t*, 97*t*
Bichloracetic acid, 333
Birt-Hogg-Dubé syndrome, 330
Bis-ethylhexyloxyphenol methoxyphenyl triazine. *See* Tinosorb S
Bismuth, 119
Blacks, 12. *See also* African Americans
    blepharoplasty in, 250–256, 251*f*, 253*f*, 254*f*, 255*f*, 256*f*
    rhinoplasty and, 257–261, 258*f*, 259*f*, 260*f*
    skin of, 20–24, 21*t*, 23*t*
Bleaching
    agents, 119, 279
    formulation, Kligman, 157
Blepharoplasty
    for Asian eyes, 243–249, 244*f*, 245*f*, 246*f*, 247*f*, 248*f*, 249*f*
    in blacks/Latinos, 250–256, 251*f*, 253*f*, 254*f*, 255*f*, 256*f*
    complications associated with, 254–255, 256*f*
    conclusions on, 256
    lower, 252–254, 253*f*, 254*f*, 255*f*
    transconjunctival lower, 252
    upper, 250–252, 251*f*
Blinding, 45
Blistering, 52
Blood vessels, 23–24, 23*t*
Body
    -contouring procedures, 268–275, 269*f*–270*f*, 271*f*, 272*f*, 273*f*, 274*t*, 275*t*
    image surgery, 38, 40
    size, 12
Body dysmorphic disorder (BDD), 39, 59
Boots Star Rating. *See* UVA: UVB ratio
Botox, 211–221, 212*t*
Botulinum toxin (BT)
    available, 211–212
    clinical use of, 211
    complications/side effects of, 221
    conclusions on, 221
    conservation/dilution/pharmacology/storage of, 212–214, 212*t*
    contraindications of, 216
    dark skinned patients and, 214–216, 214*f*, 215*f*
    injections, 15, 100, 216–220, 217*f*, 218*f*, 219*f*
    mechanisms of action, 212
    pre-/postoperative care of, 216

347

Brazil, 10, 212
Breast
    augmentation, 15, 264–267, 264f, 265f, 266f, 266t
    reduction, 262–264, 263f
Breast Chest Ratings Scale, 40t
BT. *See* Botulinum toxin
Busulfan, 119
Buttocks, contouring of, 270–271, 273f
Butyl methoxydibenzoylmethane (Avobenzone; Parsol 1789), 106t, 110

Café au lait macules (CALMs), 120–121, 122t
Caffeic acids, 111t
Cambodians, 8
Cancer Registry (Singapore), 103
Capoids, 15
Captique, 229t
Carbon dioxide (CO_2), 171–172, 171t, 324
Caribbean, 10
Carmustine, 119
Carotenoids, 111t
Catechins, 100
Caucasians, 7, 11t, 15, 237
CCCA. *See* Central centrifugal cicatricial alopecia
Cellular all-*trans* retinoic acid-binding protein (CRABP), 83
Central centrifugal cicatricial alopecia (CCCA), 287, 289–290, 289f, 293
Cephalexin, 272
Cetaphil, 127, 163
Chemical peel(s), 54
    AHAs as, 152
        complications with, 159
        contraindications for, 159
        formulations of, 157
        indications for, 157–159, 158f, 159f, 160f
    darker skin types and, 154–155, 155f, 155t
    deep, 171t, 174–178
    medium-depth, 170–174, 171t, 172f, 173f, 174f, 176–177, 177f
    microdermabrasion and, 152
    patient preparations for, 155–157, 156f
    salicylic acid as, 159–161, 162f–163f, 164f, 165f, 166–168, 167f
        advantages/disadvantages of, 163
        contraindications of, 162
        formulations of, 162
        indications of, 162
        side effects of, 161, 165f
        technique, 160–161, 162f, 163f, 164f
    superficial, 154–168, 155f, 155t, 156f, 158f, 159f, 160f, 162f–163f, 164f, 165f
China, 101
Chinese, 8
Chronic venous insufficiency (CVI), 276
Ciba Specialty Chemicals, 107
Cinnamates, 106t
Cis-urocanic acids, 105
Citric acids, 101
Clofazimine, 119
Clostridium botulinum, 211
Cobalt chloride, 53
Cobblestoning, 141
Coenzyme Q_{10} (Ubiquinone), 96t, 97–99
Collagen, 197
    fillers
        autologous, 234
        bovine, 230, 231t–234t
        other human, 234–235, 234f
        porcine, 231t, 234
    non, 235
Compression therapy, 277
Confocal laser microscopic imaging (CSLM), 66
Congoids, 15
Connective tissue-derived growth factor (CTGF), 315–316
Conney, Allan, 99

CONSORT (Consolidated Standards of Reporting Trials), 42–44, 43t–44t
Cook Islands, 12
CoolTouch lasers, 198–199
Corticosteroids, 79, 289, 325
Cosmetic research studies, 42–44, 43t–44t
    compliance and, 47
    components of good, 44–45
    conclusions on, 48
    evaluation methods for, 45–47, 46t
    maintenance treatment and, 47
    Qol and, 47
    safety and, 47, 47t
    treatment duration and, 47
Cosmetic surgery. *See also specific procedures*
    body image surgery and, 38, 40
    concerns
        cultural, 56–57
        within skin of darker racial ethnic groups, 49–57, 49t, 50f, 51f, 52f, 53f, 54f, 55f, 56f, 57f
    facial, 7–8, 16
    in U.S., 15–16, 37–38
Cosmoderm, 232t, 234
Cosmoplast, 232t, 234
CRABP. *See* Cellular all-*trans* retinoic acid-binding protein
CRBP. *See* Cytosolic retinol-binding protein
Critical wavelength (CW), 108
Cross-linking theory, 94
Crow's feet, 217
Cryosurgery, 323–324
Cryotherapy, 119
CSLM. *See* Confocal laser microscopic imaging
CTGF. *See* Connective tissue-derived growth factor
Curad Scar Therapy, 323
CVI. *See* Chronic venous insufficiency
CW. *See* Critical wavelength
Cyclophosphamide, 119
Cymetra, 231t, 234–235
Cyproterone, 288
Cysteines, 17
Cysteinyl-dopa, 17
Cytokines, 27, 53
Cytosolic retinol-binding protein (CRBP), 83

DA. *See* Deoxyarbutin
da Vinci, Leonardo, 5
DAS59. *See* Derriford Appearance Scale
Deoxyarbutin (dA), 78
Depressor anguli oris, 220
Dermabrasion, 176
Dermadeep, 229t
Dermalive, 229t
Dermasanding, 176
Dermatitis, 22, 49t
Dermatofibroma (DF), 328–329, 331t
Dermatology, 16
Dermatology Life Quality Index (DLQI), 47
Dermatosis papulosa nigra (DPN), 327–328, 328f, 329f, 331t
Derriford Appearance Scale (DAS59), 40t
Detergents, 278
Dexamethasone, 272
DF. *See* Dermatofibroma
DHICA. *See* Dihydroxyindole-2-carboxylic acid
Dichloroethyl sulfide, 22
Differin. *See* Adapalene
Dihydroxyindole, 74
Dihydroxyindole-2-carboxylic acid (DHICA), 74
Dihydroxyphenylalanine (DOPA), 74
Dioxybenzone, 106t
DLQI. *See* Dermatology Life Quality Index
DNA/genetic theory, 94
DOPA. *See* Dihydroxyphenylalanine
Dopaquinone, 17
Down syndrome, 330–331, 330f, 331t

Doxycycline, 289
DPN. *See* Dermatosis papulosa nigra
Drometrizole trisiloxane. *See* Mexoryl XL
Dyspigmentation, 52

East Indians, 8
Egypt, 3, 125
Electromagnetic radiation wavelength effects, 104–105, 104t
ELM. *See* Epiluminescence micrography
Elubiol, 54
Embilica, 74t, 80
Ensulizole. *See* Meradimate
Epiluminescence micrography (ELM), 66
Epinephrine, 250, 252, 292
EQ 5D. *See* EuroQol
Ermengen, Emile Pierre Van, 211
Erythema. *See also* Minimal erythema dosing
    irritation and, 22, 89f
    reactions, 104–105
    skin color and, 16–17
Escalol 557. *See* Octinoxate
Eskimos, 15
Esthelis, 226t–229t
Estrogen, 32
Estrogenicity, 110
Ethiopia, 3
Ethnic groups
    antioxidants and, 100
    darker racial, 12
        aging face in, 27–35, 28t, 29t, 30f, 31f, 32f, 33t, 34t, 35t
        LHR in, 303–309, 304f, 304t, 305f, 306f, 306t, 307f, 308f
        melanin and, 17–21, 17f, 18f, 19f, 20f
        skin of, 15–25, 16f, 17f, 18f, 19f, 20f, 21t, 23t
        vascular surgery in, 276–283, 277f, 279f, 280f, 281f, 282f
    definition of beauty and, 8–9, 8t, 9t, 10t, 11t
    rhinoplasty and, 257–261, 258f, 259f, 260f
    skin of
        fillers in, 225–240, 226t–229t, 230f, 231t–233t, 234f, 237f, 238f, 239f
        topical retinoids and, 82–90, 83f, 84f, 85f, 86f, 87f, 89f, 90f, 90t
    vitiligo and, 134–135
    in U.S., 12–13
Ethnicity, 15
EUK-134, 98t
Eumelanin, 17
Europeans, 8, 10, 12
EuroQol (EQ 5D), 40
Eusolex 2292. *See* Octinoxate
Evolence, 231t, 234
Eyebrow elevations, 217, 218f, 219f

Face
    aesthetic parameters of, 5–8, 5t, 6f, 7f
    aging, 189
        conclusions on, 35
        in darker racial ethnic groups, 27–35, 28t, 29t, 30f, 31f, 32f, 33t, 34t, 35t
        Glogau classification of, 27–30, 29t, 30f, 31f, 32f
        intrinsic, 31–34, 32f, 33t
    asymmetry of, 220
    measurements of, 5–8, 5t, 6f, 7f
    neoclassical canons of, 5–8, 5t, 6f
    rejuvenation of, 148
    wrinkles
        of mid, 218f, 219
        of upper, 216–217, 217f
Facelifts
    complications associated with, 193–195, 194f, 195f

composite/deep plane, 191
ethnic issues related to, 192–193, 192*f*, 193*f*
history of, 189–190
nonsurgical, 197–207, 200*f*, 201*f*, 203*f*, 204*f*, 205*f*, 206*f*
patient evaluation/selection for, 190
subcutaneous, 190
    with SMAS, 190–191
subperiosteal, 191
summary on, 195
techniques for
    minimally invasive, 191–192
    operative, 190–191
Facial Appearance Sorting Test (FAST), 40
Famciclovir, 157
Fascian, 231*t*–233*t*
FAST. *See* Facial Appearance Sorting Test
Female pattern hair loss (FPHL), 287–294, 288*f*, 288*t*
Fentanyl, 272
Ferulic acids, 98*t*, 111*t*
Fibroblasts, 23–24, 23*t*, 27
Filipinos, 8
Fillers
    collagen
        autologous, 234
        bovine, 230, 231*t*–233*t*
        other human, 234–235, 234*f*
        porcine, 234
    combination therapies and, 239–240
    conclusions on, 240
    cultural considerations with, 239
    in ethnic skin, 225–240, 226*t*–229*t*, 230*f*, 231*t*–233*t*, 234*f*, 237*f*, 238*f*, 239*f*
    hydraulic acid, 225–230, 226*t*–229*t*, 230*f*
    noncollagen, 235
    permanent, 235–236
Finasteride, 297*t*
Fitzpatrick skin type classification, 16–17, 17*f*, 59–60, 305
Fitzpatrick skin types, 152
Fitzpatrick, Thomas, 16–17
Flaps
    advancement, 341
    A-T advancement, 341, 342*f*
    bilateral/unilateral, 341, 342*f*
    island pedicle, 341–342
    rotation, 341–342, 342*f*
    transposition, 343, 343*f*
Fluocinolone acetonide, 75, 76*f*, 87–88
5-Fluorouracil (5-FU), 86, 321, 325
Folkers, Karl, 100
Follicular units, 298
Formaldehyde-releasing preservatives, 53
FP. *See* Fractional photothermolysis
FPHL. *See* Female pattern hair loss
Fractional photothermolysis (FP), 118, 118*f*
Fragrances, 110
Frankfort horizontal plane, 5*t*, 7, 7*f*
Franklin, John Hope, 15
Free-radical theory, 93
French Society of Plastic Reconstructive and Aesthetic Surgery, 273
5-FU. *See* 5-Fluorouracil

Galderma, 82
Genes
    C-Fos, 83
    C-Jun, 83
Glabellar rhytides, 217, 218*f*, 219*f*
Glabridin, 79
Glogau classification of aging face, 27–30, 29*t*, 30*f*, 31*f*, 32*f*
Glutathione, 17, 98*t*
Glycerin, 278
Glycolic acid, 54
    peels, 152
        complications with, 159

contraindications for, 159
formulations of, 157, 174
indications for, 157–159, 158*f*, 159*f*, 160*f*
as skin-lightening agent, 74*t*, 78–79
Gold, 119
Golden Proportion, 3, 5*t*, 6*f*
Grape seed (*Vitus coignetiae*; *Vitus vinifera*), 98*t*
Greeks, 3, 5, 5*t*, 6*f*
Green tea (tea polyphenols), 96*t*, 99, 108, 111*t*

Hair
    characteristics of, 290, 291*f*, 291*t*
    follicles, 24
    graft
        preparation, 293
        size of, 299, 299*f*
    induction, 306
    recipient sites for, 293, 293*t*
    removal, laser, 56
        in darker racial ethnic groups, 303–309, 304*f*, 304*t*, 305*f*, 306*f*, 306*t*, 307*f*, 308*f*
    restoration in women of color, 287–294, 288*f*, 288*t*, 289*f*, 291*f*, 291*t*, 292*f*, 293*t*
    senescence, 34–35
    surgical techniques for, 292–293, 293*t*
    transplantation
        for men, 296–302, 297*f*, 297*t*, 298*f*, 298*t*, 299*f*, 300*f*, 301*f*, 302*f*
        for women, 290
Hayflick limit theory, 94
Health Utilities Index (HUI), 40
Health-related quality of life (HRQol), 47
Helix aspersa Müller, 74*t*, 80
HETEs. *See* 12-Hydroxyeicosatetraenoic acids
Hirsutism, 308*f*, 309
Hispanic Americans, 15
Hispanics, 12–13. *See also* Latinos
    facial features of, 8–9, 8*t*
    photoaging of, 29, 35*t*
Hiwi tribe, 9
Homomenthyl salicylate. *See* Homosalate
Homosalate (Homomenthyl salicylate), 106*t*
Hori's nevi, 49*t*, 52, 123
Hormone replacement therapy (HRT), 33
HQ. *See* Hydroquinone
HRQol. *See* Health-related quality of life
HUI. *See* Health Utilities Index
Humans (homo sapiens), 15
Hume, David, 3
Hyaluronidase, 250, 252, 279
Hydraulic acids, 225–230, 226*t*–229*t*, 230*f*
Hydroquinone (HQ)
    as skin-lightening agent, 73, 74*t*, 75–77, 75*f*, 76*f*, 77*f*
    uses of, 87–88, 158, 172, 279
Hydroxy acids, 22
4-hydroxyanisol. *See* Mequinol
12-Hydroxy eicosatetraenoic acids (HETEs), 141
Hydroxycinnamic acids, 111*t*
Hylaform, 225, 226*t*–229*t*, 239
Hyperpigmentation, 75, 87–88, 87*f*
    acquired, 73, 73*t*
    causes of, 73
    laser therapies for, 117–123, 118*f*, 120*f*, 121*f*, 122*t*
    medication-induced, 119, 122*t*
    microdermabrasion and, 148–150, 149*f*
Hypertrichosis, 309
Hypertrophic scars, 293–294, 301
    occurrence of, 24, 49*t*, 54
    risks for, 197–198
Hypopigmentation, 66, 77
    complications with, 129
    conclusions on, 130–132
    micropigmentation, 130, 130*f*
    pathogenesis of, 125, 126*f*

surgical intervention for, 129–130, 130*f*, 131*t*
therapeutic approaches to
    NB-UVB as, 128, 128*f*, 131*t*
    targeted light therapy as, 128–129, 129*f*, 131*t*
    topical photochemotherapy as, 125–129, 126*f*, 127*f*, 128*f*, 129*f*, 131*t*
Hypoplasia, infraorbital, 34
Hypovitaminosis D, 110
Hypoxia hypothesis, 319

Imaging, 69. *See also* Photography; *specific imaging types*
    compression during, 65
    manipulation/storage/transmission of, 69
    photography and, 65–66, 65*t*
    resolution during, 64–65
Imiquimod therapy, 320–321
Immediate pigment darkening (IPD), 104
Immune protection factor (IPF), 110
India, 10, 101
Indonesians, 8
Infections, 141, 340
Infrared light (IRL), 104, 104*f*
Intense pulse light therapy (IPL), 105, 120, 180, 182
Interferons, 316, 320
Interleukin
    -6, 316
    -10, 104
International Agency for Research on Cancer, 103
Iodine, 278
IPD. *See* Immediate pigment darkening
IPF. *See* Immune protection factor
IPL. *See* Intense pulse light therapy
IRL. *See* Infrared light
Isoflavones, 111*t*
Isologen, 231*t*–233*t*
Isopropyl alcohol, 279
Isotretinoin, 332, 333

Japan, 101
Japanese, 8, 21, 29
Jessner's peel
    advantages/disadvantages of, 165
    contraindications for, 165
    formulations of, 161, 172
    side effects of, 165
    technique, 163, 166*f*, 173, 173*f*
Juvéderm, 225, 227*t*, 237

Keloids, 293–294, 301
    altered growth factors/cytokines and, 313–316, 313*f*, 314*f*, 315*t*
    conclusions on, 318, 325
    medical/surgical therapies for, 320–325, 321*f*, 322*f*, 323*f*, 324*f*, 325*t*
    occurrence of, 24, 54, 55, 141
    pathogenesis of, 313–318, 313*f*, 314*f*, 315*t*
    risks for, 197–198
Keratinocytes, 18, 27
Kerner, Justinus, 211
Klein tumescent solution, 271
Kligman bleaching formulation, 157
Kojic acids, 74*t*, 77, 160
Korea, 54, 101
Koreans, 8, 20–21, 29

Lactic acids, 74*t*, 96*t*, 163
Lakshmi, 3
Laser, 176
    Aramis Erbium: Glass, 198–199
    CoolTouch, 198–199
    hair removal, 56

Laser (*continued*)
light, 303, 304*f*, 304*t*
modalities and, 279–280
Smooth Beam, 198–199
surgery, 324–325
technology, 120
therapies
for hyperpigmentation, 117–123, 118*f*, 120*f*, 121*f*, 122*t*
for lentigines, 119–120, 120*f*
for melasma, 117–118, 118*f*, 122*t*
for PIH, 118–119, 122*t*
treatment, endovenous, 282
types of, 119–121, 179–185, 180*f*, 183*f*, 184*f*, 185*t*, 198–199
Laser Doppler velocimetry (LDV), 22
Laser hair removal (LHR), in darker racial ethnic groups, 303–309, 304*f*, 304*t*, 305*f*, 306*f*, 306*t*, 307*f*, 308*f*
clinical applications of, 307–309, 308*f*
complications/contraindications of, 306–307, 306*f*, 306*t*, 307*f*
practical aspects of, 305–306
Latinos, 8. *See also* Hispanics
blepharoplasty in, 250–256, 251*f*, 253*f*, 254*f*, 255*f*, 256*f*
LDL. *See* Low-density lipoprotein
LDV. *See* Laser Doppler velocimetry
Lecithins, 74*t*
Lentigines
cosmetic concerns regarding, 49*t*, 51–52, 51*f*
laser therapies for, 119–120, 122*f*
Leukodermas. *See* Hypopigmentation
Leukotrienes, 141
LHR. *See* Laser hair removal
Licorice extract, 74*t*
Lidocaine, 216, 234, 271, 292, 305
Light. *See also* Ultraviolet
devices, broadband, 199, 200–201, 201*f*
-emitting diode, 184–185
photography, polarized, 66
sunscreens against emitted, 105
therapy, targeted, 128–129, 129*f*, 131*t*
Linoleic acid, 74*t*, 80
Liposuction, 15
for abdomen, 268–270, 269*f*–270*f*
anesthesia for, 271–272, 274–275, 275*t*
for buttocks, 270–271, 273*f*
complications associated with, 274–275, 275*t*
conclusions on, 275
safety of, 272–274
for thighs, 270, 271*f*, 272*f*
Liquirtin, 74*t*, 80
Low-density lipoprotein (LDL), 100
Lycopene, 98*t*

Magnesium L-ascorbic acid-2-phosphate (MAP), 79
Malic acids, 96*t*
Mammaplasty, reduction, 262–264, 263*f*
MAP. *See* Magnesium L-ascorbic acid-2-phosphate
Marcaine, 250, 252
MASI. *See* Melasma Area Severity Index
Mast cells, 23–24, 23*t*
MED. *See* Minimal erythema dosing
Medication(s)
for acne vulgaris, 82
antiviral, 152
-induced hyperpigmentation, 119, 122*t*
side effects of, 59
Melanin
absorption spectrum, 305
amounts of, 197
content of, 17, 19*f*
effects of, 27
epidermal, 100
production of, 50–51, 74–75, 74*t*

skin of darker racial ethnic groups and, 17–21, 18*f*, 19*f*, 20*f*
Melanocyte(s)
/melanocyte suspensions, cultured epidermis with, 140–141
production of, 50
skin of darker racial ethnic groups and, 17–21, 18*f*, 19*f*, 20*f*
suspension, noncultured, 138
Melanoma, malignant, 335–336, 337*f*
Melasma, 88
cosmetic concerns regarding, 49*t*, 50–51, 51*f*
laser therapies for, 117–118, 118*f*, 122*t*
post, 105
Melasma Area Severity Index (MASI), 46, 88, 158
MELASQOL, 47
Melatonin, 74*t*, 79–80, 98*t*
Melomental folds, 220
Membrane theory of aging, 94
Men, hair transplantation for, 296–302, 297*f*, 297*t*, 298*f*, 298*f*, 299*f*, 300*f*, 301*f*, 302*f*
Mental crease, 220
Menthyl anthranilate. *See* Meradimate
Meperidine, 272
Mequinol (4-hydroxyanisole), 74*t*, 79
Meradimate (Menthyl anthranilate; Ensilizole), 106*t*
Methionine, 98*t*
8-Methoxypsoralen, 125–126
Methotrexate, 119, 323
Methoxsalen, 127, 128
Methylarbutin, 77
Meximeter MX 16, 17, 17*f*
Mexoryl SX (Terephthalylidene trisiloxane; Silatriazole), 107*t*
Mexoryl XL (Drometriazole trisiloxane; Silatriazole), 107*t*
Microdermabrasion
advantages of, 152
aluminum oxide crystals and, 152–153
chemical peels and, 152
complications/side effects of, 152
contraindications to, 153
hyperpigmentation and, 148–150, 149*f*
indications of, 149*f*, 150*f*, 148–150
procedure, 147–148, 148*f*, 148*t*
skin response after, 150–152
summary on, 153
Micrografts, 299
Micropigmentation, 130, 130*f*
Microthermal treatment zones (MTZs), 118
Midazolam, 272
Minimal erythema dosing (MED), 16, 105
Minimum melanogenic dosing (MMD), 16
Minoxidil, 287–288, 297*t*
Mitochondrial decline theory, 93–94
MMD. *See* Minimum melanogenic dosing
MMS. *See* Moh's micrographic surgery
Mofty, El, 125
Moh's micrographic surgery (MMS), 344
Mongoloids, 15
Mouth frown, 220
M-plasty, 339, 340*f*
MSBRQ. *See* Multidimensional Body-States Relations Questionnaire
MTZs. *See* Microthermal treatment zones
Multidimensional Body-States Relations Questionnaire (MSBRQ), 40

NA-CAP. *See* N-acetyl-4-S-cystalminylphenol
N-acetyl-4-S-cystalminylphenol (NA-CAP), 79
N-acetylcysteine, 108
NADH. *See* Nicotinamide adenine dinucleotide
Naphthoic acid, 82
Narrowband UVB (NB-UVB), 128, 128*f*, 131*t*
Native Americans, 8
NB-UVB. *See* Narrowband UVB

Neck, 220
Nefertiti, 3, 4*f*
Negroids. *See* Congoids
Neoglycoproteins, 74*t*
Nerve injuries, 195
Neuroendocrine theory, 94
Nevus
acquired bilateral, 122–123, 122*t*
of Ota, 121–122, 121*f*, 122*t*
New England Journal of Medicine, 42
Newsweek, 13
Niacin, 79
Niacinamide, 74*t*, 79
Nicotinamide adenine dinucleotide (NADH), 98*t*
Nitrogen, liquid, 119
NMSC. *See* Nonmelanoma skin cancer
Nonmelanoma skin cancer (NMSC), 335
Nonsteroidal anti-inflammatory drugs (NSAIDs), 193–194
North American Hair Research Society, 289
Noses, 257–261, 258*f*, 259*f*, 260*f*
NSAIDs. *See* Nonsteroidal anti-inflammatory drugs

Obesity, 263, 276
Ochronosis, 77
Octinoxate (Parsol MCX,Octylmethoxycinnamate; Escalol 557; Eusolex 2292), 106*t*, 110
Octisalate (Octyl salicylate), 106*t*
Octocrylene Ensulizole, 106*t*
Octyl salicylate. *See* Octisalate
Octyldimethyl PABA. *See* Padimate O
Octylmethoxycinnamate. *See* Octinoxate
Oleic acid, 80
Oligomeric proanthocyanidins (OPCs), 98*t*
Oligosaccharides, 111*t*
OPCs, Oligomeric proanthocyanidins
Optical profilometry, 37
Oral contraceptives, 288
Orbicularis oculi muscles, 217–219
Ortho Pharmaceuticals, 82
Ortho-hydroxybenzoic acid. *See* Salicylic acid
Osmotic agents, 278
Oxybenzone, 106*t*, 110

Padimate O (Octyldimethyl PABA), 106*t*, 110
Paper mulberry, 74*t*, 79
PAR-2. *See* Protease-activated receptor-2
Paraguay, 9
Para-phenylenediamine, 53
Parsol 1789. *See* Butyl methoxydibenzoyl methane
Parsol MCX. *See* Octinoxate
Patch, 110
Patients, informed consent and
background of, 59
causation of, 60
damages and, 60
documentation and, 61, 61*t*
exceptions and, 60
requirements of, 59–60
summary on, 61
PDGF. *See* Platelet-derived growth factor
Pearson, Lester B., 13
Peau d'orange chin, 220
Pentoxifylline (Trental), 321
Perlane, 226*t*–229*t*
Persistent pigment darkening (PPD), 104
PFA. *See* Protection factor against UVA
PFB. *See* Pseudofolliculitis barbae
PFV. *See* Protection factor against visible light
Phenol-Bakers, 157
Phenols, 170, 174
Phenothiazines, 119
Pheomelanin, 17
Phi, 5
Phidias, 5